Current Topics in Pathology

Ergebnisse der Pathologie

Edited by

E. Grundmann · **W. H. Kirsten**
Münster · *Chicago*

Advisory Board

Volume 60

With 74 Figures

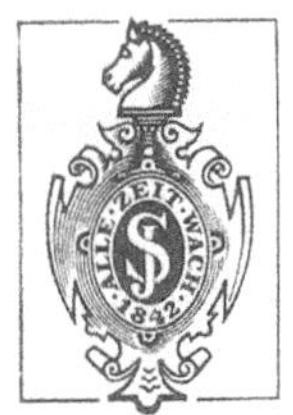

Springer-Verlag Berlin · Heidelberg · New York 1975

ISBN-13: 978-3-642-66217-1   e-ISBN-13: 978-3-642-66215-7
DOI: 10.1007/ 978-3-642-66215-7

Typesetting: Universitätsdruckerei H. Stürtz AG, Würzburg

Contents

List of Contributors

G. ALTSHULER, Department of Pathology, Children's Hospital Medical Center, Cincinnati, Ohio 45229, USA

N. BÖHM, Pathologisches Institut der Universität, Albertstraße 19, D-7800 Freiburg, Germany

K. BÜRKI, Pathologisches Institut der Universität, Freiburgstraße 30, CH-3000 Bern, Switzerland

T. FRANKEN, Pathologisches Institut der Universität, Moorenstraße 5, D-4000 Düsseldorf, Germany

P. GRÉTILLAT, Pathologisches Institut der Universität, Freiburgstraße 30, CH-3000 Bern, Switzerland

F. HUTH, Pathologisches Institut der Universität, Moorenstraße 5, D-4000 Düsseldorf, Germany

M. KOJIMAHARA, Pathologisches Institut der Universität, Moorenstraße 5, D-4000 Düsseldorf, Germany

H. MITSCHKE, Pathologisches Institut der Universität, Martinistraße 52, D-2000 Hamburg 20, Germany

P. RHEDIN, Pathologisches Institut der Universität, Moorenstraße 5, D-4000 Düsseldorf, Germany

K. A. ROSENBAUER, Pathologisches Institut der Universität, Moorenstraße 5, D-4000 Düsseldorf, Germany

P. RUSSELL, Department of Pathology, Children's Hospital Medical Center, Cincinnati, Ohio 45229, USA

W. SAEGER, Pathologisches Institut der Universität, Martinistraße 52, D-2000 Hamburg 20, Germany

W. SANDRITTER, Pathologisches Institut der Universität, Albertstraße 19, D-7800 Freiburg, Germany

J. C. SCHAER, Pathologisches Institut der Universität, Freiburgstraße 30, CH-3000 Bern, Switzerland

R. SCHINDLER, Pathologisches Institut der Universität, Freiburgstraße 30, CH-3000 Bern, Switzerland

Institute of Pathology, University of Düsseldorf (Director: Prof. Dr. H. Meessen)
Institute of Anatomy, University of Düsseldorf (Director: Prof. Dr. K. A. Rosenbauer)

Aortic Alterations in Rabbits Following Sheathing with Silastic and Polyethylene Tubes*

F. Huth, M. Kojimahara, T. Franken, P. Rhedin, K. A. Rosenbauer

With 17 Figures

Contents

Introduction and Survey of Literature

Disturbances and qualitative alterations of the liquid flow within the vascular wall have been discussed among the pathogenetic factors influencing human arteriosclerosis. Ribbert (1904) and Adami and Aschoff (1906) postulated a direction of the liquid flow within the vascular wall from the inner to the outer vessel layers; their conception was followed by the infiltration theory of Anitschkow (1913/14). Insudative processes with and without preceding lesions of the endothelium have been demonstrated especially in atheromatous alterations of the vascular walls (Duff, 1935; Gofman et al., 1950; Prior and Hartmann, 1956; Still et al., 1962/1968; Haust, 1962 to

---

* Herrn Prof. Dr. med. Dr. h.c. H. Meessen zum 65. Geburtstag gewidmet.

1970; Adams, 1964; Haust and More, 1965/1972; Still and Dennison, 1967). A liquid flow in the other direction is shown by the existence of the vasa vasorum. It cannot be stated definitely that the liquid flow from the inside to the outside has any significance in the induction of atherosclerotic changes. A liquid flow penetrating the vascular wall in a longitudinal direction as discussed by Linzbach (1957) and Doerr (1958/1963) could become effective pathogenetically by blocking the vascular drainage. An aortic lesion that could be interpreted in this sense was produced by Cremer and Müller (1973) following ligature of the thoracic duct.

Pathogenetic considerations on the importance of liquid flow within arterial walls induce the question for the drainage of the liquids along the outer vascular wall structures. Factors affecting the drainage of the vascular wall should also influence the nutrition of the arterial wall from outside to inside at least secondarily. In that respect the plexus of lymphatics have to be taken into consideration as well as the vasa vasorum of the adventitia and the media. At the suggestion of Prof. Meessen and stimulated by his methodological advice we tried to develop an experimental model which would lead to a blockage of nutrition and drainage on the outside of the aortic wall. Within the experimental procedure compression of the vascular wall and especially stenosis of the vascular lumen should be avoided. Comparable investigations have been performed by only a few authors. Table 1 shows a survey of experimental work with comparable experimental procedures.

Table 1. Earlier experiments with sheathing of arteries

Lange (1924)	wax plates	rabbits	carotis, aorta
Wilens (1942)	silver cuffs	rabbits	femoralis, carotis
Nylander and Olerud (1961/62)	polyethylene	dogs	aorta
Takeda (1961)	acrylic resin	rabbits, rats, mice	carotis
Iijima (1964)	rubber, acrylic resin, silver cuffs	rabbits	carotis
Suzuki (1967)	silver cuffs	rabbits	carotis, femoralis, aorta
Mizukawa (1969)	metal cuffs etc.	rabbits, guinea pig	carotis
Zellweger et al. (1970)	siliconized synthetic rubber	dogs	aorta

Zellweger and coworkers (1970), Nylander and Olerud (1961/62) induced constrictions of the vessels by sheathing them with siliconized rubber or polyethylene. Suzuki (1967) also caused vascular constrictions by using silver cuffs. Similar effects have to be assumed for the method of Lange (1924) and Wilens (1942). Quick hardening acrylic resin as used by Iijima (1964) and TAKEDA (1961) should also cause constrictions. The results of multiple sheathing of the aorta and large arterial vessels within the same animal and corresponding comparisons have yet to be published. Our experimental model with multiple sheathings of vessels without vascular compression and subsequent comparison by light-, transmission-, electron-, and scanning electron-microscopic investigations ought to reveal the effects of nutritional and drainage blocking of the vascular wall. The alterations of the vascular segments within the cuffs should be compared. In addition, the model should make it possible to compare the vascular segments above the cuffs with the segments within a defined intermediate vascular segment between the cuffs. The alterations of the "bare" segments should be compared with those within the cuffs.

Material and Methods

Eighty male and female rabbits from the same stock weighing an average of 2.3 kg were operated on under sterile conditions in anaesthesia with ether. Following laparatomy by a pararectal incision of 15 cm the aorta was prepared beneath the celiac trunc and above the inferior mesenteric artery. The renal arteries were prepared accordingly. The dissected vascular segments of 25 rabbits were sheathed in cuffs of silastic measuring 1 mm in thickness. The cuffs were either carefully contracted with 2 threads of silk or with small skin clamps around the circumference of the vascular segments, avoiding constriction of the vessels. In 53 animals the cuffs for the vascular sheathing were made out of polyethylene tubes of different diameters. Silk threads were woven within the cuffs which allowed tight enclosure of the vascular segments by the cuffs. Further, in 60 animals the renal arteries were also sheathed. The sheathed segments are demonstrated in Scheme 1.

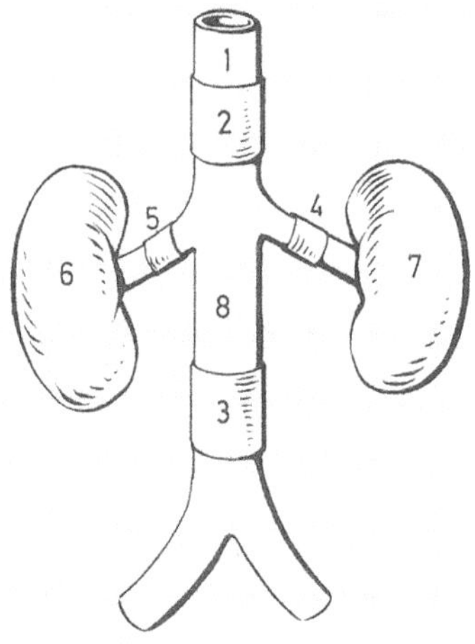

Scheme 1

In 4 control animals sheathing was done without knotting the threads around the constriction. In 2 additional control animals the aortic segments were only dissected but not sheathed by cuffs. There were 3 normal rabbits that had not been operated on as controls. Following the sheathing of the vascular segments renal perfusion and the distal blood supply were checked. The surgical wounds were sutured layer by layer and covered with sterile material. The duration of the operations could be limited to 30 or 40 min after a series of preliminary experiments.

Thirty-six animals were thoracotomized in anesthesia with ether at intervals as follows: 30 and 60 min, 3 and 24 h, 2, 3, 4, and 5 days, 1, 2, 3, 5, and 6 weeks, 2, 3, 4, 5, and 6 months. Perfusion was performed with physiological sodium chloride for 2 min, immediately followed by an injection of 2% buffered glutaraldehyde in the upper descending aorta. The pressure in the perfusion system was maintained at a level of 60 to 80 mm Hg. In the remaining rabbits fixation was done by perfusion or by immersion in 10% neutral formalin. Corresponding to Scheme 1, the following organs and tissues were dissected out for further investigation: both kidneys (6, 7), the aorta above the cuffs (1), the aorta within the cuffs (2, 3), the intermediate segment of the aorta between the cuffs (8), and both sheathed renal arteries (5, 4). Tissues fixed by perfusion with glutaraldehyde were cut into 1 mm strips. These strips were postfixed in osmium tetroxide and embedded in araldite. The ultrathin sections were treated with uranyl acetate and lead citrate to enhance the contrast. The transmission electron microscopy was performed with Siemens-E-microscope 101. For scanning electron microscopic investigations the vascular tissue, fixed in glutaraldehyde, was mounted on cork sheets and dehydrated by alcohol in ascending concentrations. Drying of the specimens was carried out either by a method developed by Rosenbauer and Schlösser (1973) or according to the critical-point procedure. Subsequently, the specimens were mounted with conducting silver and coated in a JEOL vacuum vaporizer JEE-4 B with carbon and gold. The investigations and photographic documentation were performed with the scanning electron microscope JSM-U-3 (JEOL) fitted with devices for preventing distortion (LWU-Kontron) and for controlling the electronic image (SDT-monitored signal processing). The photographs were taken at an accelerating voltage of 15 and 25 kV.

For the light-microscopic investigations, vascular segments, embedded in paraffin, were cut into longitudinal and transverse sections. These sections were stained with hematoxylin–eosin, ironhematoxylin-van Gieson combined with resorcin, Goldner's modification of Masson's trichrome stain, and the PAS reaction. The vascular segments as well as the kidneys, heart, liver, and lungs of most of the animals were examined light microscopically.

In 36 animals a 12-point measurement of all vascular segments was made with the aid of the Reichert Visopan microscope. Two examiners independently measured and counted the thickness of the intima, the media and the total vascular wall, and the number of elastic units. The 7000 measurements were subjected to correlated calculations with the aid of an electronic calculator Olivetti P 102. Mean values and standard deviations of measurable alterations were reproduced graphically for the purpose of comparison. The mean values of each vascular segment and of the layers of the vascular wall were adjusted according to the duration of the experiments. Significance was calculated according to Student's t distribution.

Observations During the Experiments

During the operations 14 rabbits died; in 4 cases due to the anesthesia and the rest from bleeding due to ruptures of the celiac trunk, of the renal arteries or an aortic rupture. Twenty six animals died postoperatively following surgical shock, peritonitis, abscesses of the abdominal wall and pneumonia. A further 8 animals developed hypertension due to constrictions of the abdominal aorta or of the renal arteries within the cuffs. In one animal thrombi were found in both cardiac auriculars with also multiple pulmonary infarctions.

Macroscopic Findings

The macroscopic findings differed with duration of experiment and type of sheathing cuff. Following the tightening of the cuffs by skin clamps, huge foreign-body granulomas containing old necroses of fatty tissue were frequently observed. Tubular cuffs of polyethylene with enwoven threads induced only mild foreign-body reaction. The cuffs were found to be encapsulated in dense connective tissue as early as 4 weeks. The superficial serosa was intact. Adhesions of the abdominal organs were rarely found, and there were no signs of bacterial peritonitis in the surviving rabbits. Within the cuffs the outer aortic wall was surrounded by a greyish-yellowish smear of debris. After a certain period the sheathed vascular segments became sclerosed. After 2 to 3 months an almost parchment-like transparence occurred. Pulvinate intimal thickenings could barely be seen with the naked eye. In 6 animals, the cuffs were too tightly constricted by the threads, resulting in stenosis of the renal arteries; signs of hypertension and myocardial hypertrophy were noticed in these cases. Two further animals developed complete thrombotic obliteration and partial fibrosis of the renal arteries. The corresponding kidneys had undergone sclerotic atrophy. These 8 animals were not taken into consideration in further investigations. Neither the intermediate segment (8) between the aortic cuffs nor the aorta superior to the cuffs showed macroscopically detectable inflammatory or sclerotic alterations.

Light-Microscopic Findings

In spite of the expected differences resulting from each method of sheathing, the histological alterations of the aorta within the cuffs were found to be almost identical; therefore the findings will be presented as a whole and individual deviations will be pointed out. We shall confine our demonstration of light- and electron-microscopic findings to alterations of the aortic segments. Those of the renal arteries will be discussed later.

Three hours after application of the cuff the desquamation of some endothelial cells was observed. The outer medial musculature and the adventitial connective tissue were slightly edematous. After 24 h some leukocytes were observed in the subendothelial space of the intima.

After 3 to 4 days the intima was broadened by edema containing leukocytic infiltrations. At this time, the medial muscle was strongly distorted by edema. In some areas, both the media and the adjacent adventitial connective tissue underwent necrotic changes. Necroses of muscle cells were mainly limited to the outer media; only occasionally could total necrosis of the media be demonstrated (Fig. 1a).

After 5 days the dissociation of the elastic laminae and the necroses of the medial muscle cells with clotting of nuclei were enhanced. Lipophagous granuloma arose in the adventitial tissue.

After 10 to 14 days proliferations of intimal cells became visible with staining properties resembling those of smooth muscle and a fine network of collagenous fibers. Elastic laminae did not at this time develop within the intima. The elastic laminae of the media were often collapsed and condensed to thick dark bundles (Fig. 1b). Capillaries with wide lumina were observed between necrotic parts and lipophagous granulomas of the adventitia.

After 4 weeks the proliferation of smooth muscle cells continued in the intima with numerous elastic laminae maturing between the muscle cells. There were fewer inflammatory alterations of the intima. Adjacent to the necrotic and partly fibrotic layers in the media, spindle-like strips of hyperregenerative muscle were also seen (Fig. 1c).

After 6 weeks the proliferations of intimal muscle cells were partly replaced by a dense and relatively homogeneous connective tissue. Fibrosis of the necrotic medial layers was still proceeding. Lipophagous granuloma were continuously present within the adventitial connective tissue (Fig. 1d).

After 3 months, regardless of the type of cuff, the sclerotic reconstruction was almost totally completed within the vascular segments. In some cases the thin residuals of the aortic wall, rich in collagen, resembled the mural structures of chronic vascular aneurysms. Within the aortic segments enclosed by polyethylene tubes, small remnants of medial muscle could be demonstrated between the outer and inner collagenous mural layers, even after 5 or 6 months (Fig. 2b). In other areas, especially following tightening of the silastic cuffs by skin clamps, the medial remnants consisted of dense bundles of collapsed elastic fibers (Fig. 2a). Occasionally irregular edematous disintegration of the sclerosed aortic wall continued even after 4 to 6 months.

The alterations described above could be observed only within the sheathed vascular segments. The proliferative and sclerotic reconstructive processes ceased abruptly at the ends of the cuffs. Very high proliferations of the intima were sometimes seen above the edges of the cuffs.

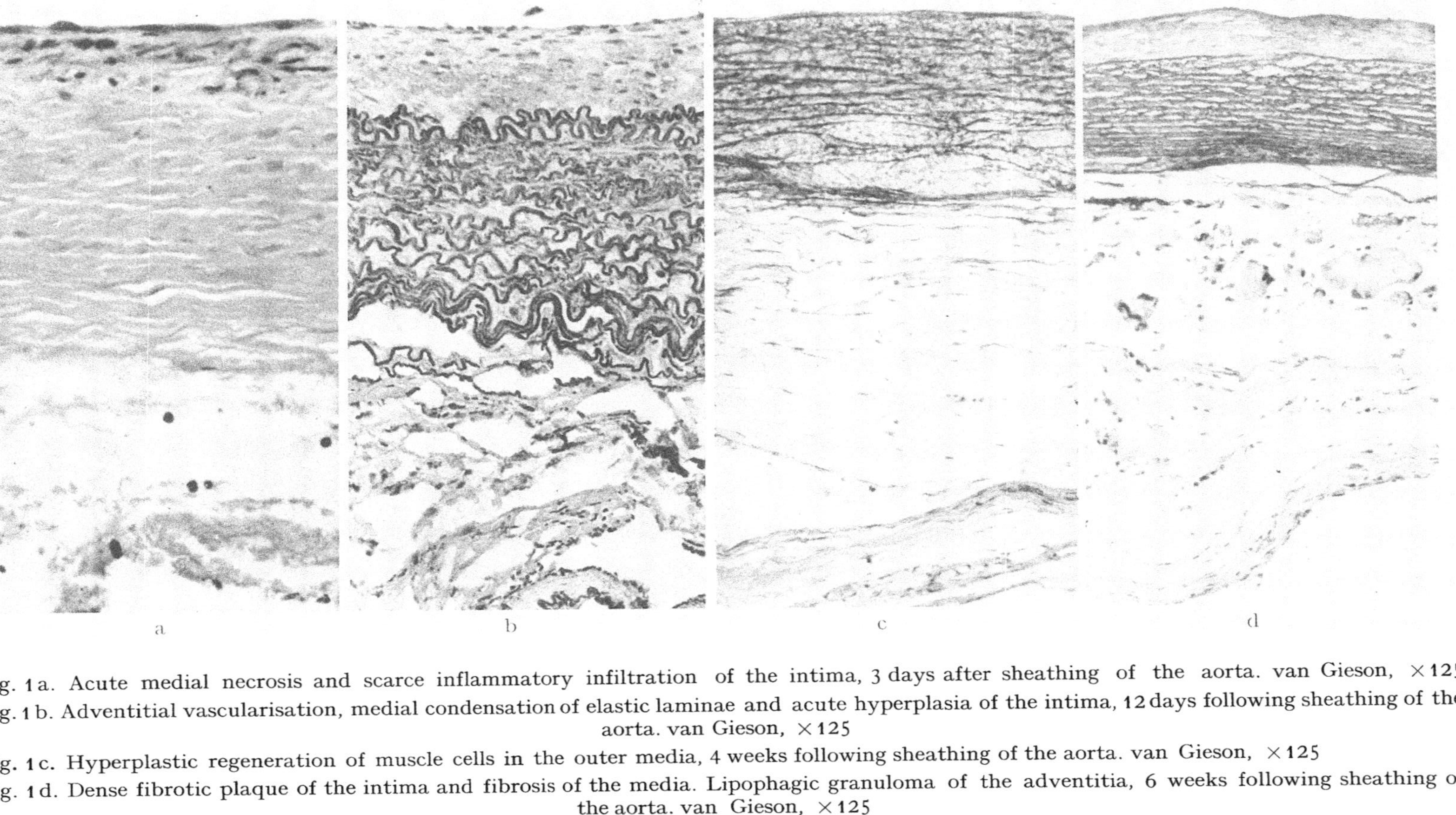

Fig. 1a. Acute medial necrosis and scarce inflammatory infiltration of the intima, 3 days after sheathing of the aorta. van Gieson, ×125
Fig. 1b. Adventitial vascularisation, medial condensation of elastic laminae and acute hyperplasia of the intima, 12 days following sheathing of the aorta. van Gieson, ×125

Fig. 1c. Hyperplastic regeneration of muscle cells in the outer media, 4 weeks following sheathing of the aorta. van Gieson, ×125
Fig. 1d. Dense fibrotic plaque of the intima and fibrosis of the media. Lipophagic granuloma of the adventitia, 6 weeks following sheathing of the aorta. van Gieson, ×125

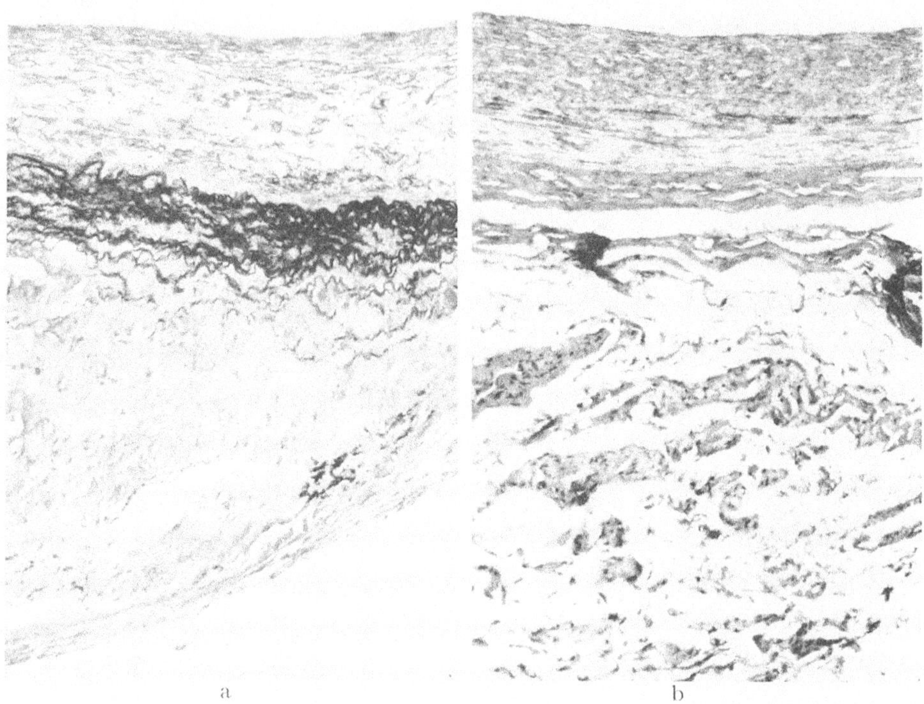

Fig. 2a. Fibrous thickening of the intima and patchy hyperelastosis of the sclerosed media, $3^1/_2$ months following sheathing of the aorta. van Gieson, ×125

Fig. 2b. Diffuse fibrotic hypertrophy of the intima, fibrosis and partial atrophy of the media, condensed and capillarized adventitia, 6 months following sheathing of the aorta. van Gieson, ×125

The vascular walls that were enclosed by plastic tubes without tightening threads showed alterations mostly confined to proliferations of the intimal cells at the edges of the cuffs. In addition, these tubes enclosed fibrotic adventitia. Necroses of the medial cells were nonexistent.

Cranial to the cuffs no pathologic alterations occurred in the aortic wall. The intermediate segment of the aorta (8) between the sheathed segments of the aorta and the renal arteries occasionally presented a slight fibrosis of the intima and the media; this, however, was not a constant finding but was always present to a minor degree. Comparable slight alterations were observed within those segments that were only dissected but not sheathed by a cuff. The layering of the medial muscle cells and the elastic units appeared unaltered within the dissected segments not sheathed by a cuff.

Scanning-Electron-Microscopic Findings

Due to the experimental procedure, only the secondary electron micrographs allow conclusions to be drawn from the properties of the intimal

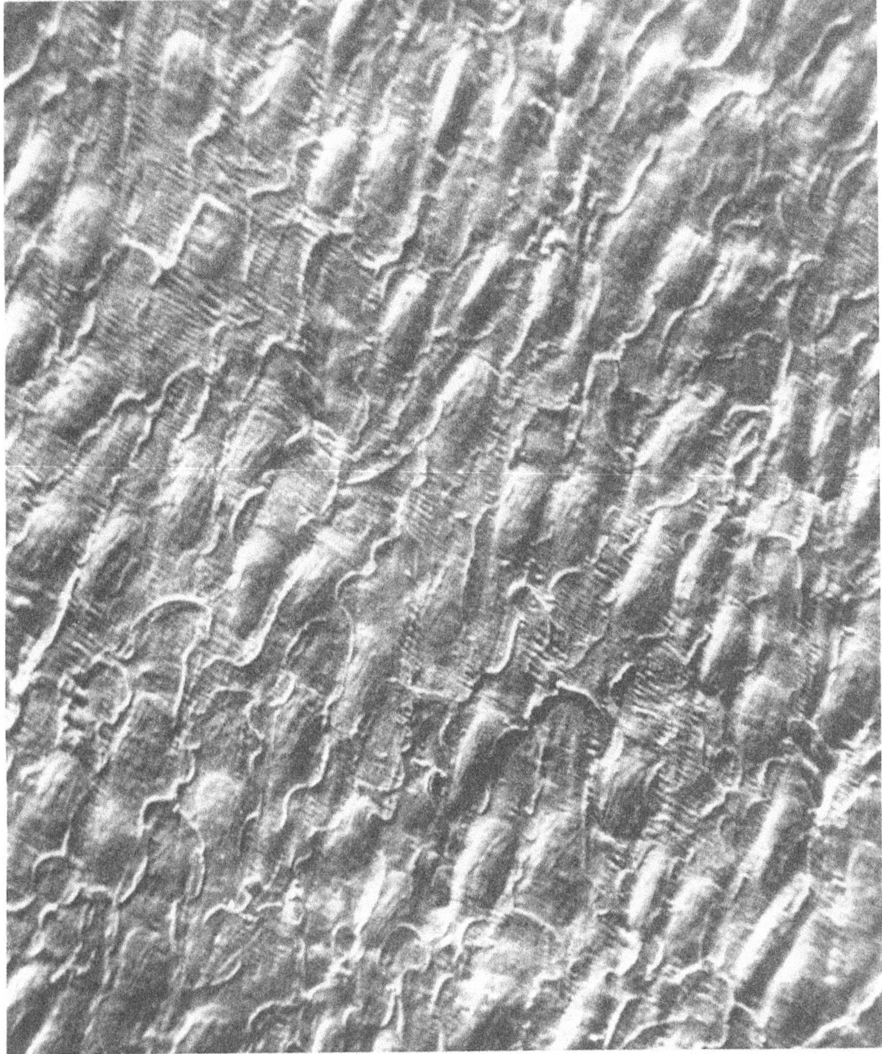

Fig. 3. Scanning electron microscopic survey of the intimal surface with normal nuclei population. ×800

surface. The normal endothelium of the rabbit aorta consists of irregular flat cells with well-defined cell borders (Fig. 3). Roundish stigmata (cf. BJÖRKERUD *et al.*, 1972) appear in varying density between the borders of the endothelial cells (Fig. 5). The endothelial cells bulge into the vascular lumen to a varying degree, probably correlated with the state of fixation, tension, and dryness of the specimens. On the 3rd to 5th postoperative day mainly small (Fig. 4a) but sometimes quite larger intimal defects became visible (Fig. 4b). The small endothelial lesions were covered by thrombocytic aggregates. Different cell types adhered to the rough surface of the vascular layers beneath the endothelial defects. In some places leukocytes and erythrocytes predominated.

     F. Huth *et al.*:

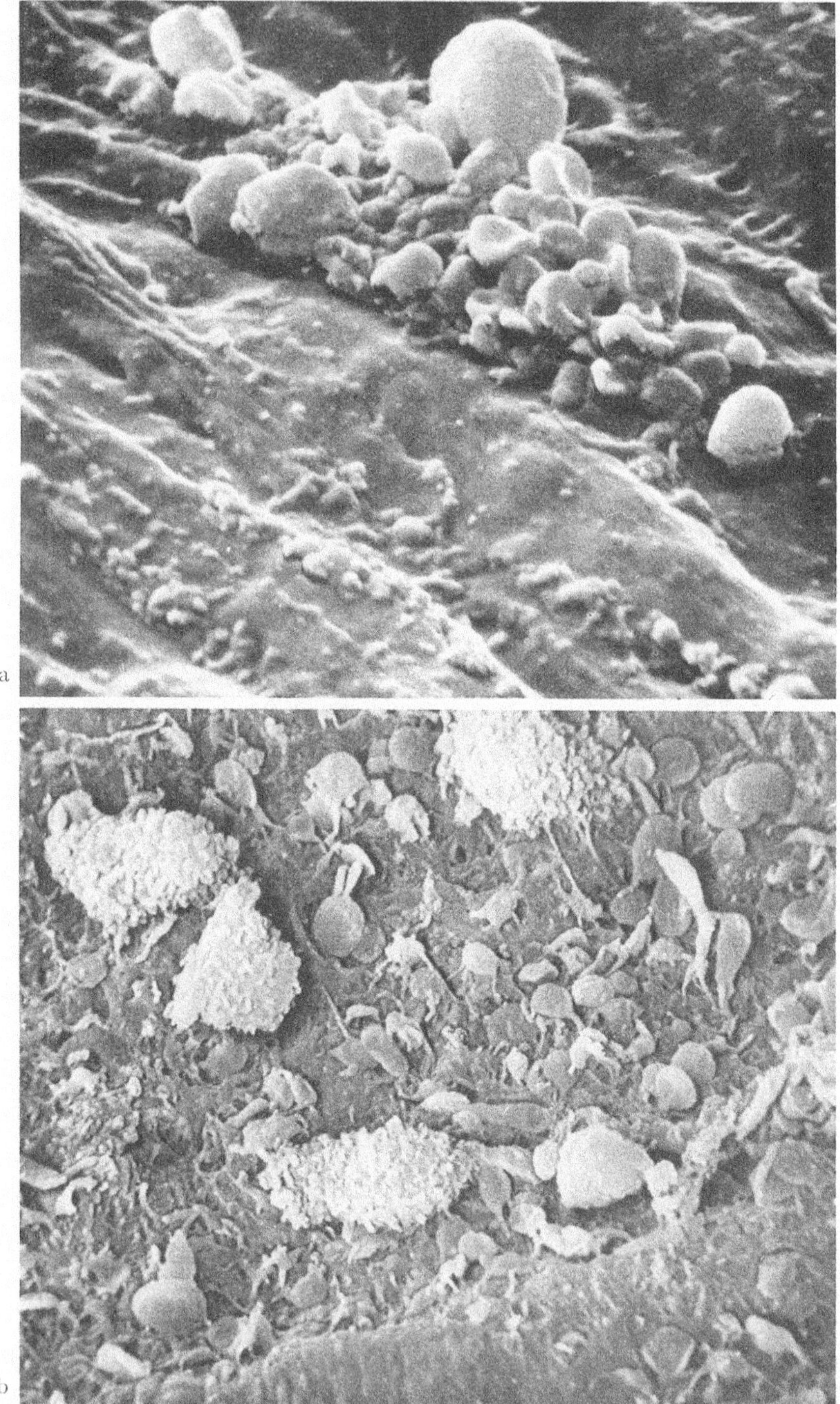

Fig. 4a, b

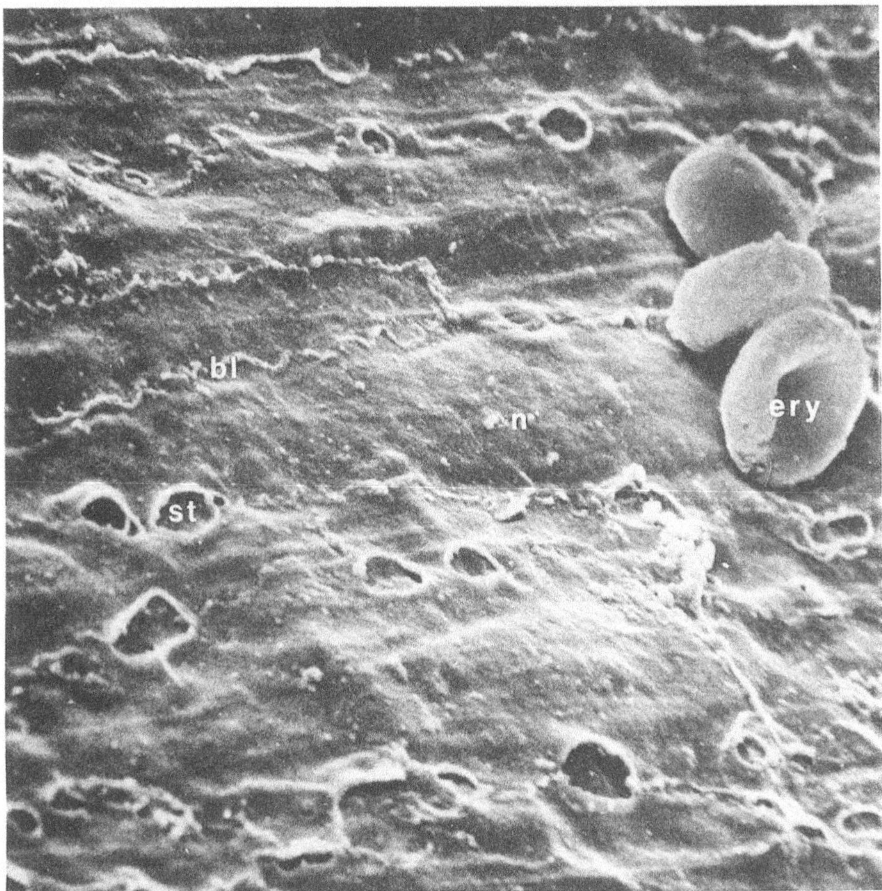

Fig. 5. Numerous stigmata (*st*) between the cell borders of the endothelial cells with prominent nuclei (*n*), well-defined cellular borders (*bl*), and 3 erythrocytes (*ery*), 6 months following sheathing of the aorta. ×4000

Mostly, however, the endothelial defects were also coated by thrombocytes (Fig. 4a, b). Remnants of endothelial cells and fibrillar structures could also be seen. The remaining intima did not differ from normal endothelial surface images.

After about $3^1/_2$ weeks following the vascular sheathing the number of stigmata appeared to have increased (Fig. 5). Even after 6 months this finding was still present in some specimens.

Fig. 4a. Circumscribed endothelial defect with aggregates of thrombocytes and erythrocytes, 5 days following sheathing of the aorta. ×4500

Fig. 4b. Extensive endothelial defect 3 days after sheathing of the aorta, beside thrombocytes, erythrocytes and fibrillar structures residual endothelial cells with microvillar protrusions on the surface. ×2600

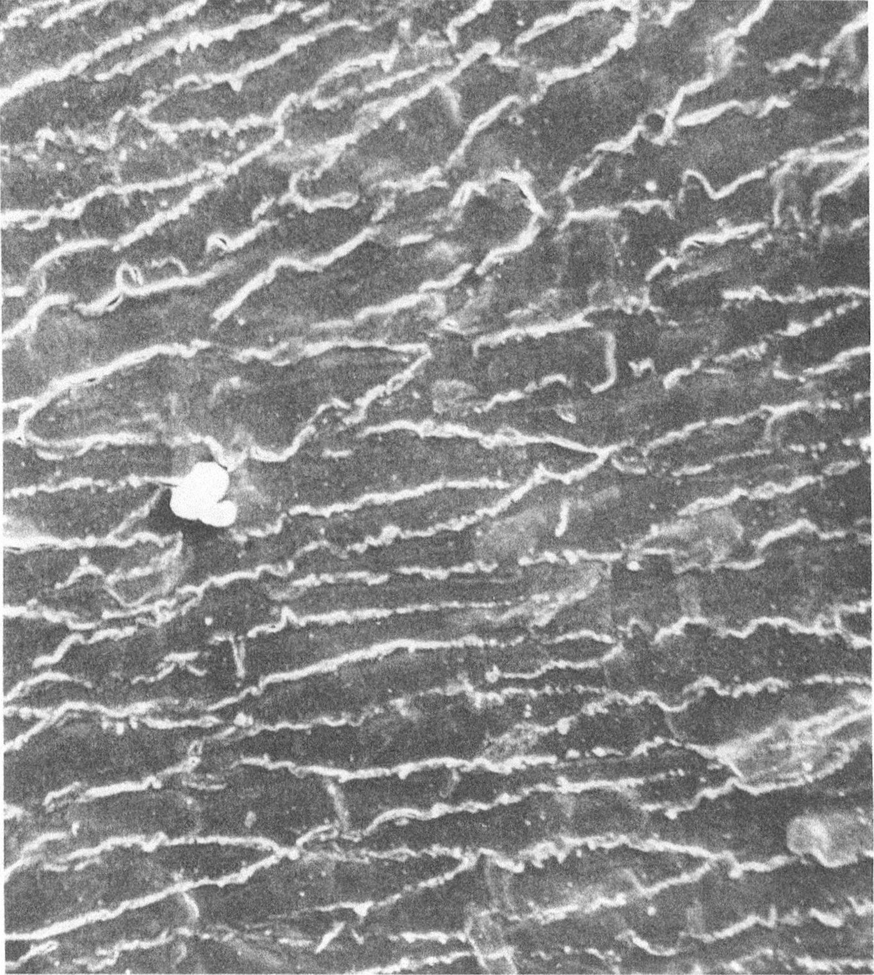

Fig. 6. Survey of the intimal surface with prominent cell borders 6 months following sheathing of the aorta, decrease of amount of cells per surface unit in comparison to normal endothelium (cf. Fig. 3). ×800

After 3 months the endothelial nuclei appeared large and plump. An analysis of the nuclear and cellular counts in the scanning electron micrographs revealed fewer endothelial cells per surface unit, sometimes only one third of the normal cell count (Fig. 6).

Transmission-Electron-Microscopic Findings

Studies of aortic segments by the transmission electron microscope did not reveal essential differences in the chronological or topographical manifestations of alterations with regard to the different methods of sheathing. Therefore, the observed changes will again be discussed with respect to their chronologic course.

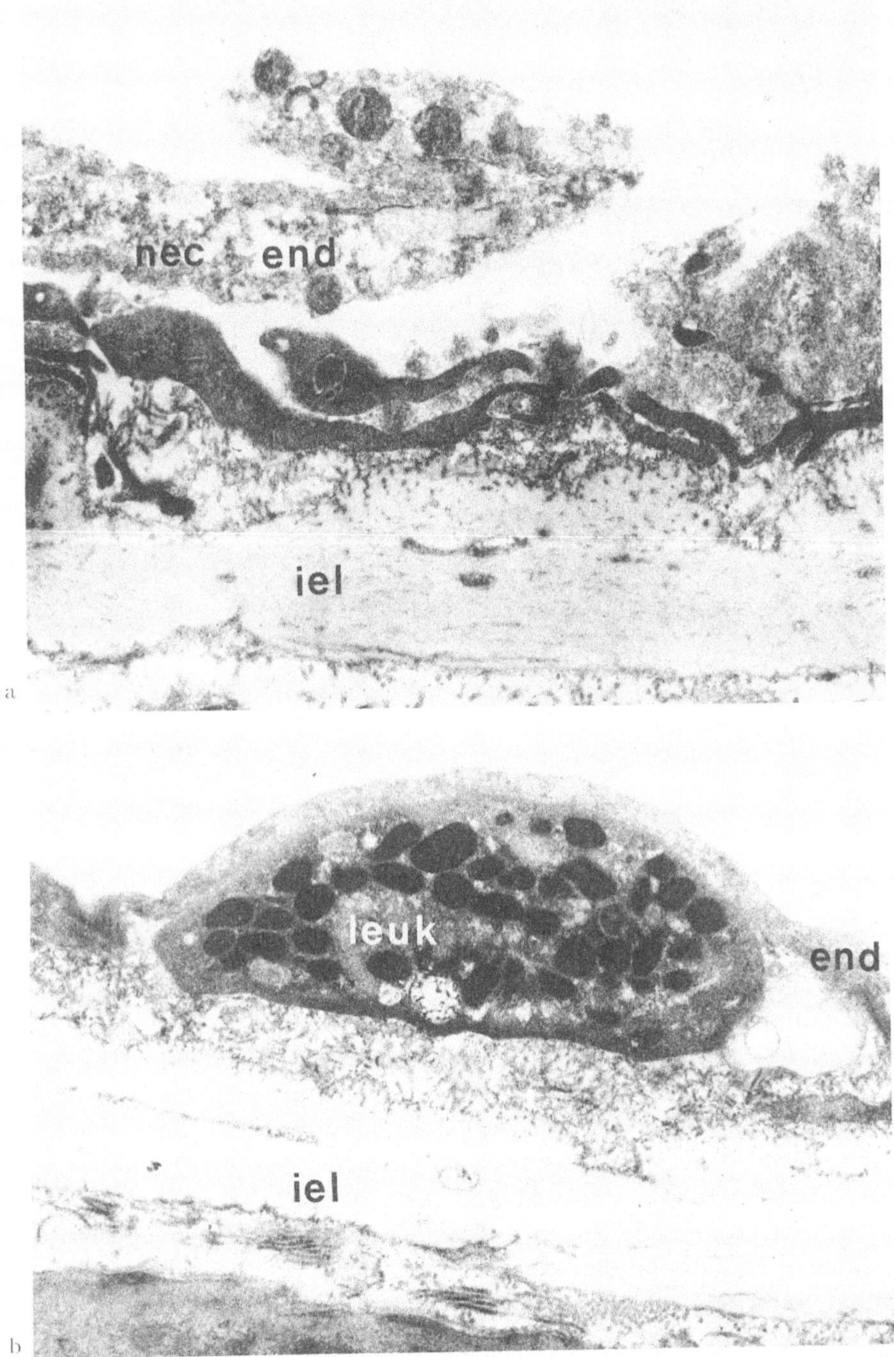

Fig. 7a. Acute endothelial lesion (*nec end*) 3 h after the sheathing of the aorta (*iel* = internal elastic lamina). ×17000

Fig. 7b. Leukocyte (*leuk*) beneath flattened endothelium (*end*), 3 h after sheathing of the aorta. ×12750

The intima was broadened by edema 3 h after the enclosure of the aortic segments. Some endothelial cells were desquamating. Fibrin occurred in some areas below the detaching endothelial cells. Polymorphonuclear leukocytes

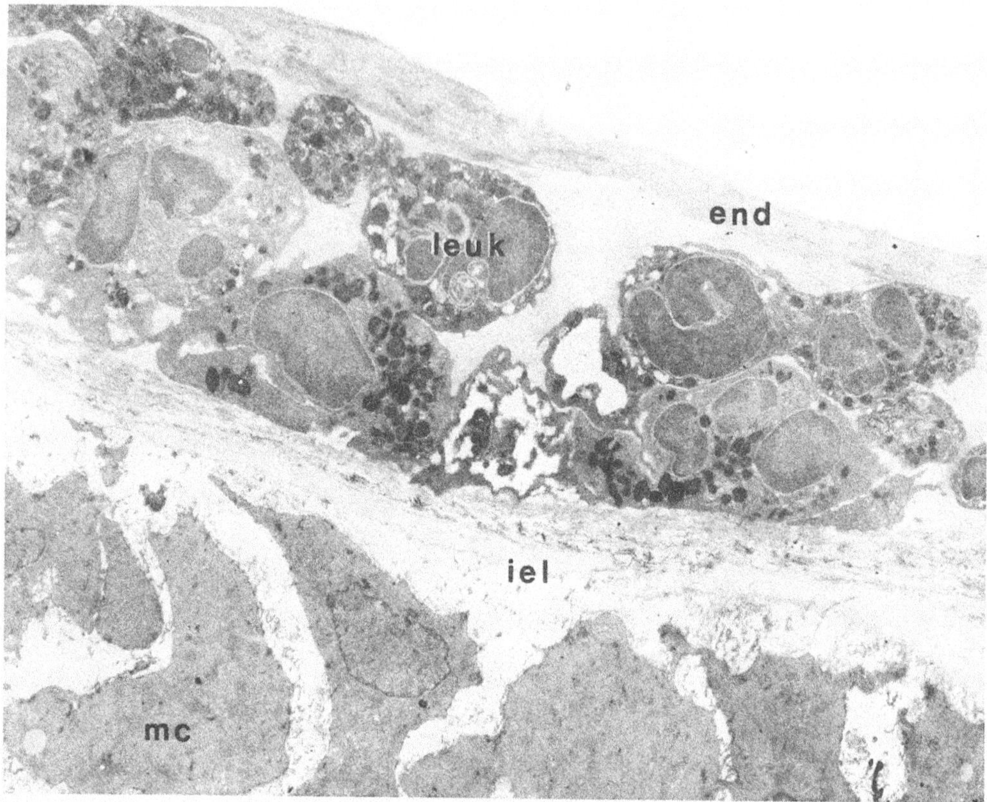

Fig. 8. Leukocytic infiltration (*leuk*) beneath flattened endothelium (*end*) above internal elastic lamina (*iel*), 3 days following sheathing of the aorta. ×15000

were found in the subendothelial intimal space, beneath the still intact endothelial cells as well as within the endothelial defects (Fig. 7a, b). The media was still intact at that time, and a limited number of leukocytes were visible between the smooth muscle cells. The edematous adventitial connective tissue was also invaded by leukocytes. After 2 days the endothelial and subendothelial intimal cells were enlarged, and the subendothelial intimal cells were quite often transformed to large "blasts" with irregularly invaginated cell membranes. The ground substance of the media was somewhat swollen in addition to being partly loosened by edema. Colliquative necroses, with degeneration of at least 3 elastic units, took place within the outer media.

After 3 days the subendothelial edema of the intima developed strongly, and focal concentrations of numerous leukocytes became apparent within it (Fig. 8). One or two layers of large subendothelial intimal cells with numerous mitochondria, as well as pronounced ergastoplasm and myofilaments filled up the intimal tissue (Fig. 9). Some intimal cells rich in ergastoplasm were enlarged with greater vacuoles. The vacuoles within these cells could not be clearly classified as being part of the ergastoplasm. Giant phagosomes oc-

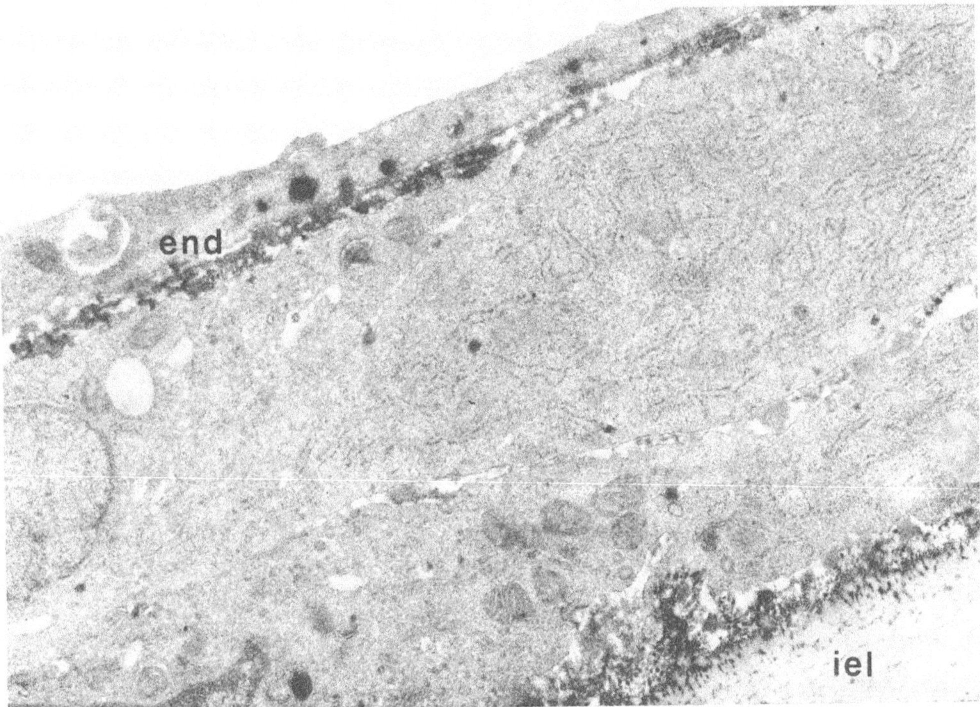

Fig. 9. Proliferation of subendothelial intimal cells above internal elastic lamina (*iel*) 3 days following sheathing of the aorta. ×17000

casionally appeared in the intimal cells (Fig. 10), and coagulation necroses were then prominent among the smooth muscle cells of the outer media. The ground substance and the collagenous fiber network were dissociated. The ergastoplasm was increased within the surviving smooth muscle cells (Fig. 11). In addition to the coagulation necroses, cytolytic figures with formations of huge vacuoles appeared. Within some specimens the acute necroses of smooth muscle cells reached the internal elastic lamina. In these areas the media was sparsely infiltrated by polymorphonuclear leukocytes.

One to 2 weeks later the huge subendothelial intimal cells were replaced by modified flat smooth muscle cells lying in up to 10 layers. These proliferations of intimal cells were especially well developed above the holes of the internal elastic lamina (Fig. 12). The proliferated cells were separated by numerous fibers of collagen and elastic microfibrils. In addition, a lamellar system of newly formed elastic laminae developed (Fig. 13). Leukocytic infiltrations were rare in this phase. The media revealed atrophic spindle-shaped smooth muscle cells between the broadened elastic fiber structure and collagen fibrils. A condensation of the collagenic fiber network and infiltrates of histiocytes, lymphocytes, and leukocytes also became evident in the adventitia. The adventitial blood capillaries were occasionally dilated to lacunae.

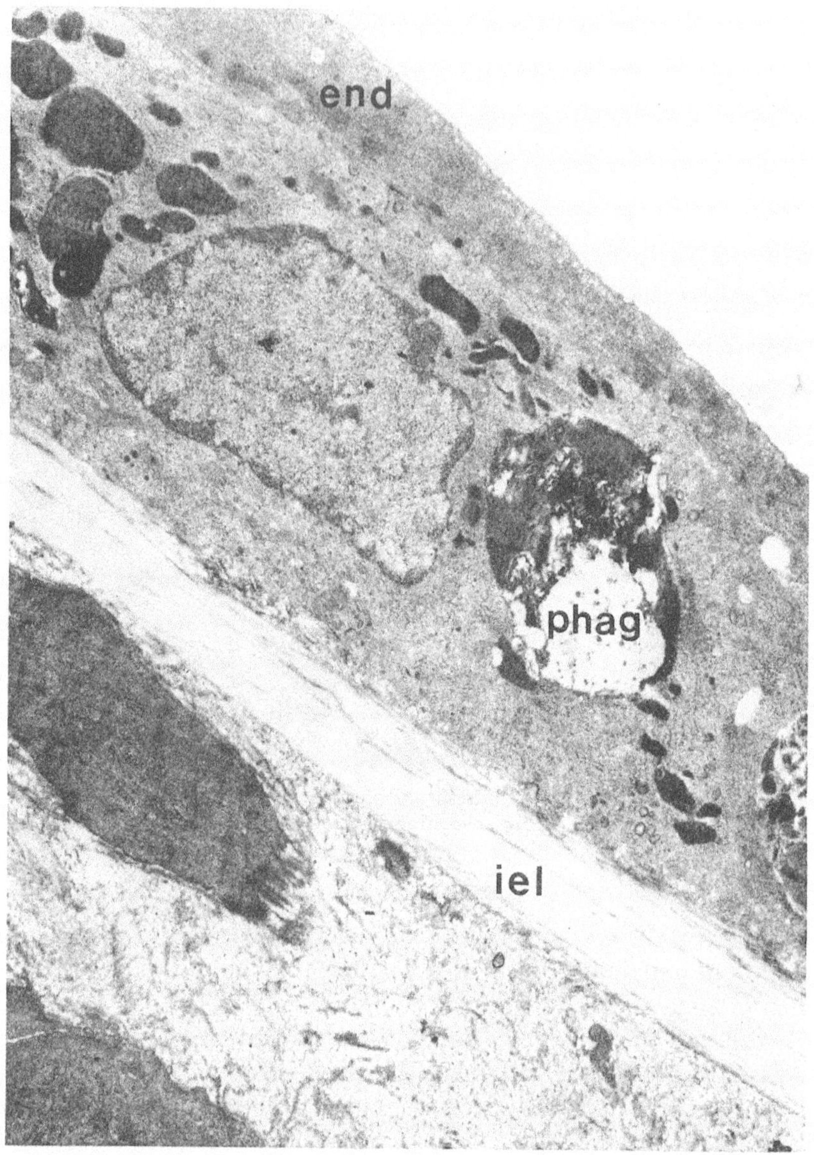

Fig. 10. Phagocytosing subendothelial intimal cells, 3 days after sheathing of the aorta.
×10200

After a period of from 4 to 6 weeks the intimal plaques consisted of longitudinal endothelial cells and a proliferation of up to 10 layers of smooth muscle cells. As previously stated, the lengthened cytoplasm of the muscle cells contained different cellular organelles and numerous myofilaments (Fig. 14). Mature elastic and collagenous fibrils almost reached the endothelium; increased collagenous fibrils were found between the regular muscle cells. Large myoblasts with plump cellular processes were lying in the outer media (Fig. 15). Up to 3 units of muscle cells and the elastic laminae were dissociated by protein-rich edema at the medial-adventitial border. In the adjacent adventitial connective tissue bundles of collagenous fibrils predominated, enclosing edematous streaks.

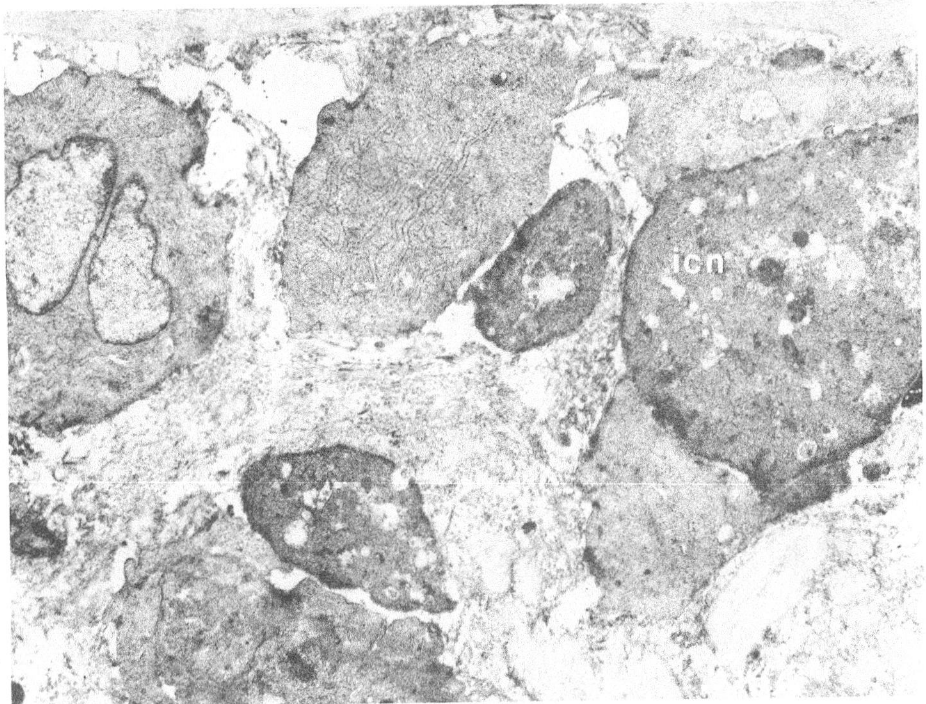

Fig. 11. Partial intracellular necroses of muscle cells (*icn*) in the media, 3 days following sheathing of the aorta. ×10000

After 2 or 3 months the endothelium was flattened; the endothelial cells were connected by small zonulae occludentes. New elastic laminae were formed within the dense ground substance and between the subendothelial collagenous fibrils. In some areas of the media several laminar units were replaced by an increased ground substance as well as by numerous collagenic fibrils (Fig. 16). By this time the adventitial connective tissue was uniformly sclerosed.

After 4 to 6 months smooth muscle cells and elastic laminae had been largely replaced by fibrosis within the intimal plaques. Only a few atrophic muscle cells with long cellular processes could be found between the condensed elastic laminae and the collagenous fiber bundles of the media (Fig. 17).

Morphometric Results

The thickness of the intima, media, and entire sheathed aortic wall were measured separately and the number of elastic units counted. One of the side-effects of sheathing was widespread disintegration of the adventitial connective tissue, which made a statistical evaluation of the adventitial data virtually impossible. With the aid the Olivetti's P 102 the mean values of the intimal thickness and of the medial thickness were determined for aortic segments (2) and (3), corresponding to chronological phases I through IV.

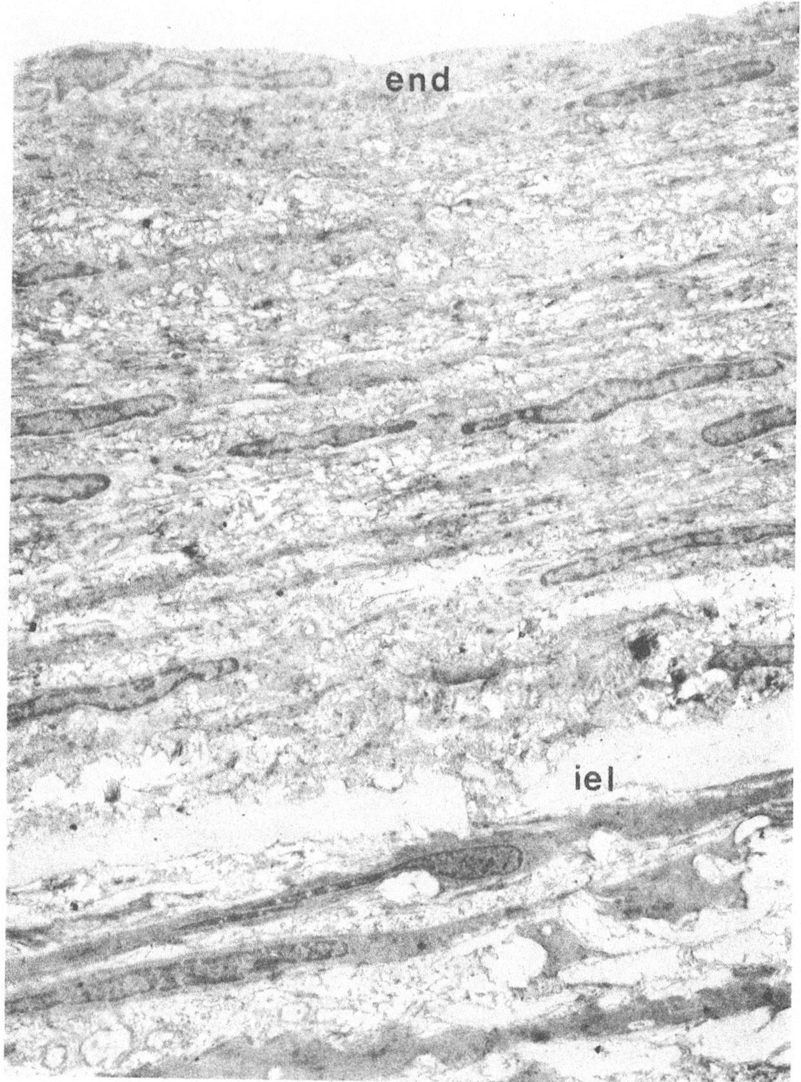

Fig. 12. High proliferation of intimal cells between endothelium (*end*) and internal elastic lamina (*iel*), 14 days following sheathing of the aorta. ×6800

The calculations also included comparisons with the normal values. The results of the calculations can be found in Table 2. Cases that developed hypertension, due to constrictions from the cuffs were discarded. Significance was calculated according to Student's t distribution.

For exact measurement, strictly transverse sections of the vascular wall are essential. Sections of the bigger arterial vessels can be taken only in preparations that still have regular layering of the vascular wall in addition to maintaining the regular elastic units of the media. Within the group of vascular segments with cuffs this condition was fulfilled only in control

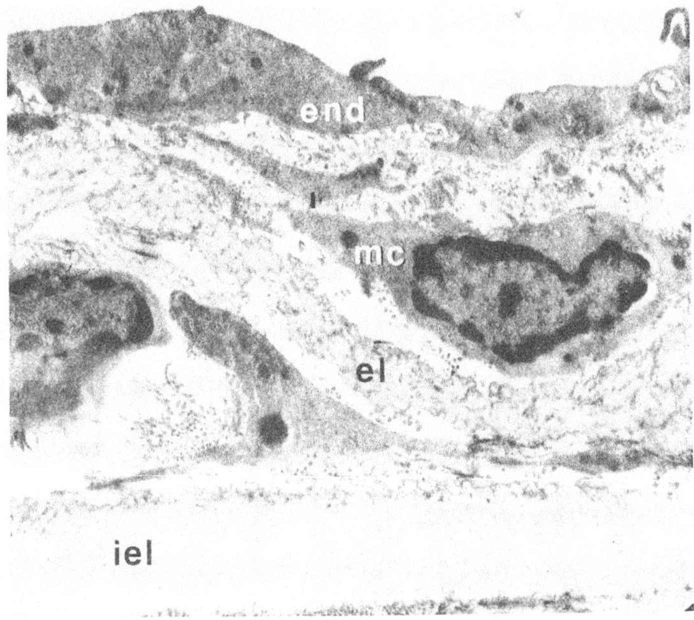

Fig. 13. Intima with proliferation of muscle cells (*mc*) and formation of new elastic laminae (*el*) above the internal elastic lamina (*iel*), 14 days after sheathing of the aorta. ×11 900

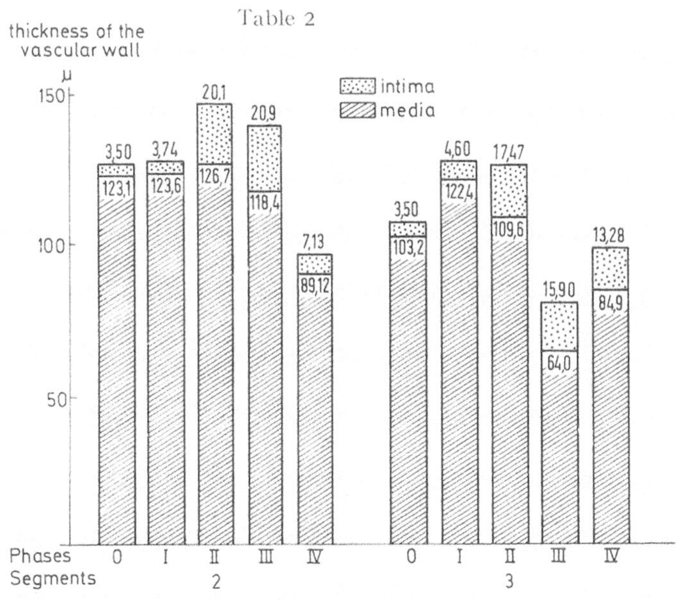

Table 2

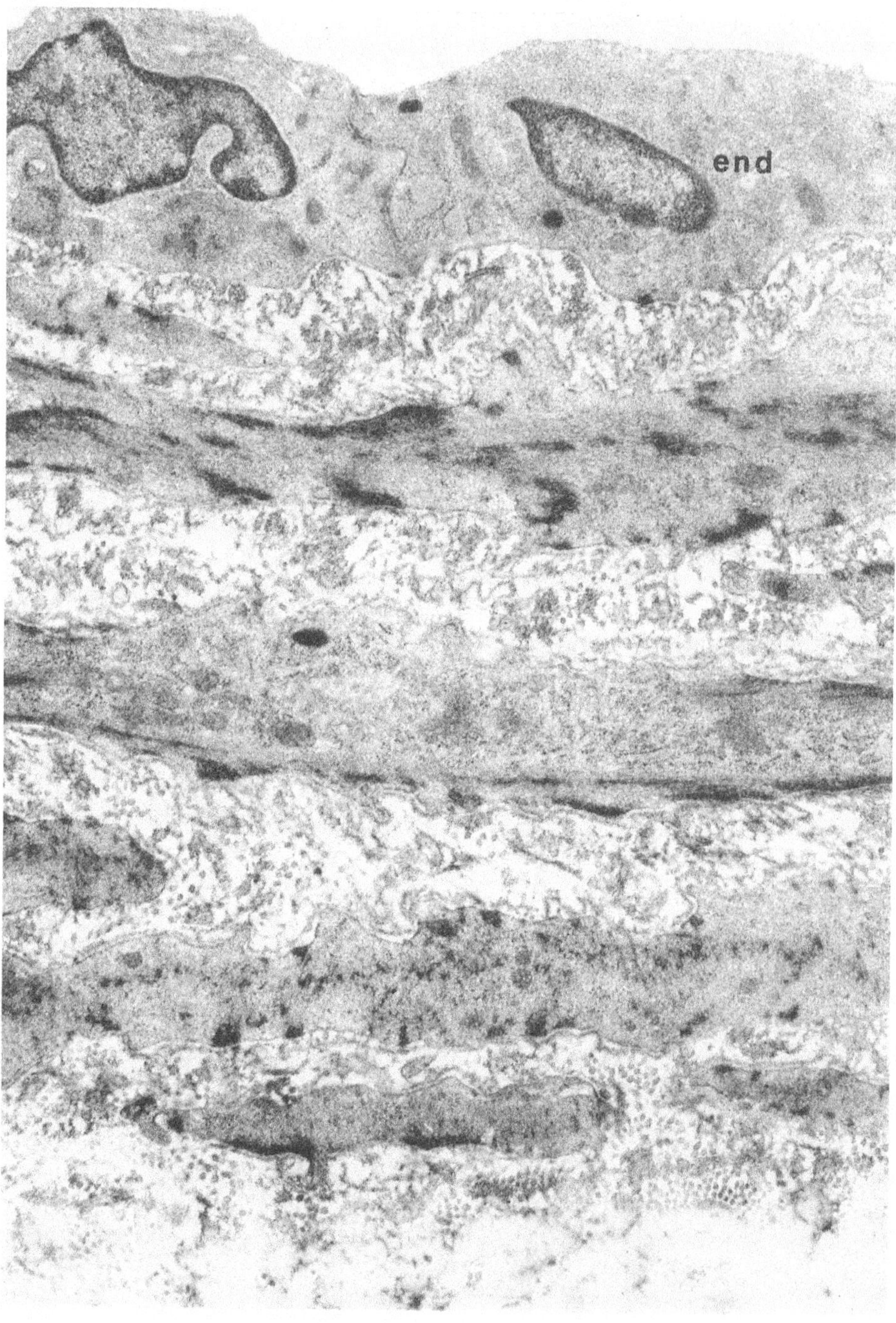

Fig. 14. Broad endothelium (*end*) and proliferated subendothelial intimal cells with myofilaments and high developed ergastoplasm, in between elastic laminae, 4 weeks after sheathing of the aorta. ×17000

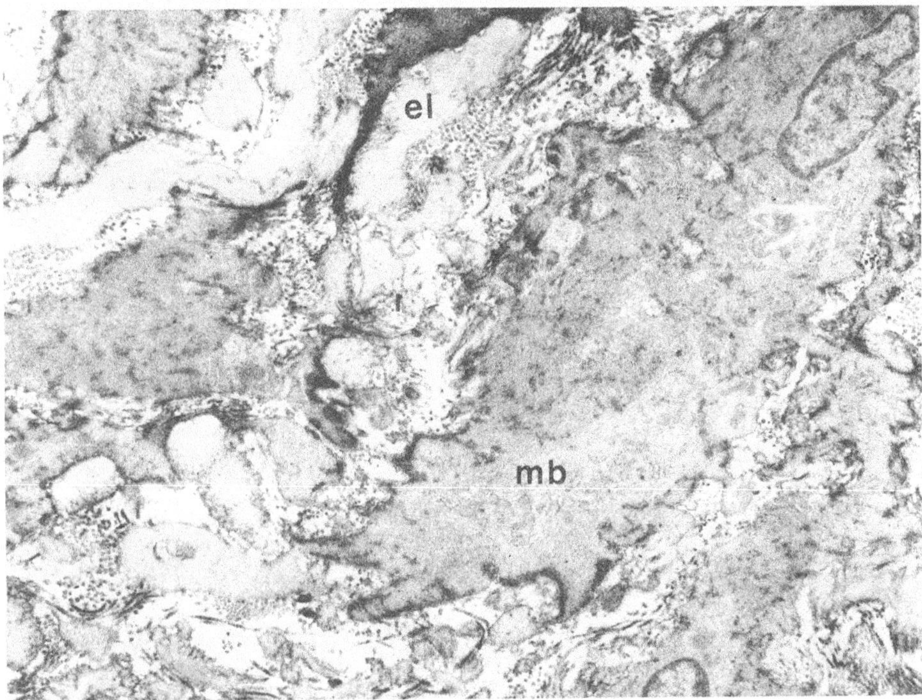

Fig. 15. Partly collapsed elastic laminae (*el*), atrophic muscle cells and myoblasts (*mb*) in the outer media, 4 weeks following sheathing of the aorta. ×10 200

segments or during the first experimental phase (6 days after sheathing). Exact orthograde sections reveal 17 to 19 medial elastic units within the aorta of rabbits. These ideal transverse sections give the following mean values for the media and intima: 89.12 μ medial and 3,74 μ intimal thickness within the upper aortic cuff (2), as well as 78.80 μ medial and 4.60 μ intimal thickness in the lower sheathed segment (3).

Since the dissociation of the aortic vascular structures prevented the identification of ideal transverse sections during phase II, we were unable to make measurements and calculations in absolute transverse sections. Thus the values had to be calculated by numerous measurements of the vascular mural cross-sections, ranging from the thinnest to the thickest. Under these conditions the following average relative values have been calculated:

In control animals and control segments (0) the intima measures 3.5 μ and the media 123.1 μ within segment 2 and in segment 3 the thickness of the intima is 3.5 μ and of the media 103.2 μ.

Within segment 2 during phase I (up to 6 days survival) the media thickness was 123.6 μ and that of the intima 3.74 μ. The corresponding values for the lower segments are 122.4 μ and 4.6 μ respectively.

In phase II (after 2 to 3 weeks) a mean medial thickness of 126.9 μ and an increase of the intimal thickness up to 20.1 μ were measured within the

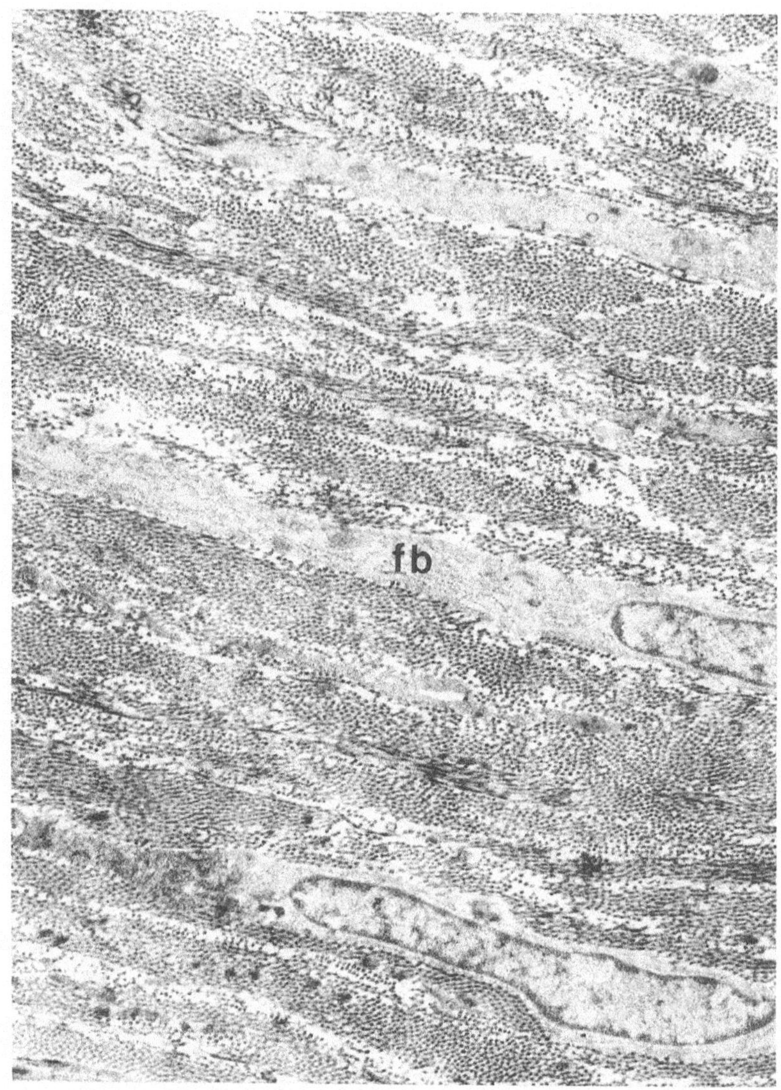

Fig. 16. Dense collagenous fibrous network and fibroblasts (*fb*) of the adventitia, 11 weeks following sheathing of the aorta. ×10200

upper cuff. The values for segment 3 ranged around 109.6 μ for the media and 17.5 μ for the intima.

During phase III (1 to 3 months survival) the mean values of the media were 118.5 μ and of the intima 20.8 μ in the upper segment (2). Since 3 animals of this group developed a total sclerosis of the vascular wall and thus prevented differentiated measurement of the layers in the vascular wall, these values are based only on individual measurements.

The corresponding values of the lower segment (3) were 64.0 μ for the media and 15.1 μ for the intima.

During phase IV (up to 6 months) the medial thickness decreased to 89.1 μ in the upper segment (2) and 84.8 μ in the lower segment (3). Intimal averages were 7.1 μ in segment 2 and 13.3 μ in segment 3.

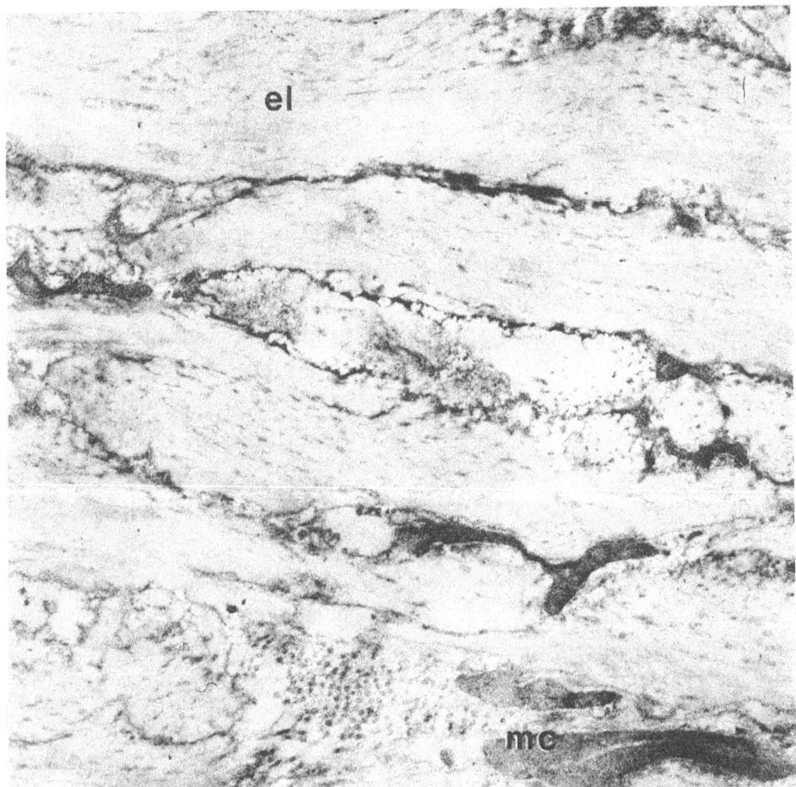

Fig. 17. Elastic laminae (*el*) and highly atrophic muscle cells (*mc*) of the media, 5 months following sheathing of the aorta. ×19 500

The results of the count of all elastic laminae can be summarized as progressive reduction of medial elastic laminae within the sheathed segments over the duration of the experiment. Exact counts were not possible during the later experimental phases, because the strongly sclerosed aortic segments contained only remnants of collapsed elastic laminae. The newly formed elastic laminae within the proliferated intima cannot be counted exactly due to a wide variety of staining qualities and different stage of maturity.

Discussion of the Experimental Methods

Previously published experimental investigations with vascular sheathing, as shown in Table 1, demonstrated that the experimental model can be performed surgically. The model also showed that the plastic cuffs used can prevent foreign-body reactions that could dominate the proliferative and sclerotic reconstructive processes of the vascular wall. Therefore, we focused the light- and electron-microscopic investigations on animals which showed the lowest degree of foreign body reaction in the macroscopic and light-microscopic preparations. The silastic cuffs were inert, whereas the skin clamps used for tightening the cuffs induced intensive formation of granulomata. Following application of polyethylene tubes, the foreign-body reaction was limited to the adventitial tissue actually sheathed by the cuff.

Going beyond the published experimental models, the authors sheathed more than one vascular segment, simultaneously applying cuffs around the upper abdominal aorta between the superior mesenteric artery and the renal arteries as well as around both renal arteries, and approximately 3 mm distal to them on the lower abdominal aorta. Such multiple sheathing allows a comparison of the different enclosed vascular segments within the same animal. Furthermore, the demonstrated method of multiple sheathing creates an intermediate segment (8) of the abdominal aorta between the two aortic cuffs and those round the renal arteries. The alterations in such an intermediate segment are especially interesting because of a potential disturbance of the flow of liquid through the aortic wall in either a longitudinal or an oblique direction. Squeezing of vascular layers by constricting threads or temporary ligature of the vessels is not comparable with the demonstrated sheathing, since circumscribed strangulations or stronger compressions of the vascular wall lead to traumatic lesions and change the intravascular pressure with varying consequences (Kunz *et al.*, 1967; Hoff and Gottlob, 1968; Hoff, 1970; Ts'ao, 1970). It should be mentioned in a critical review of our experimental model that the vascular sheathing was sometimes not complete enough to obtain total enclosure of the vascular segment by the cuff. In addition, the desired slight compression of the adventitial tissue tended to vary. Such incomplete sheathing as against total blockage of vascular nutrition and drainage could explain the individual variations in the vascular alterations. The achieved blockage of the vascular drainage to the outside cannot be compared with pure lymphostasis of the aortic wall. Jellinek, Veress and their coworkers (1961/1966) did induce experimental sclerosis of coronary and pulmonary arteries by mediastinal lymphostasis, but comparable sclerosing processes have been observed following venous stasis, as has already been pointed out by Johnson (1969). An experimental lymphostasis should have subsided within 2 to 3 weeks.

The additional morphometric interpretations of the vascular sclerosis in this series of investigations allow comparisons of vascular reaction within the different sheathed segments. Furthermore, the degree of the sclerosis is more apparent due to the morphometric means. The fixation applied, as well as the morphometric methods do not allow the data to be recorded as absolute values. Since the conditions were held constant throughout the entire series of experiments, it seems legitimate to make a statistical calculation of the morphometric data and to interpret them collectively. The demonstrated scanning-electron-microscopic results complement earlier findings in transmission electron microscopy and with ultrathin sections. The scanning-electron-microscopic images of the intimal surface allow a comparison with the so-called "Häutchenpräparate" as, for instance, obtained by SUZUKI (1967) following vascular sheathing. In addition, surface images allow one to estimate the density of the endothelial cells in the various phases of the experiments, as well as to the amount and size of the interendothelial stigmata. The variety of tensional conditions that occur in the fixed and dried preparations, as frequently noted, has to be regarded as a limiting factor for the reliability of conclusions drawn from scanning-electron-micrographs.

Discussion of the Findings

Sheathing of the aortic segments by cuffs of different plastic materials leads to degenerative and proliferative alterations of the aortic wall. These can be roughly divided into four phases according to their chronological development:

1. Up to 6 days after sheathing: small endothelial defects arise, partly coated by aggregates of thrombocytes. Plasmatic insudation, precipitation of fibrin, and focal leukocytic infiltrates occur within the intima. Several layers of smooth muscle cells become necrotic in the outer media. A slight foreign-body reaction can be observed within the partially squashed adventitia.

2. Two weeks after sheathing: some intimal cells are proliferating. The necrotic muscle cells of the media are partly replaced by proliferations of muscle cells. The adventitial foreign-body reaction remains moderate.

3. One to three months after sheathing: the proliferated intimal cells undergo progressive narrowing. The myofilaments become more apparent. New elastic laminae and collagenous fibrils of increasing maturity develop between the muscle cells. The muscle cells become partly replaced by fibroblast-like cells. Elastic laminae become rarer or collapse increasingly. Dense bundles of collagenous fibrils predominate within the adventitia.

4. Up to 6 months after sheathing: the fibrotic alterations proceed throughout all mural layers. The muscle cells of the vascular wall remain atrophic and fibrocytoid with an increasing density of long cellular processes between the fibrillar network. After 4 to 6 months the sclerosis of the vascular wall has developed so far that the total aortic wall consists of a uniform tube of connective tissue with only a few scattered cells and dense collagen. The mural structure sometimes resembles that of chronic arterial aneurysms. During this phase occasional new endothelial lesions can be demonstrated with the aid of scanning electron microscopy.

None of the phases revealed atheromatous alterations. Concerning the above classification into four phases, it should be emphasized that the described findings cannot be sharply separated. Overlapping of alterations in chronological pathogenesis always occur. The primary proliferative and secondary sclerotic mural reconstruction following the first traumatic lesion resulting from the surgical procedure corresponds to a parabolic increase and decrease of the intimal thickness. As demonstrated by morphometry, it also corresponds to a decrease of the medial thickness during the third and fourth phases.

A comparison between our results and those reported in the literature on experimental atherosclerosis of rabbits clearly demonstrates that feeding of cholesterol and mechanical mural lesions like overstretching and endothelial damage, were preferred as a model of human atherosclerosis (PRIOR and HARTMANN, 1956; HEPTINSTALL and PORTER, 1957; BUCK, 1958; WILLIAMS, 1961; STILL, 1963; BAUMGARTNER and STUDER, 1963; PARKER and ODLAND, 1966; GETZ *et al.*, 1969; SHIMAMOTO *et al.*, 1971; KNIERIEM, 1970/1973). CONSTANTINIDES (1965) regarded rabbits as especially suitable for comparative investigations of atherogenesis. He claimed that thrombocytes do not play an atherogenous role in acute intimal lesions; this explained why thrombosis could be observed relatively seldom, and why no influence of thrombotic processes on the proliferative and sclerotic mural changes of vessels could be found. This method does not allow a comparison with experiments in which aortic segments are stretched by balloon catheters with regard to either the procedure of the effects obtained (STUDER and LOREZ, 1967; HELIN *et al.*, 1971). In the demonstrated method of aortic sheathing, traumatic stretching and corresponding mural lesions cannot be completely excluded; for the sheathing procedure the aorta has to be pulled out of its surrounding tissue in a longitudinal direction. Comparable intimal thickenings induced by vascular sheathing were reported earlier by LANGE (1924), TAKEDA (1961), IIJIMA (1964), and ZELLWEGER *et al.* (1970). A local intimal plaque at the end of the cuffs, as demonstrated by sheathing without tightening by enwoven threads, has been described similarly by WILENS (1942), SUZUKI (1967), and MIZUKAWA (1969). With the exception of LANGE (1924), these authors all mentioned medial necroses following sheathing. The acute traumatic lesion of the aortic wall can account for such early findings as endothelial defects, insudation of plasm, leukocytic infiltrates, and necroses of medial cells. These changes appeared as early as 30 to 100 min after sheathing, which is in agreement with published findings. The further development of proliferative and sclerotic processes in the intima and media cannot normally be considered to be the result of a single stretching of the vascular wall. Following a single traumatic lesion of the intima and outer media proliferative intimal plaques arise which can secondarily undergo sclerotic changes accompanied by medial scars (WILLIAMS, 1956; DUNCAN, 1963; STILL and DENNISON, 1967; BJÖRKERUD, *et al.*, 1972; HOFF and GOTTLOB, 1968). HASS (1955) regarded the traumatic stretching of the vascular wall with resulting ruptures of the internal elastic lamina as the cause of reactive intimal proliferations. The progression of the proliferative and sclerotic vascular alterations can, however, be explained only by additional stress factors, assumed to be due to the experimental procedure. Control investigations with similar traumatic stretching of the vessels, but without subsequent sheathing did not lead to a progressive sclerosis of the vessels. The blockage of nutritional vessels in the adventitia and the interruption of the adventitial drainage of the aortic wall by the cuffs are considered important additional stress factors. The importance of the slight adventitial compression due to the cuffs is clear from our experience of animals operated on with only loosely applied tubes around their vessels. Only a few of these animals showed small proliferative plaques of the intima at the edge of the tubes, and definite sclerotic alterations did not occur inside the loosely ensheathed vascular segments.

Vasa vasorum are not a constant constituent of the rabbit aorta. According to LINZBACH (1957) arterial walls do not contain medial vasa vasorum below a thickness of 500 μ. However, a rather dense adventitial plexus of vessels exists in the outer aortic wall with definite nutritional functions (HUNDEIKER, 1970; HAUST and MORE, 1972). In addition to the nutritional vessels, a system of lymphatics and small collecting lymph vessels has been described in the aortic adventitia. The blockage of these vessels has been discussed as an atherogeneous factor (JOHNSON and BLAKE, 1965; HUNDEIKER, 1970). Among the investigation results presented, the recurrent necroses of the muscle cells in the outer media in particular can be explained by nutritional deficiency. The type of necroses of the medial cells observed including the necroses of circumscribed cytoplasmic parts of medial muscle cells is well known to be a hypoxic effect due to various conditions like shock and collapse (MEESSEN, 1939; HUEPER, 1944/45; LOPEZ DE FARIA, 1955; SORGER, 1968). TAKEDA (1961), IIJIMA (1964), and SUZUKI (1967) pointed out that a moderate increase of mural permeability is to be expected in all vascular layers rather than an oxygen deficiency. These factors lead to a vicious circle of hypoxia—increase of permeability—mural edema—condensation of ground substance—elongation of the distance for diffusion—hypoxia. However, hypoxia cannot be regarded as the only important factor, since other severe signs of hypoxic damage, such as fatty degeneration of vascular mural constituents, are completely lacking.

A condensation of ground substance in intima and media following the acute mural edema can be regarded under the conditions used in the experiment primarily as an effect of blockage of the vascular drainage from the inside to the outside. The progressive replacement of degenerating medial muscle cells by connective tissue as well as the extensive fibrillogenesis within the dense ground substance can be interpreted as a formation of a protein-rich matrix which enables fibrogenous elements to grow inwards. Such fibrotic processes have been induced in several organs by the interruption of the lymphatic outflow and development of edema rich in protein (RUSZNYÁK et al., 1969). A blockage of lymphatic drainage from the aortic adventitia can be expected, since a reactive outgrow of lymph vessels has often been observed in the surrounding tissue of the cuffs.

Concerning the morphological appearance of the induced vascular sclerosis, it should be emphasized once more that no atheromatous component arose in contrast to the spontaneous arteriosclerosis in rabbits and in other types of experimental arteriosclerosis of rabbits described by other authors due to different experimental methods (CONSTANTINIDES, 1965; KNIERIEM, 1970;

Knieriem *et al.*, 1973). Thus, the experimental methods presented and the sclerotic changes provoked can be regarded as a model of a pure proliferative sclerosing type of arteriosclerosis.

The vascular alterations demonstrated were strictly limited to the segments within the cuffs. Even in the intermediate segment (8) between the cuffs of the aorta and those of the renal arteries no atheromatous alterations occurred, and no sclerosis developed. Therefore, it may be presumed that the effect of the pathogenetic factors discussed was limited to the vascular segments within the cuffs. It may be concluded accordingly that liquid flow in a longitudinal or oblique direction through the aortic wall, as deduced by Linzbach (1957) and Doerr (1958), cannot play an important role in the species investigated. A blockage of such longitudinal or oblique liquid flow by the cuffs would have induced alterations at least in the vascular parts adjacent to the cuffs. The fact that proliferative and sclerotic alterations were lacking in the intermediate segment (8) and in the cranial control segment (1) proves that no hypertonic effect arose and that the cuffs did not cause hypertension due to vascular constriction. The development of the mural alterations of the vessels and the pathogenetic factors influencing these developments are shown in Scheme 2.

The experimental model presented invokes questions concerning analogous stress factors in human vessels. Sheathing of intact vessels with plastic

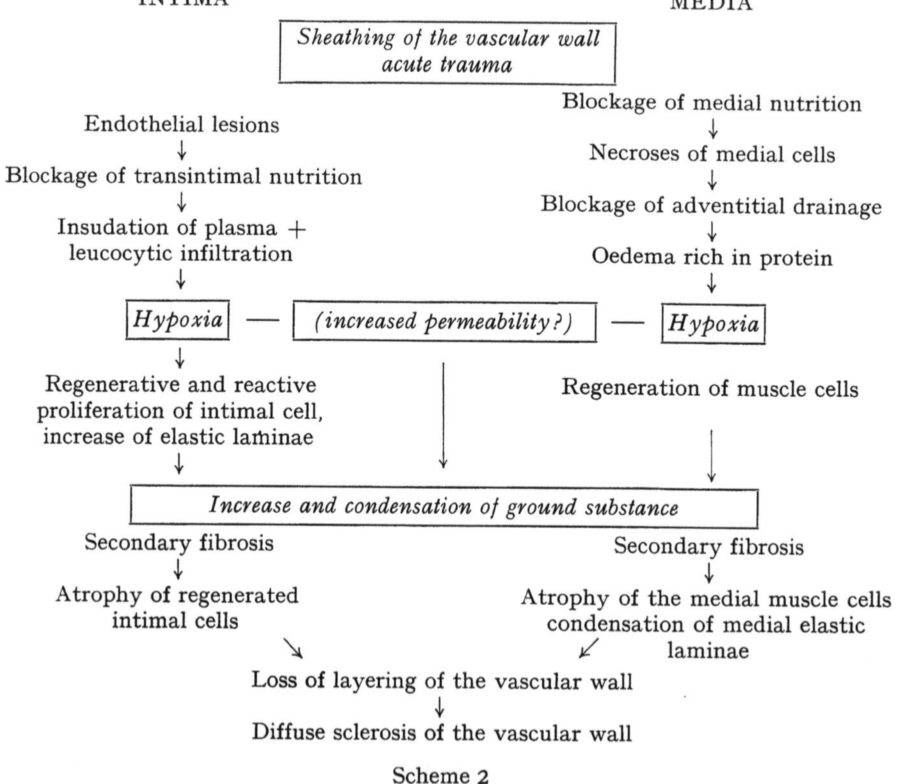

Scheme 2

materials is unlikely to have any importance in human medicine. A blockage of adventitial nutritional or draining vessel is, however, conceivable. Such manifestations as venous stasis, primary or secondary dynamic insufficiency of the lymph vessel system, tumorous encapsulation of the aorta or a lymphangiosis carcinomatosis, sclerosing processes of the mediastinal or retroperitoneal space and the effects of irradiation have been discussed (ZINSERLING, 1934/35; CONSTANTINIDES *et al.*, 1958; THOMAS and FORBUS, 1959; HOLLE, 1962; PESCH and KRACHT, 1963; DOERR, 1963). It remains open to discussion how far senile lymphangiosclerosis (BORCHARD *et al.*, 1972; OTTO *et al.*, 1973) can promote secondary arteriosclerotic vascular alterations.

The experimental procedure developed and the model of pure proliferative sclerotic arteriosclerosis will allow further studies of arteriosclerotic changes. In addition, the method of vascular sheathing could be combined with other factors thought to be concerned in the pathogenesis of arteriosclerosis and atherosclerosis.

Summary

Sheathing of the upper and lower abdominal aorta of rabbits by cuffs of plastic material leads to acute necroses of the outer media and the adventitial connective tissue. Simultaneously the acute traumatic stress of the vascular segments causes focal endothelial lesions with subsequent insudation of plasma and leukocytic infiltration of the intima. After 3 days occasional hyperregenerative proliferations of medial muscle cells and subendothelial intimal cells occur. After 2 to 6 weeks a progressive fibrosis of all mural layers develops within the sheathed aortic segments, accompanied by an outgrowth of mature collagenous connective tissue between the intimal and medial smooth muscle cells. Following the progressive fibrosis the muscular elements of the vascular wall appear increasingly atrophic. After 2 to 4 months the vascular wall has undergone complete sclerosis.

For the induced vascular alterations the following pathogenetic factors have been discussed: acute trauma by vascular stretching, blockage of the medial nutrition from the outside, blockage of the transintimal nutrition, obstruction of the adventitial drainage, a subsequent mural edema rich in protein, and hypoxia of the vascular wall leading to increased permeability as well as to an increase in and condensation of the ground substance.

The proliferative and secondary sclerotic alterations of the vessels are limited to the sheathed segments. Atheromatous changes do not develop. The combined sheathing and the subsequent alterations of the aortic wall introduced above as a model of a non-atheromatous, pure proliferative sclerosing experimental arteriosclerosis allow speculations as to the pathogenesis of sclerotic vascular processes in man. In addition, the experimental model presented could be combined with other stress factors known to induce arteriosclerosis or atherosclerosis.

References

Adami, I. G., Aschoff, L.: On the myelins, myelin bodies and potential fluid crystals of the organism. Proc. roy. Soc. B **78**, 359 (1906).

Adams, C. W. M.: Passage of cholesterol through the arterial wall. Proc. roy. Soc. Med. **57**, 789 (1964).

Anitschkow, N.: Über die Veränderungen der Kaninchenaorta bei experimenteller Cholesterinsteatose. Beitr. path. Anat. **56**, 379–404 (1913).

Anitschkow, N.: Über die Atherosclerose der Aorta beim Kaninchen und über deren Entstehungsbedingungen. Beitr. path. Anat. **59**, 308–348 (1914).

Baumgartner, H. R., Studer, A.: Controlled over-dilation of the abdominal aorta in normo- and hypercholesterinemic rabbits. Path. et Microbiol. (Basel) **26**, 129–148 (1963).

Björkerud, S.: Über die Heilung experimenteller Intimaläsionen und ihre Beziehung zur Genese der Atheromatose und Arteriosklerose. Klin. Wschr. **47**, 1322 (1968).

Björkerud, S.: Atherosclerosis initiated by mechanical trauma in normolipidemic rabbits. J. Atheroscler. Res. **9**, 209 (1969).

Björkerud, S., Hanson, H. A., Bondjers, G.: Subcellular valves and canaliculi in arterial endothelium and their equivalence to so called stigmata. Virchows Arch. Abt. B **11**, 19–23 (1972).

Borchard, F., Borchard, H., Huth, F.: Beitrag zur lymphvasculären Sklerose des Ductus thoracicus. Beitr. path. Anat. **146**, 145–161 (1972).

Buck, R. C.: The fine structure of the aortic endothelial lesions on experimental cholesterol atherosclerosis of rabbits. Amer. J. Path. **34**, 879 (1958).

Constantinides, P.: Experimental atherosclerosis in the rabbit. In: Comparative atherosclerosis (ed. Roberts and Straus), p. 276–290. New York: Harper & Row 1965.

Constantinides, P.: Experimental atherosclerosis. Amsterdam-London-New York: Elsevier 1965.

Constantinides, P., Gutmann-Auersperg, N., Hospes, D.: Acceleration of intimal atherogenesis through prior medial injury. Arch. Path. **66**, 247–254 (1958).

Cremer, H., Müller, N.: Histological findings in the aorta of rats after experimental ligature of the thoracic duct. Folia angiol. (Pisa) **21**, 270–273 (1973).

Doerr, W.: Über Aortensklerose. Studien zur Pathogenese. Klin. Wschr. **36**, 1087 (1958).

Doerr, W.: Pathologie der herznahen großen Gefäße. In: Bargmann, W., Doerr, W.: Das Herz des Menschen, Bd. II, S. 894–979. Stuttgart: Thieme 1963.

Doerr, W.: Perfusionstheorie der Arteriosklerose. Stuttgart: Thieme 1963.

Duff, G. L.: Experimental cholesterol arteriosclerosis and its relationship to human arteriosclerosis. Arch. Path. **20**, 81–123, 123–304 (1935).

Duncan, L. E.: Mechanical factors in the localisation of atheromata. In: Evolution of the atherosclerotic plaque (ed. Jones, R. J.), p. 171–182. Chicago: University Press 1963.

Getz, G. S., Vesselinovitch, D., Wissler, R. W.: A dynamic pathology of atherosclerosis. Amer. J. Med. **46**, 657–673 (1969).

Gofman, J. W., Lindgren, F., Elliott, A., Mantz, W., Hewitt, J., Strisower, B., Hetting, V., Lyon, T. P.: The role of lipids and lipoproteins in atherosclerosis. Science **111**, 166–171 (1950).

Hass, G. M.: Observations on vascular structure in relation to human and experimental arteriosclerosis. In: Symposium on Atherosclerosis, p. 24. Nat. Acad. Sci. Nat. Res. Counc. Publ. 338, Washington D.C. (1955).

Haust, M. D.: Injury and repair in the pathogenesis of atherosclerotic lesions. In: Atherosclerosis (ed. Jones, R. J., p. 12–20). New York-Heidelberg-Berlin: Springer 1970.

Haust, M. D., More, R. H.: Spontaneous lesions of the aorta in the rabbit. In: Comparative atherosclerosis (ed. Roberts and Straus), p. 255–275. New York: Harper & Row 1965.

Haust, M. D., More, R. H.: Development of modern theories on the pathogenesis of atherosclerosis. In: The pathogenesis of atherosclerosis (ed. Wissler, R. W., Geer, J. C.), p. 1–19. Baltimore: Williams & Wilkins 1972.

Haust, M. D., More, R. H., Balis, J. U.: Electron microscopic study of intimal lipid accumulations in human aorta and their pathogenesis. Circulation **26**, 656–657 (1962).

HELIN, P., LORENZEN, I., GARBASCH, C., MATTHIESSEN, M. E.: Arteriosclerosis in rabbit aorta induced by mechanical dilatation. Atherosclerosis 13, 319–331 (1971).

HEPTINSTALL, R. H., PORTER, K. H.: The effect of a brief period of high blood pressure on cholesterol-induced atheroma in rabbits. Brit. J. exp. Path. 38, 55–61 (1957).

HOFF, H. F.: Studies on the pathogenesis of atherosclerosis with experimental model systems. Virchows Arch. Abt. A 351, 179–192 (1970).

HOFF, H. F., GOTTLOB, R.: Ultrastructural changes of large rabbit blood vessels following mild mechanical trauma. Virchows Arch. Abt. A 345, 93–106 (1968).

HOLLE, G.: Falten und Leisten in der Aortenwand infolge abnormer Krümmung des Gefäßrohres oder durch Narbenzug. Virchows Arch. path. Anat. 335, 617–625 (1962).

HUEPER, W. C.: Arteriosclerosis. A general review. Arch. Path. 38, 162, 245, 350 (1944); 39, 51, 117, 187 (1945).

HUNDEIKER, M.: Zur Darstellung der Vasa vasorum in der Tunica media der Arterienwand. Angiologica 7, 1–7 (1970).

IIJIMA, Y.: Experimental studies on the arteriosclerosis in rabbits. Kitakanto med. J. 14, 36–70 (1964).

JELLINEK, H., FÖLDI, M., BÜKY, B., MESZAROS, S.: Some data concerning the problem of interconnections between intraadventitial spaces of the pulmonary arteries and the lymph vessels. Acta morph. Acad. Sci. hung. 11, 41–46 (1961).

JOHNSON, R. A.: Lymphatics of blood vessels. Lymphology 2, 2, 44–56 (1969).

JOHNSON, R. A., BLAKE, T. M.: Lymphatics of arteries. Circulation (Suppl. II) 32, 119 Ref. (1965).

KNIERIEM, H. J.: Elektronenmikroskopische Untersuchungen zur Bedeutung der glatten Muskelzellen für die Pathogenese der Arteriosklerose. Beitr. path. Anat. 140, 298–332 (1970).

KNIERIEM, H. J.: Immunhistochemische Untersuchungen zur Bedeutung der glatten Muskelzellen für die Pathohistogenese der Arteriosklerose des Menschen. Beitr. path. Anat. 141, 4–18 (1970).

KNIERIEM, H. J., BONDJERS, G., BJÖRKERUD, S.: Electron microscopy of intimal plaques following induction of large superficial mechanical injury (transverse injury) in the rabbit aorta. Virchows Arch. Abt. A 359, 261–282 (1973).

KUNZ, J., KRANZ, D., KEIM, D.: Autoradiographische Untersuchungen zur Synthese von DNS, Kollagen und Mucopolysacchariden bei der experimentellen Proliferation der Aortenintima. Virchows Arch. path. Anat. 342, 345–352 (1967).

LANGE, F.: Studien zur Pathologie der Arterien, insbesondere zur Lehre von der Arteriosklerose. Virchows Arch. path. Anat. 248, 463–604 (1924).

LINZBACH, A. J.: Vergleich der dystrophischen Vorgänge an Knorpel und Arterien als Grundlage zum Verständnis der Arteriosklerose. Virchows Arch. path. Anat. 311, 432–508 (1944).

LINZBACH, A. J.: Die Bedeutung der Gefäßwandfaktoren für die Entstehung der Arteriosklerose. Verh. dtsch. Ges. Path. 41, 24–41 (1957).

LOPEZ DE FARIA, J.: Medionekrose der großen und mittelgroßen Arterien nach orthostatischem Kollaps des Kaninchens. Beitr. path. Anat. 115, 373–404 (1955).

MEESSEN, H.: Experimentelle Untersuchungen zum Collapsproblem. Beitr. path. Anat. 102, 191–267 (1939).

MIZUKAWA, H.: Experimental studies on the morphogenesis of arteriosclerosis. Kitakanto med. J. 19, 475–496 (1969).

NYLANDER, G.: Morphologic changes in the experimentally compressed aortic wall in the dog. Acta chir. scand. 123, 92–103 (1962).

NYLANDER, G., OLERUD, S.: The vascularization of the abdominal aorta of the dog after experimental compression. Angiology 12, 2–11 (1961).

OTTO, P. CH., BORCHARD, F., HERBERTZ, G., HUTH, F.: Morphometrische Untersuchungen der Hauptlymphstämme des Halses. Beitr. path. Anat. 148, 55–66 (1973).

PARKER, F., ODLAND, G. F.: A correlative histochemical, biochemical and electron microscopic study of experimental atherosclerosis in the rabbit with special reference to the myointimal cell. Amer. J. Path. 48, 197–239 (1966).

PARKER, F., ODLAND, G. F.: A light microscopic, histochemical and electron microscopic study of experimental atherosclerosis in rabbit coronary and a comparison with rabbit aorta atherosclerosis. Amer. J. Path. 48, 451–481 (1966).

Pesch, K. J., Kracht, J.: Retroperitoneale Fibrose bei Myxödem. Frankfurt. Z. Path. **73**, 97–110 (1963).

Prior, J. T., Hartmann, W. H.: Effect of hypercholesterinemia upon intimal repair aorta of rabbit following experimental trauma. Amer. J. Path. **32**, 417–431 (1956).

Ribbert, H.: Über die Genese der arteriosklerotischen Veränderungen der Intima. Verh. dtsch. Ges. Path. **7**, 168–177 (1904).

Rosenbauer, K. A., Schlösser, H.-W.: Raster-elektronenmikroskopische Untersuchungen an Tube und Ovar. Verh. anat. Ges. (Jena) **67**, 625–631 (1973).

Rusznyák, I., Földi, M., Szabo, G.: Physiologie und Pathologie der Lymphgefäße und des Lymphkreislaufs. Stuttgart: G. Fischer 1969.

Shimamoto, T., Yamashita, Y., Numano, F., Sunaga, T.: Scanning and transmission electron microscopic observations of endothelial cells in the normal condition and in initial stages of atherosclerosis. Acta path. japon. **21**, 93–119 (1971).

Sorger, K.: Über die Veränderungen der Vasa vasorum bei Medionekrosis aortae. Virchows Arch. Abt. A **345**, 107–120 (1968).

Still, W. J. S.: Electron microscopic study of cholesterol atherosclerosis in the rabbit. Exp. molec. Path. **2**, 491–502 (1963).

Still, W. J. S.: The pathogenesis of the intimal thickening produced by hypertension in large arteries in the rat. Lab. Invest. **19**, 84–91 (1968).

Still, W. J. S., Dennison, S. M.: Reaction of the arterial intima of the rabbit to trauma and hyperlipemia. Exp. molec. Path. **6**, 245–253 (1967).

Still, W. J. S., O'Neil, R. M.: Electron microscopic study of experimental atherosclerosis in the rat. Amer. J. Path. **40**, 21–35 (1962).

Studer, A., Lorez, H. P.: Spätveränderungen nach Überdehnung der Aorta abdominalis des Kaninchens bei gleichzeitiger distaler Stenosierung. Path. et Microbiol. (Basel) **30**, 129–138 (1967).

Şuzuki, K.: Experimental studies on morphogenesis of arteriosclerosis, with special reference to relation between hemodynamic change and developments of cellulo-fibrous intimal thickening and atherosclerosis. Gunma J. med. Sci. **16**, 185–243 (1967).

Takeda, F.: Morphogenesis of arteriosclerosis. Trans. Soc. Path. Jap. **50**, 367–393 (1961).

Thomas, E., Forbus, W. D.: Irradiation injury to the aorta and the lung. Arch. Path. **67**, 256–263 (1959).

Ts'ao, Ch.: Graded endothelial injury of the rabbit aorta. Arch. Path. **90**, 222–229 (1970).

Veress, B., Jellinek, H., Hüttner, I., Kerenyi, T., Sotti, F., Iskum, M., Hartai, A., Nagy, J.: Über die Morphologie der lymphstauungsbedingten Koronarveränderungen. Frankfurt. Z. Path. **75**, 331–335 (1966).

Wilens, S. L.: The distribution of intimal atheromatous lesions in the arteries of rabbits on high cholesterol diets. Amer. J. Path. **18**, 63–77 (1942).

Williams, A. W.: Relation of atheroma to local trauma. J. Path. Bact. **81**, 419–422 (1961).

Williams, G.: Experimental studies in arterial ligation. J. Path. Bact. **72**, 569–574 (1956).

Zellweger, J. P., Chapuis, G., Mirkovitch, V.: Consequences morphologiques de l'emballage de l'aorte du chien dans une membrane de caoutchouc silicone. Virchows Arch. Abt. A **350**, 22–35 (1970).

Zinserling, W. D.: Vergleichende Untersuchungen über die Arterienpathologie bei Mensch und Tier. Beitr. path. Anat. **94**, 20–50 (1934/35).

Department of Pathology, University of Bern, Switzerland

Radioactively Labeled Iododeoxyuridine in the Study of Experimental Liver Regeneration*

K. Bürki, J. C. Schaer, P. Grétillat and R. Schindler

With 9 Figures

Contents

A. Labeled Iododeoxyuridine as a DNA Precursor

Since its introduction by Taylor *et al.* (1957) and by Verly and Hune-belle (1957), tritiated thymidine has been used extensively as a precursor of DNA in the autoradiographic and biochemical analysis of proliferating cell systems. In place of thymidine, the deoxyribonucleosides of certain halogenated pyrimidines, such as 5-iodo-2′-deoxyuridine (IDU) may be incorporated into DNA. IDU contains an iodine atom in place of the methyl group of thymidine (Fig. 1). Due to this isosteric substitution, IDU resembles thymidine in being a highly specific precursor of DNA (Eidinoff *et al.*, 1959; Cheong *et al.*, 1960; Prusoff *et al.*, 1960; Hughes *et al.*, 1964). Accordingly, it is incorporated exclusively by DNA-synthesizing cells (Commerford, 1965; Feinendegen *et al.*, 1966a).

---

* This work was supported by the Swiss National Science Foundation.

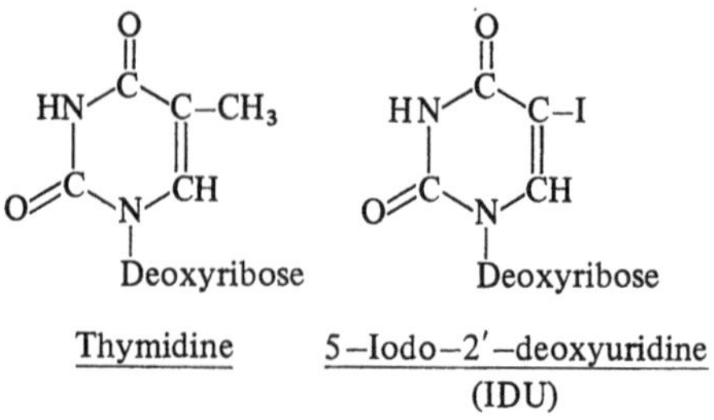

Thymidine   5–Iodo–2′–deoxyuridine
                          (IDU)

Fig. 1. Chemical structure of thymidine and of 5-iodo-2′-deoxyuridine. The iodine atom may be labeled by ^{125}I or ^{131}I

Within a few minutes after a single intravenous injection, IDU is distributed in the tissues of the organism and, as thymidine, it is incorporated quite rapidly into cellular DNA (HAMPTON and EIDINOFF, 1961; HUGHES *et al.*, 1964). Of the injected IDU, however, only a relatively small proportion is incorporated into DNA (PRUSOFF, 1960; HUGHES *et al.*, 1964; Fox and PRUSOFF, 1965), e.g. about 5 to 10% of IDU injected into mice is used for DNA synthesis (HUGHES *et al.*, 1964), whereas approximately 50% of thymidine is incorporated under comparable conditions (POTTER, 1959; STEEL and LAMERTON, 1965). This difference appears to be attributable, at least in part, to less efficient conversion of IDU monophosphate than of thymidine monophosphate to the corresponding triphosphate (BAUGNET-MAHIEU and GOUTIER, 1968).

After being incorporated into DNA, IDU is metabolically stable and remains in the nucleus until cell death (HUGHES *et al.*, 1964; COMMERFORD, 1965; FEINENDEGEN *et al.*, 1966a). Conversely, any IDU that is not incorporated into DNA is rapidly catabolized. The metabolic fate of IDU, as well as the kinetics of elimination of labeled IDU and products of its catabolism have been studied extensively (PRUSOFF *et al.*, 1960; HUGHES *et al.*, 1964; O'FARRELL and DUNAWAY, 1967). The biochemical pathways involved in the incorporation of iodine-labeled IDU into DNA and the metabolic degradation of this iodinated nucleoside are summarized in Fig. 2. The main labeled product of catabolism of iodine-labeled IDU is inorganic iodine; of this, a large proportion is excreted by the kidneys. In the mouse, IDU exhibited a biological half-life of approximately 3 min. In fact, after injection of ^{125}IDU, degradation of the nucleoside as well as excretion of the radioactive isotope were found to occur more rapidly than after administration of ^{3}H-thymidine (Fox and PRUSOFF, 1965). In the mouse, the liver seems to be the main site of IDU catabolism, as judged from differences in labeling patterns after injection of labeled IDU into the portal vein or the vena cava (HUGHES *et al.*, 1964).

As a result of the relatively inefficient incorporation of IDU into DNA and the rapid catabolism of this unnatural precursor, the extent of reutilization by DNA-synthesizing cells of IDU liberated from DNA of disintegrating cells

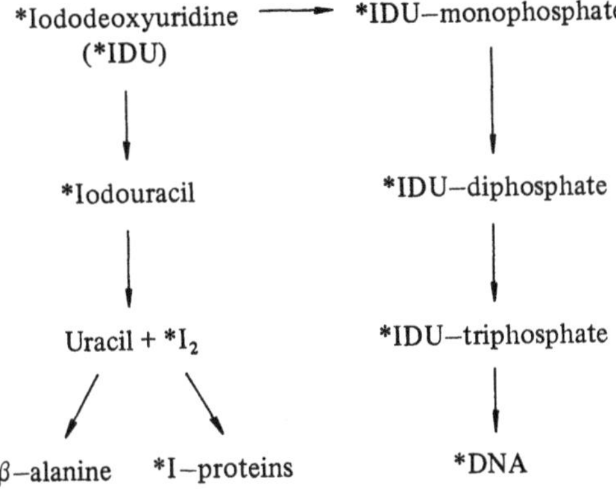

Fig. 2. Metabolic pathways involved in incorporation of iodine-labeled IDU into DNA, degradation of this labeled precursor and in subsequent labeling of proteins, as proposed by PRUSOFF et al. (1960)

is lower than that of thymidine (COMMERFORD, 1965; FEINENDEGEN et al., 1966b; BAUGNET-MAHIEU and GOUTIER, 1968; DETHLEFSEN, 1970). The use of labeled IDU instead of thymidine minimizes the difficulties of estimating the relative contribution of reutilization to labeling of cells (BRYANT, 1962, 1963; FEINENDEGEN et al., 1966b; HEINIGER et al., 1971a) so that the decrease in radioactivity of organs and tissues may be used as a convenient measure of loss of labeled cells. This technique has also been successfully applied to neoplastic cell populations (HOFER et al., 1969a, b; PORSCHEN and FEINENDEGEN, 1969; HOFER, 1970; HOFER and HUGHES, 1970; HOFER et al., 1970; DETHLEFSEN, 1971; HOFER and HOFER, 1971).

Another advantage of IDU compared with thymidine is that labeling can be done with either ^{131}I or ^{125}I. Both isotopes emit gamma radiation of sufficient energy to permit measurement in intact tissues or the entire organism without time-consuming procedures involving biochemical fractionation and/or autoradiography (CALABRESI et al., 1961; HAMPTON and EIDINOFF, 1961; ROTENBERG et al., 1962; HUGHES et al., 1964; COMMERFORD, 1965; FEINENDEGEN et al., 1966b; O'FARRELL and DUNAWAY, 1967, 1969).

Like tritiated thymidine, ^{125}IDU may also be used as a DNA precursor in autoradiographic studies. ^{125}IDU is better suited than ^{131}IDU for autoradiographic analysis of cells and tissues; decay of ^{125}IDU results in emission of Auger and IC electrons with a short range. Resolution of autoradiograms after ^{125}IDU labeling is similar to that after labeling with ^{3}H-thymidine, and the results of autoradiographic analysis after labeling with these two precursors in appropriate doses have been shown to be comparable (APPELGREN et al., 1963; MAK and TILL, 1963; FORBERG et al., 1964; FEINENDEGEN et al., 1966a; SEEMAYER et al., 1966). IDU labeled with ^{125}I may therefore be used for studies of cell proliferation in which autoradiographic analysis is combined with measurements of gamma radiation of intact tissues or organs.

On the other hand, certain limitations inherent in the use of labeled IDU should be kept in mind:

a) After incorporation of halogenated pyrimidines, DNA is chemically modified. This may result in cell damage, particularly after prolonged exposure of cells *in vitro* to these analogs of thymidine at relatively high concentrations (Mathias *et al.*, 1959; Cheong *et al.*, 1960; Djordjevic and Szybalski, 1960; Prusoff *et al.*, 1960; Calabresi *et al.*, 1961). In addition, radiation from the labeled iodine contained in IDU may have harmful effects. In fact, Hofer and Hughes (1971) using L 1210 ascites cells as a model system, showed that ^{131}IDU, after being incorporated into cellular DNA, exhibited only slightly higher radiotoxicity per disintegration per cell than ^{3}H-thymidine, whereas under the same conditions the radiotoxicity of ^{125}IDU was higher by approximately one order of magnitude. On the other hand, no radiation artifacts after were observed after administration of doses of ^{131}IDU as high as 10 µCi per mouse (Hughes *et al.*, 1964). It is, however, of interest that cells containing halogenated pyrimidines in their DNA exhibit increased sensitivity to ionizing radiation (Djordjevic and Szybalski, 1960; Erikson and Szybalski, 1963).

b) The specificity of incorporation into DNA of labeled IDU preparations is affected by radioactive impurities. Such impurities may be formed by radiochemical decomposition of IDU (Hughes *et al.*, 1964). Furthermore, metabolic degradation of labeled IDU (Prusoff, 1960) results in iodine-containing organic products of low molecular weight and inorganic iodine which, in turn, may be incorporated into cellular constituents other than DNA, such as proteins (Prusoff *et al.*, 1960; Hughes *et al.*, 1964; Fox and Prusoff, 1965). It has been shown that in animals given drinking water containing iodide, incorporation of labeled iodine from IDU into proteins is markedly reduced due to dilution of the isotope (Prusoff *et al.*, 1960; Hughes *et al.*, 1964).

c) Since a major part of parenterally administered IDU is catabolized, low-molecular-weight products will remain in the organism for a certain time. If measurements of radioactivity are carried out within short periods after injection of labeled IDU, these products of IDU degradation make a marked contribution to total tissue radioactivity (Hampton and Eidinoff, 1961; Hughes *et al.*, 1964; Fox and Prusoff, 1965; O'Farrell and Dunaway, 1967).

After injection of labeled IDU, total radioactivity in liver and other tissues is thus affected by a number of factors such as purity and metabolic fate of the labeled nucleoside. Furthermore, possible artifacts due to pharmacological and/or radiotoxic effects of IDU should be taken into consideration.

B. The Regenerating Rat Liver as a Model System

Among model systems of experimental liver regeneration, the rat liver regenerating after resection of two thirds of the organ (Higgins and Anderson, 1931) has been studied most extensively, and several reviews on various aspects of this subject are available (Bucher, 1963, 1967; Grundmann and

SEIDEL, 1969; SCHINDLER, 1969; BUCHER and MALT, 1971). The liver of rodents exhibits a relatively homogeneous parenchymal cell population and is composed of only a few cell types; it thus appears well suited for biochemical analysis of the processes involved in regeneration. Hepatocytes are characterized by a long lifespan and do not emigrate from the liver; other cell types may, however, migrate into and out of the liver. In addition, cell death may occur in the liver after partial hepatectomy (ALTMANN, 1966). Since the liver plays an important role in the catabolism of IDU (HUGHES et al., 1964), the distribution of radioactivity between DNA and low-molecular-weight substances in liver after injection of labeled IDU may differ from that in other tissues. In addition, this distribution may undergo changes during liver regeneration.

In rats subjected to partial hepatectomy, DNA synthesis in the remaining liver lobes usually begins to increase after a time lag of 12 to 18 h. This time lag was demonstrated by cytophotometric determination of DNA content of parenchymal liver cells (GRUNDMANN and BACH, 1960), by measuring the incorporation of labeled thymidine into liver DNA (BUCHER and SWAFFIELD, 1964; BUCHER et al., 1964; STÖCKER, 1966), and by autoradiographic analysis of liver tissue after injection of thymidine-^{3}H (GRISHAM, 1962; STÖCKER, 1966).

After this time lag, the rate of DNA synthesis and the number of DNA-synthesizing liver cells increase, and peak values are generally observed between 18 and 26 h after partial hepatectomy. Variations with time depend, however, on experimental conditions; this is due, at least in part, to the diurnal periodicity of DNA synthesis and mitotic activity in regenerating rat liver. Animals may be subjected to partial hepatectomy at different times in order to be sacrificed at a fixed time of day. Under these conditions, a single peak in the number of DNA synthesizing liver cells and in thymidine incorporation is usually observed (GRISHAM, 1962; BUCHER et al., 1964); in young rats, this may be followed by a smaller, second peak (BUCHER et al., 1964). If, however, partial hepatectomy is performed at a given time, the number of DNA-synthesizing hepatocytes, after reaching a first maximum, exhibits a cyclic pattern with a 24-h rhythm (RABES, 1967; BARBIROLI and POTTER, 1971). Similar observations have been reported with respect to mitotic activity (JAFFE, 1954; GÜNTHER et al., 1968; KLINGE and MATHYL, 1969). In rats, high proliferative activity generally occurs at night. Variations with time after partial hepatectomy of mitotic activity and DNA synthesis of liver parenchymal cells thus depend on the time of the day at which the operation is performed.

Differences in the time course of DNA synthesis in regenerating rat liver depending on the time of surgery were also observed when ^{131}IDU was used as DNA precursor (BÜRKI et al., 1971b). This phenomenon is illustrated in Fig. 7, which shows incorporation of ^{131}IDU into liver of partially hepatectomized rats as a function of time after the operation. Whereas the latency period between surgery and the onset of clearly increased ^{131}IDU incorporation was approximately 14 h in both animals partially hepatectomized in the morning and those subjected to the operation in the evening, subsequent changes with time of [131]IDU incorporation were different in the two groups of animals. If partial hepatectomy was performed in the morning, [131]IDU incorporation exhibited a first maximum between 20 and 22 h after surgery, decreased to a minimum at around 28 h, and underwent a second increase. On the other hand, in animals partially hepatectomized in the evening, [131]IDU incorporation after the lag period of 14 h increased more slowly, reaching a maximum between 30 and 34 h, with a possible shoulder at around 26 h.

C. Materials and Methods

In the authors' studies described below, the following materials and methods were used.

Animals. Male rats of CFN strain were obtained from the Animal Breeding Institute of the University of Zürich, Switzerland. At the time of partial hepatectomy, average age of the animals was 7 weeks and average weight 180 g. From at least 5 days before the start of the experiments, the animals were maintained at a constant room temperature of 23°C and under an artificial diurnal rhythm of light and darkness (light from 6 a.m. to 8 p.m.). They had free access to food and water. Three days before partial hepatectomy, 0.1% sodium iodide was added to the drinking water of rats to be operated and of control animals; both groups were offered drinking water containing sodium iodide until sacrifice. The results of preliminary experiments had shown that addition of sodium iodide to the drinking water for even 8 days had no detectable effect on the growth and well-being of the animals.

Partial Hepatectomy. Partial hepatectomy (removal of approximately 66% of total liver mass) was performed under ether anesthesia according to the procedure originally described by HIGGINS and ANDERSON (1931). Unless otherwise stated, the operation was carried out between 9 and 11 a.m.

Injection of Labeled IDU. [131]IDU was obtained from the Radiochemical Centre, Amersham, England, at specific activities of 0.14 to 0.16 Ci/mmole, or from the Swiss Federal Institute for Reactor Research, Würenlingen, Switzerland, at a specific activity of 1.4 Ci/mmole. [125]IDU was obtained from the Radiochemical Centre, Amersham, England, at a specific activity of 2 Ci/mmole. The animals were injected intramuscularly or intraperitoneally with a single dose of 0.02 or 0.04 μCi of [131]IDU per g of body weight or, alternatively, with 1 μCi of [125]IDU per g of body weight. Injections of labeled IDU were given to control rats not subjected to partial hepatectomy at the same time of the day as to partially hepatectomized animals.

Processing of Organs and Tissues for Radioactivity Measurements. At various times after injection of [131]IDU the animals were sacrificed by exsanguination under ether anesthesia, and a sample of liver tissue was weighed and its radioactivity determined by measuring radiation in the range 270 to 420 keV in a gamma-well spectrometer. In addition, in a series of experiments, approximately 300 mg of liver tissue was weighed, homogenized and fractionated according to the procedure of SCHMIDT and THANNHAUSER (1945) as modified by SCHNEIDER (1946). This permitted the separation of acid-soluble materials, lipids, RNA, DNA and protein, and determination of radioactivity in these fractions. The remaining liver tissue was cut into fragments approximately 1 mm in diameter and fixed for at least 48 h in neutral, phosphate-buffered, 10% formalin. During this time, the formalin was changed twice, and before radioactivity was measured, the tissue fragments were rinsed with tap water for approximately 12 h. Similarly, the spleen, kidneys and right tibia of each animal were treated with formalin and subjected to radioactivity determinations as described above. Formalin was obtained from the Siegfried Laboratories, Zofingen, Switzerland, as an aqueous 38% formaldehyde solution [Pharmacopoea Helvetica V (Ph.H.V)] and diluted with 2.6 volumes of tap water. This solution was brought to pH 7 by adding 8.1 g $Na_2HPO_4 \cdot 2\,H_2O$, 2.74 g KH_2PO_4 and 0.56 g $CaCO_3$ per liter. All results were corrected for decrease of radioactivity with time due to decay of the isotope.

Autoradiography. For autoradiographic studies, animals were injected intramuscularly with [125]IDU. Tissue was taken from each liver lobe, fixed in formaldehyde solution, and embedded in paraffin. Histological sections 4 µm thick were subjected to autoradiography, using Kodak NTB_2 emulsion. Autoradiographic exposure at 4°C was carried out for 65 days. The developed and fixed preparations were stained with nuclear fast red through the film.

Histological Examinations. For morphological studies, paraffin sections 4 µm thick were prepared from liver tissue and stained with hemalum-eosin, PAS, or hematoxylin (Böhmer)-EA (Papanicolaou). Mitotic index determinations were done on preparations stained with hemalum-eosin.

D. Labeling of Liver Tissue and its Biochemical Subfractions after Administration of [131]IDU

1. Radioactivity in Normal and Regenerating Liver and its Biochemical Subfractions at Different Times after [131]IDU Injection

Measurements of gamma radiation emitted from unfractionated tissue after injection of labeled IDU do not permit estimation of radioactivity incorporated into DNA unless the amounts of label in other biochemical fractions are relatively small. Previous studies have shown that a certain time is required for the elimination of label contained in fractions other than DNA; in rodents, it takes at least 16 h before the major part of the radioactivity remaining in the tissue is representative of IDU incorporated into DNA (PRUSOFF *et al.*, 1960; HUGHES *et al.*, 1964; FOX and PRUSOFF, 1965; O'FARRELL and DUNAWAY, 1967).

To enable us to study the distribution of radioactivity in biochemical fractions of normal and regenerating liver as a function of time after [131]IDU administration, rats were given an i.m. injection of [131]IDU 22 h after partial hepatectomy; a similar dose was injected into non-operated control animals. Groups of rats were sacrificed at various times after injection, and radioactivity of liver tissue and of its biochemical subfractions was determined as described under Methods.

The results, as presented in Table 1, indicate that radioactivity per g of tissue fell rapidly during the first 24 h after injection of labeled precursor; this is in agreement with previous observations (HUGHES *et al.*, 1964). A further fall in radioactivity was, however, found during the time interval between 24 and 48 h in both intact and regenerating liver.

In regenerating liver, some at least of this continued decrease in radioactivity may be attributed to liver growth resulting in smaller amounts of label per g of tissue. On the other hand, as illustrated in Fig. 3, the distribution of radioactivity between the acid-soluble fraction and DNA changed during both the first and the second 24 h period after injection of [131]IDU. Label in the acid-soluble fraction underwent a continued decrease during the observation period of 48 h in normal as well as regenerating liver. In contrast, radioactivity in the DNA fraction exhibited relatively minor changes with time between 2 and 48 h after injection of the labeled precursor. Table 1 also summarizes the relative contributions of biochemical subfractions of liver to total tissue radioactivity at different times after injection of [131]IDU. It is seen that 2 h after the injection label in the acid-soluble fraction represented the major portion of total radioactivity in liver and, even at 24 h, radioactivity in the acid-soluble fraction of non-regenerating liver was higher than that in DNA. At 48 h, however, label in DNA represented the major portion of total radioactivity in both normal and regenerating liver. Throughout the observation period of 48 h radioactivity was rather low in fractions other than the acid-soluble fraction and DNA.

Table 1. *Radioactivity in normal and regenerating rat liver and its bio-*
(reproduced in part from

	Time after injection of [131]IDU h	Number of animals	Radioactivity (% of injected dose)	
			per liver	per g of liver tissue $\times 10^3$
Non-operated control animals	2	5	1.74 ± 0.13[a]	155.7 ± 1.6[a]
	24	12	0.10 ± 0.02	9.6 ± 1.4
	48	5	0.07 ± 0.01	5.9 ± 1.4
Partially hepatectomized animals[b]	2	5	0.70 ± 0.02	185.2 ± 9.9
	24	10	0.15 ± 0.03	34.5 ± 4.8
	48	5	0.13 ± 0.02	28.1 ± 2.2

[a] Standard errors.
[b] [131]IDU was injected 22 h after partial hepatectomy.

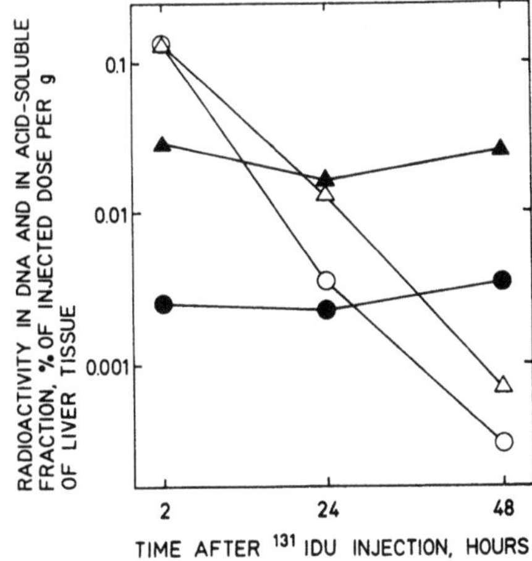

Fig. 3. Radioactivity in the acid-soluble fraction (open symbols) and in DNA (closed symbols) per g of normal and regenerating rat liver at different times after an i.m. injection of ^{131}IDU. (From Bürki *et al.*, 1971a.) ○ ● Non-operated control animals. △ ▲ Partially hepatectomized animals injected with ^{131}IDU 22 h after the operation

Total radioactivity in DNA of regenerating liver underwent a statistically significant decrease ($P < 0.05$) between 2 and 24 h after injection of ^{131}IDU (see Fig. 9). As discussed below, this decrease may be attributed to loss of labeled hepatocytes by cell death. The increase in radioactivity of total DNA of regenerating liver between 24 and 48 h after injection of ^{131}IDU is compatible with immigration of labeled mesenchymal cells into the growing liver during this time interval. It should also be noted that radioactivity in the protein fraction per g of regenerating liver was higher by factors of 2.7 to 4.3 than in normal, non-regenerating liver, at least up to 48 h after injection

chemical subfractions at different times after an i.m. injection of ^{131}IDU
Bürki *et al.*, 1971a)

Radioactivity in biochemical fractions (% of total liver radioactivity)

DNA	Acid-soluble fraction	Lipids	RNA	Protein
2.0 ±0.2[a]	93.8 ±0.8[a]	2.3 ±0.0[a]	1.1 ±0.1[a]	0.8 ±0.5[a]
31.2 ±2.2	45.3 ± 3.3	6.1 ± 1.0	5.3 ±0.4	11.7 ±2.1
67.5 ±7.1	7.6 ±1.2	1.9 ±0.2	11.0 ±1.6	12.7 ±6.5
16.4 ±0.4	77.3 ±0.6	1.7 ±0.2	1.7 ±0.1	2.9 ±0.4
50.5 ± 2.9	34.1 ± 3.3	1.9 ± 0.4	4.8 ± 0.4	8.7 ± 1.7
81.8 ± 3.9	3.3 ± 1.1	1.2 ± 0.3	6.1 ±0.8	7.8 ± 2.2

of [131]IDU. That this difference was not the result of incomplete hydrolysis of DNA during the fractionation procedure was shown by radioactivity determinations of the protein fraction after repeated hydrolysis of tissue samples.

2. Effect of Partial Hepatectomy on the Fate of IDU

The liver appears to be an important site of IDU catabolism. For instance, interruption of portal blood flow for 10 min after i.v. injection of labeled IDU resulted in prolongation of the time of IDU availability and augmented incorporation of precursor into organs and tissues outside the portal system (HUGHES *et al.*, 1964). It should, therefore, be remembered that partial hepatectomy may cause changes in the relative proportion of anabolic and catabolic reactions, as previously reported for natural nucleic acid precursors such as uracil and thymine (CANELLAKIS *et al.*, 1959; FRITZSON, 1962, 1964).

In order to study the effects of partial hepatectomy on the fate of labeled IDU, we determined the rate of elimination of radioactivity from the acid-soluble fraction of liver as a function of time after surgery and compared it with that in non-operated controls. Groups of partially hepatectomized rats were given an i.m. injection of [131]IDU immediately after, 10 h, or 22 h after the operation. Non-operated animals were similarly injected. At various time intervals after injection of [131]IDU, groups of animals were sacrificed, and radioactivity was determined in the different biochemical fractions of liver.

At 2 h after injection of the labeled precursor, essentially the same proportion of injected radioactivity, i.e. 0.123 to 0.146%, was recovered from the acid-soluble fraction of 1 g of liver tissue in all groups of animals. The results obtained in the acid-soluble and DNA fractions at later time intervals after [131]IDU injection are summarized in Fig. 4. It can be seen that at both 24 h and 48 h after labeled precursor injection, the radioactivity of the acid-soluble fraction was lower in control animals than in partially hepatectomized rats. This indicates that in the operated group the rate of elimination of label from the acid-soluble fraction was slower. In particular, partially hepatectomized animals injected with [131]IDU immediately or 10 h after the operation had about 6 times more radioactivity in the acid-soluble fraction of 1 g of liver at 24 h after precursor injection than non-operated controls.

This lower rate of elimination is not necessarily indicative of a change in the rate of IDU catabolism after partial hepatectomy. In addition to modification of metabolic functions of the liver, there may be a decrease in elimination of label due to impaired kidney function. Irrespective of the underlying mechanism, the lower rate of elimination of radioactivity from the acid-soluble fraction observed after partial hepatectomy has practical consequences. It means that, in partially hepatectomized animals, the contribution of acid-soluble products of IDU degradation to total liver radioactivity will be more important than under control conditions. A comparison of radioactivity in the acid-soluble fraction with that incorporated into DNA

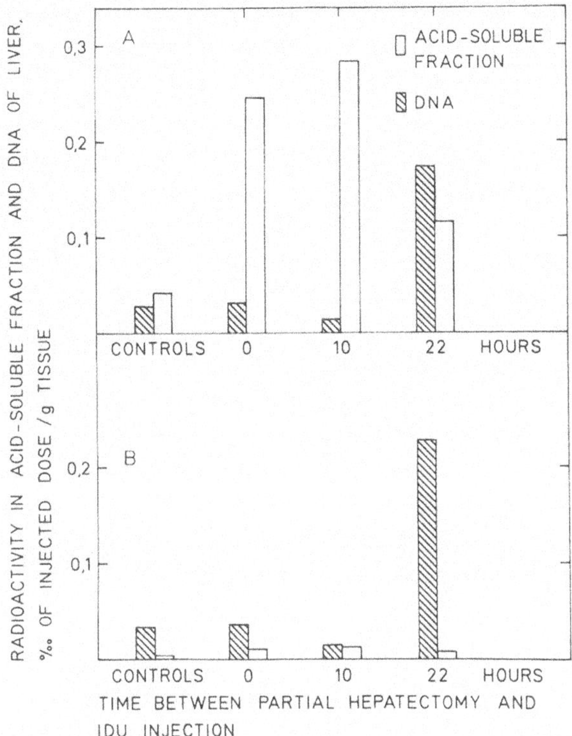

Fig. 4A and B. Distribution of radioactivity between DNA and the acid-soluble fraction in liver tissue of non-operated control animals and of partially hepatectomized rats injected with [131]IDU at different times after the operation. A Sacrifice of animals at 24 h after [131]IDU injection. B Sacrifice of animals at 48 h after [131]IDU injection

under various experimental conditions is presented in Fig. 4. It is apparent that 24 h after [131]IDU injection, radioactivity in the acid-soluble fraction may markedly exceed that in DNA, e.g. in liver tissue of animals that received [131]IDU immediately or 10 h after partial hepatectomy. Comparable amounts of label were found in both fractions in control animals and in animals injected with [131]IDU 22 h after partial hepatectomy, i.e. at the peak of DNA synthetic activity. In animals sacrificed 48 h after [131]IDU injection, radioactivity in liver DNA clearly exceeded that in the acid-soluble fraction, except in partially hepatectomized rats that had been injected with the labeled precursor 10 h after surgery.

These results indicate that radioactivity is eliminated from the acid-soluble fraction relatively slowly, and that it takes at least 48 h after injection of [131]IDU before the radioactivity retained by liver tissue is representative of the IDU incorporated into DNA. Similar results reported for mouse mammary tumors demonstrate that even 72 h after injection of [125]IDU approximately 10% of total tumor radioactivity was in the acid-soluble fraction (DETHLEFSEN, 1969). If time-consuming biochemical fractionation procedures are to be avoided, animals should therefore be sacrificed not less than 48 h after injection of labeled IDU in order to ensure that the measured radioactivity is representative of label incorporated into liver DNA.

On the other hand, the possibility of loss during this rather long time interval of radioactivity incorporated into regenerating liver DNA due to cell death cannot be excluded. In addition, there may be immigration of labeled cells into the regenerating liver. The assumption that these processes cannot be neglected is supported by the fact that the observed decrease of radio-activity in liver DNA during the first 24 h after ^{131}IDU injection is followed by an increase during the second 24 h period (see Fig. 9). In addition, results of autoradiographic analysis indicate that death of labeled parenchymal cells takes place in regenerating liver, as discussed below. A method permitting determination of ^{131}IDU incorporation into liver DNA at short time intervals after administration of the labeled precursor and without the necessity of time-consuming biochemical fractionation procedures thus appears highly desirable. As described below, extraction of liver tissue with formalin prior to measurement of radioactivity represents a simple means of removing the label contained in the acid-soluble fraction.

3. Effect of Formalin Fixation on Radioactivity in Liver Tissue and its Biochemical Subfractions

Changes of radioactivity in liver tissue as a function of time of extraction with formalin were determined as follows. A series of 5 different samples of liver tissue obtained from animals injected with ^{131}IDU at various times after partial hepatectomy was subjected to extraction with neutral, phosphate-buffered, 10% formalin. The fixing solution was changed every 12 h and the radioactivity remaining in the tissue samples was determined at the times indicated in Fig. 5. Label was extracted rapidly during the first 24 h and more slowly during the following 24 h, remaining essentially constant after a total extraction time of 48 h.

The same time course of extraction was observed with samples of liver tissue obtained under a variety of experimental conditions and exhibiting markedly different ratios of radioactivity in DNA and in the acid-soluble fraction. On the other hand, the proportion of total radioactivity removed from the samples by repeated formalin extraction exhibited large differences, depending on the experimental conditions chosen. In particular, radioactivity extracted by formalin was rather high at short time intervals after ^{131}IDU injection. This suggests that formalin treatment may result in a selective extraction of radioactivity contained in the acid-soluble fraction.

In order to test this hypothesis, we compared radioactivity measured in various biochemical fractions of liver before and after extraction with formalin. In this series of experiments, ^{131}IDU was injected i.m. into non-operated controls and into partially hepatectomized animals 10 and 22 h after surgery. Liver tissue was collected 2 h after ^{131}IDU injection, i.e. at a

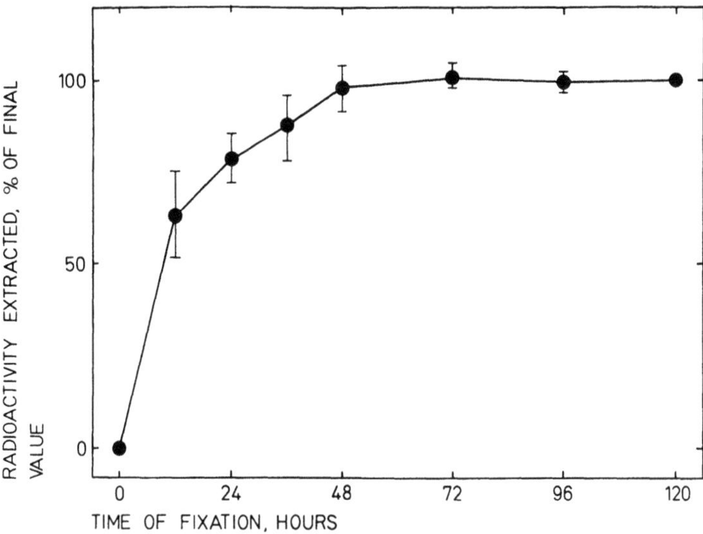

Fig. 5. Loss of radioactivity from liver tissue of partially hepatectomized rats injected with [131]IDU as a function of time of treatment with formalin. Mean values with standard errors are indicated

time when a large proportion of total radioactivity is found in the acid-soluble fraction.

The results are presented in Fig. 6. Whereas more than 99% of radioactivity present in the acid-soluble fraction was removed by formalin treatment, radioactivity incorporated into DNA was retained under these conditions. A major portion of the radioactivity present in the lipid fraction was extracted, while most of the label in the RNA and protein fractions was resistant to extraction by formalin. As previously reported, the radioactivity retained after formalin extraction correlated well with that in the combined DNA, RNA and protein fractions (BÜRKI et al., 1971 a).

After formalin treatment, a considerably higher proportion of total radioactivity was in the DNA fraction than in native tissue (Table 2). In liver of rats injected with [131]IDU 22 h after partial hepatectomy and sacrificed 2 h later, 88% of the radioactivity retained in the tissue after formalin treatment was in the DNA fraction but only 17% in native tissue. In the liver of animals injected with the labeled precursor 10 h after partial hepatectomy, only 0.6% of total radioactivity of fresh tissue was in DNA as compared to 44% after formalin extraction.

In conclusion, formalin treatment appears to be a simple method of removing radioactivity contained in the acid-soluble fraction. Of the radioactivity retained in liver tissue after formalin extraction, the major part is in the DNA fraction (BÜRKI et al., 1971 a). HUGHES et al. (1964) proposed that catabolic products of injected IDU might be removed by extraction of homogenized tissues with 10% trichloroacetic acid; this procedure was shown to be useful for extracting low-molecular-weight substances from mouse leukemia

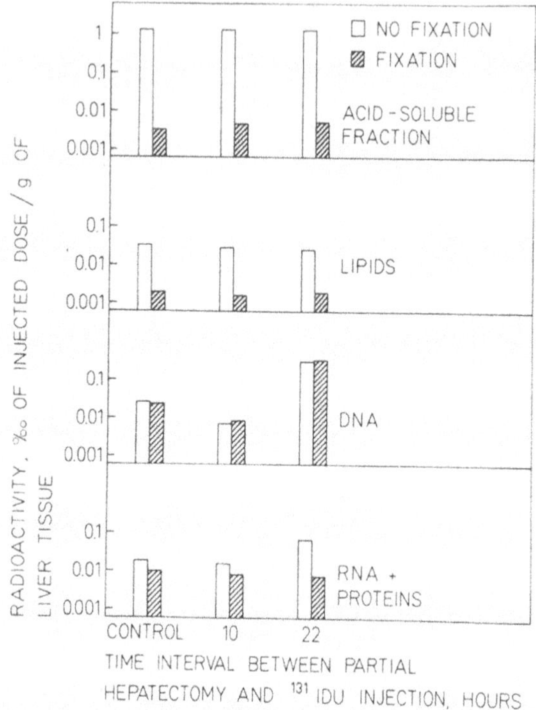

Fig. 6. Effect of formalin treatment on radioactivity measured in various biochemical fractions of liver of control animals and of partially hepatectomized rats injected with [131]IDU 10 or 22 h after the operation. Animals were sacrificed for analysis of liver tissue 2 h after [131]IDU injection

Table 2. *Effect of formalin extraction on radioactivity in DNA of 1 g of liver tissue*

Formalin treatment	Radioactivity in DNA of 1 g of tissue[a]	
	% of injected dose $\times 10^3$	% of total liver radioactivity
	Non-operated control animals	
—	2.6 (2.2–3.0)[b]	1.8 (1.6–2.8)[b]
+	2.4 (2.3–2.4)	64.0 (61.5–66.4)
	Partially hepatectomized animals ([131]IDU injected at 10 h after the operation)	
—	0.8 (0.6–0.9)	0.6 (0.4–0.8)
+	0.9 (0.8–1.1)	44.1 (41.8–46.4)
	Partially hepatectomized animals ([131]IDU injected at 22 h after the operation)	
—	29.2 (26.0–32.1)	16.6 (15.4–17.2)
+	30.2 (27.2–33.2)	88.4 (87.5–89.3)

[a] At 2 h after injection of [131]IDU.
[b] Range of values obtained from 2 to 5 animals per group.
Data presented in this table were obtained with other animals and with another preparation of [131]IDU than those summarized in Table 1.

cells in which a major proportion of total radioactivity was associated with DNA (HOFER and HUGHES, 1970). The results of our experiments indicate that, even under conditions providing for only a small extent of DNA labeling, a rather high specificity of [131]IDU as a DNA precursor is obtained if liver

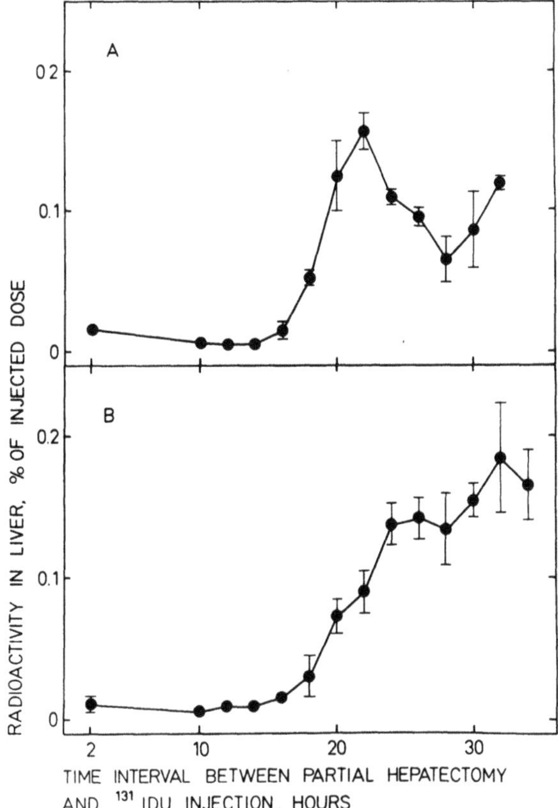

Fig. 7A and B. Incorporation of ^{131}IDU into rat liver as a function of time after partial hepatectomy. Animals were sacrificed 2 h after ^{131}IDU injection, and radioactivity was determined in formalin-fixed liver tissue. (From Bürki *et al.*, 1971 b.) A Partial hepatectomy between 9 and 11 a.m. B Partial hepatectomy between 5 and 7 p.m. Standard errors are presented where they exceed the radius of circles

tissue is treated with formalin prior to measurement of radioactivity. As shown previously by autoradiography, the proportion of isotope from nucleic acid precursors that is retained in a tissue depends on the type of fixation used (Blank *et al.*, 1951; Feinendegen *et al.*, 1960; Kopriwa and Leblond, 1962). Neutral formalin appeared preferable to other fixing solutions with respect to stability of label incorporated into nucleic acids of various tissues (Schneider and Maurer, 1963).

An application of the method of formalin extraction to liver tissue after labeling with ^{131}IDU is illustrated in Fig. 7. One group of animals was partially hepatectomized between 9 and 11 a.m., while a second group was subjected to this operation between 5 and 7 p.m. At different times after surgery, the animals were given a single i.m. injection of ^{131}IDU; 2 h later, they were sacrificed, and radioactivity retained in liver after formalin extraction was determined. As can be seen, up to 14 h after partial hepatectomy incorporation of label was quite low and exhibited small standard errors. After this time lag, incorporation increased by a factor of 10 to 20, thus permitting a rather precise determination of the time interval between partial hepatectomy and the onset of increased DNA synthesis. In addition, there are clear differences in the time course of [131]IDU incorporation between animals subjected to partial hepatectomy in the morning and those operated on in the evening.

4. Differences in Fate of Labeled IDU Depending on Site of Injection

HUGHES *et al.* (1964) demonstrated that, in mice, the relative extent of incorporation of labeled IDU into different organs and tissues depends on the site of injection of the labeled precursor. After injection into the portal vein, incorporation into intestine, spleen and skeleton was approximately 50% lower than after injection into the vena cava. On the other hand, radioactivity incorporated into liver was higher by a factor of nearly 2 after injection into the portal vein. These findings support the assumption that IDU is catabolized preferentially in the liver. According to the estimate of HUGHES *et al.* (1964), in mice about 50% of IDU is catabolized during each passage through the liver. After s.c. or i.m. injection of IDU, this precursor is absorbed relatively slowly from the injection site. After i.m. injection of [125]IDU, radioactivity at the site of injection had a half-life of approximately 30 min (CLIFTON *et al.*, 1963). Under these conditions, the time of availability of labeled IDU may be somewhat prolonged. The extent of labeling of mouse tissues after s.c. injection of [125]IDU was nearly the same as after i.v. or i.p. administration, with the exception of ascites tumor cells (HOFER and HUGHES, 1970).

We compared the fate of [131]IDU after i.m. injection with that after i.p. administration in normal and partially hepatectomized rats; labeled IDU was injected into the latter group 22 h after surgery. The animals were sacrificed 24 h after administration of the labeled precursor and radioactivity was determined in formalin-treated tissues. As shown in Table 3, the radioactivity measured in normal and regenerating liver after i.p. injection was significantly higher than after i.m. injection of [131]IDU. On the other hand, the radioactivity incorporated into spleen, tibia, and kidneys tended to be higher after i.m. injection. These results should be interpreted with caution because the relative importance of precursor uptake from the peritoneal cavity via the lymph

Table 3. Incorporation of [131]IDU after intraperitoneal, as compared to that after intramuscular injection

Site of injection	Number of animals	Radioactivity (% of injected dose)[a]				
		Regenerating liver[b]	Normal liver	Spleen	Kidneys	Tibia
Intraperitoneal	7	3.60 ±1.56[c]	0.85 ±0.18[c]	0.28 ±0.08[c]	0.12 ±0.03[c]	0.08 ±0.02[c]
Intramuscular	7	1.26 ±0.56	0.42 ±0.12	0.31 ±0.05	0.27 ±0.01	0.15 ±0.03

[a] Animals were sacrificed at 24 h after [131]IDU injection, and organs were subjected to formalin extraction prior to determination of radioactivity. Results for spleen, kidneys and tibia were obtained from animals not subjected to partial hepatectomy.
[b] [131]IDU was injected at 22 h after partial hepatectomy.
[c] Standard deviations.

Table 4. Radioactivity in liver, its acid-soluble and DNA fraction at 24 h after i.m. or i.p. injection of [131]IDU

Site of injection	Number of animals	Total liver radioactivity $^0/_{00}$ of injected dose	Radioactivity in	
			DNA, % of total liver radioactivity	acid-soluble fraction, % of total liver radioactivity
Non-operated control animals				
i.m.	12	1.0 ±0.2[a]	31.2 ±2.2[a]	45.3 ±3.3[a]
i.p.	4	0.7 ±0.1	53.3 ±1.5	28.7 ±2.3
Partially hepatectomized animals[b]				
i.m.	10	1.5 ±0.3	50.5 ±2.9	34.1 ±3.3
i.p.	4	1.7 ±0.4	71.0 ±5.5	13.5 ±6.8

[a] Standard errors.
[b] [131]IDU was injected at 22 h after partial hepatectomy.

vessels, as compared to that via the portal vein, is not known. Nevertheless, our observations seem to be in qualitative agreement with those reported by HUGHES *et al.* (1964) for injection into the vena portae vs. the vena cava. Reproducibility of incorporation was found to be similar after i.m. and i.p. injection, as is clear from standard deviations of radioactivity in different tissues following these two types of injection (Table 3).

Although the efficiency of labeling of liver DNA was found to be higher after i.p. injection of [131]IDU, i.m. injection may be preferable for two reasons. (1) Partial hepatectomy results in an increase in portal pressure (ALSTON and THOMSON, 1963) which may cause differences in kinetics of absorption of labeled precursor from the peritoneal cavity of normal and partially hepatectomized animals; (2) partial hepatectomy may cause peritoneal irritation and exudation with concomitant changes in absorption of labeled IDU.

A comparison was also made between i.m. and i.p. injection with respect to radioactivity in DNA and the acid-soluble fraction of normal and regenerating liver. As can be seen from Table 4, a smaller proportion of total radioactivity was found in DNA after i.m. than after i.p. injection, while more label was found in the acid-soluble fraction after i.m. injection of [131]IDU. These observations support the assumption that the kinetics of incorporation of IDU into DNA and metabolic degradation of this precursor depend on the site of its injection.

E. Cell Kinetics in Regenerating Liver as Studied by Labeling with [125]IDU

1. Initial Labeling of Different Cell Types as a Function of Time after Partial Hepatectomy

During the first 10 to 12 h after partial hepatectomy, the number of DNA-synthesizing cells in liver, as determined by [125]IDU labeling, decreased to

30 to 50% of control values. Similar observations were made after labeling with ^{3}H-thymidine (EDWARDS and KOCH, 1964). This decrease may possibly represent a late effect of surgery; in fact, a decrease of the labeling index after partial hepatectomy was also observed in tubular epithelial cells of the kidney (STÖCKER and HEINE, 1965; STÖCKER, 1968).

In order to determine changes in the relative number of DNA-synthesizing cells in regenerating liver, both controls and partially hepatectomized rats were given an i.m. injection of [125]IDU. The animals were sacrificed 2 h later, and the liver tissue was processed for autoradiography. Relative numbers of labeled parenchymal and non-parenchymal liver cells, as determined by evaluation of 70000 cells per animal, are presented in Table 5.

Table 5. Initial labeling indices and average labeling intensities of different cell types in normal and regenerating rat liver after injection of [125]IDU

Time interval between partial hepatectomy and [125]IDU injection h	Initial labeling index (%)		Mean no. of grains per labeled cell	
	Hepatocytes	Other nucleated cells in liver	Hepatocytes	Other nucleated cells in liver
	Non-regenerating liver			
—	2.9 ±0.6[a]	2.3 ±0.7[a]	23.0 ± 1.8[a]	12.7 ±1.2[a]
	Regenerating liver			
22	34.0 ±2.9	6.4 ±0.7	38.1 ±4.2	13.7 ±1.7
42	18.5 ± 3.1	23.6 ±2.8	32.1 ± 5.1	14.0 ±2.1

[a] Standard errors of mean values each of 4 animals.

In agreement with previous reports based on labeling with ^{3}H-thymidine (GRISHAM, 1962; FABRIKANT, 1968), the labeling index of parenchymal cells was found to have markedly increased 22 h after partial hepatectomy, whereas a high labeling index of other cells in regenerating liver was observed 42 h after the operation. With respect to labeling intensity, the grain count data presented in Table 5 suggest that the average incorporation of [125]IDU by DNA-synthesizing hepatocytes exceeds that by non-parenchymal cells. Differences in average grain counts may, however, also be due to differences in the geometry of cells and nuclei. The average labeling intensity of parenchymal cells is higher in regenerating than in normal liver; this finding is in agreement with a report by STÖCKER (1966) that the duration of the S period of hepatocytes is approximately 50% shorter in regenerating than in non-regenerating liver.

Fig. 8A—C. Autoradiograms of liver tissue of partially hepatectomized rats injected with [125]IDU. Sections were stained with nuclear fast red. (×490.) A Animal injected with [125]IDU 22 h after partial hepatectomy and sacrificed 2 h later. B Animal injected with [125]IDU 22 h after partial hepatectomy and sacrificed 24 h later. C Animal was injected with [125]IDU 42 h after partial hepatectomy and sacrificed 2 h later

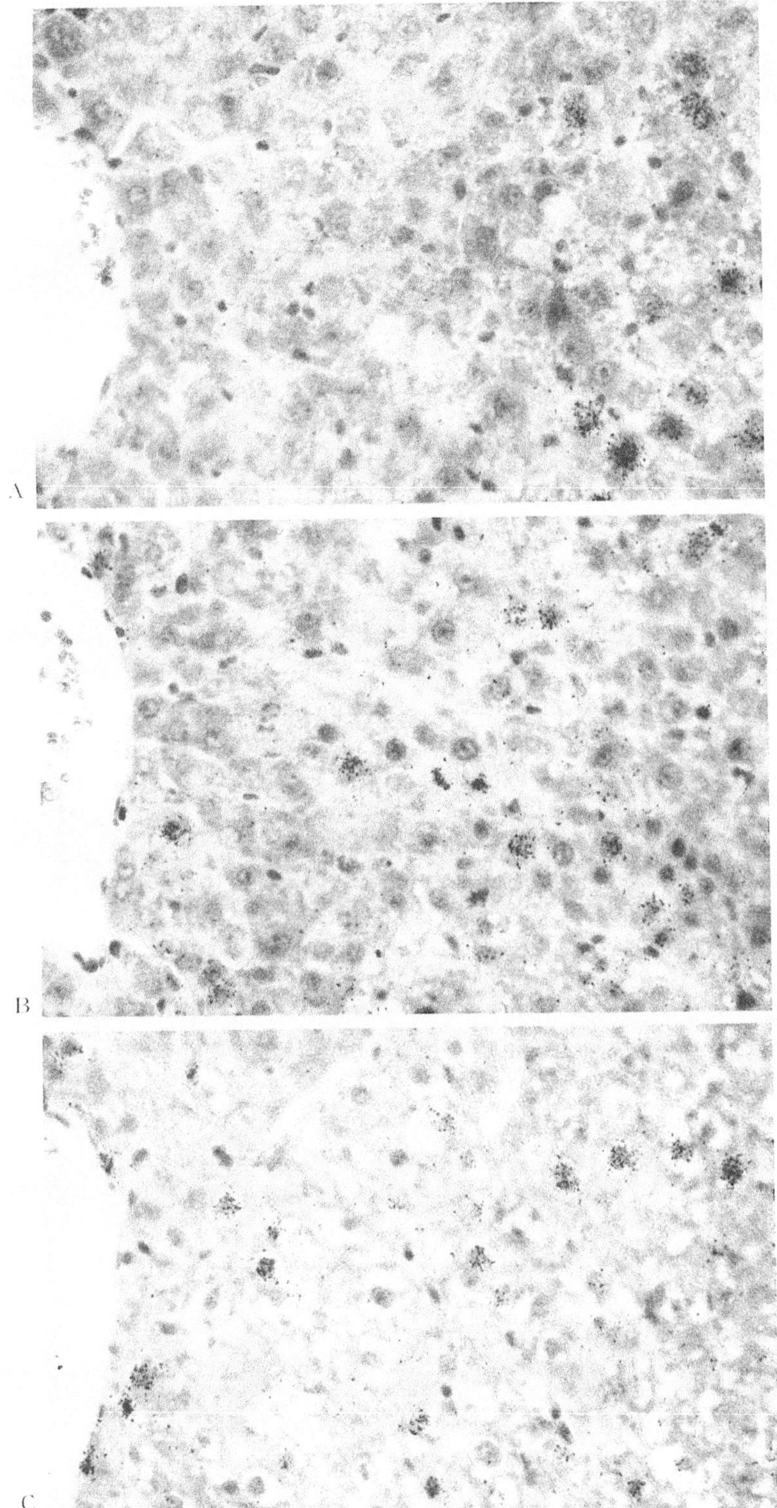

Fig. 8A-C

The results presented in Table 5 support the conclusion that the increased incorporation of labeled IDU in regenerating liver reflects both an increase in the number of DNA-synthesizing cells and a higher labeling intensity of individual parenchymal cells. This had previously been demonstrated by labeling with ^{3}H-thymidine (LOONEY *et al.*, 1967; FABRIKANT, 1968).

2. Localization of Labeled Cells within Liver Lobules

At 22 h after partial hepatectomy, rats were given an i.m. injection of [125]IDU. Groups of animals were sacrificed 2, 24, or 48 h after the injection, and liver tissue was processed for autoradiography. As Fig. 8A shows, 2 h after precursor injection, labeled parenchymal cells were located in the peripheral region of liver lobules, but labeled Kupffer cells and endothelial cells, although few in number, were distributed more or less evenly within lobules.

At 24 h after [125]IDU labeling, as shown in Fig. 8B, labeled parenchymal cells were also observed in the central region of liver lobules. In interpreting this observation, it should be noted that IDU is available for labeling for only a short period after injection and that the reutilization of IDU from disintegrating cells is sufficiently small to be negligible. The results obtained indicate, therefore, that a certain number of parenchymal cells located in the peripheral region of liver lobules at the time of labeling migrated to more central regions during the subsequent 24 h period. These findings confirm earlier observations based on ^{3}H-thymidine labeling (GRISHAM, 1962). On the basis of ^{3}H-thymidine labeling, migration of cells from peripheral to central regions of liver lobules was also found to occur at later times after partial hepatectomy (SCHERER and FRIEDRICH-FREKSA, 1970). Because of the low degree of reutilization of labeled IDU, however, the possibility that the appearance of labeled cells in central regions may be attributable to reutilization of label can be ruled out with more confidence in studies in which IDU is used as DNA precursor.

In a third group of animals, [125]IDU was injected 42 h after partial hepatectomy, and animals were sacrificed 2 h later. As can be seen in Fig. 8C, DNA-synthesizing parenchymal cells were present in all regions of liver lobules. In agreement with previous reports (GRISHAM, 1962; RABES, 1967; FABRIKANT, 1968; RABES and TUCZEK, 1970), these results support the conclusion that, after partial hepatectomy, DNA synthesis is initiated in parenchymal cells located in peripheral regions of liver lobules, whereas at later times after the operation, hepatocytes located in more central regions also enter the S period.

F. Correlation of Cell Kinetics with Radioactivity in Liver DNA

After partial hepatectomy, abnormal mitotic figures are usually observed in relatively large numbers (CURTIS, 1964; ALTMANN, 1966). Such disorders

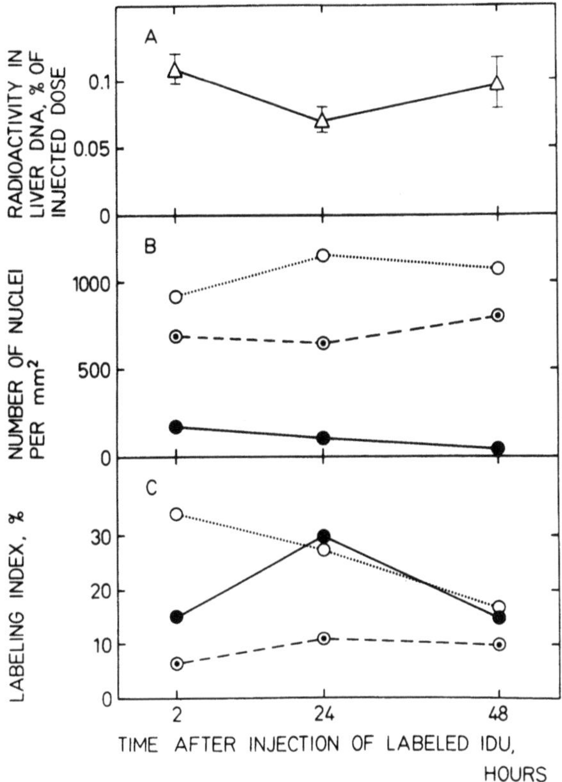

Fig. 9A—C. Radioactivity in liver DNA of partially hepatectomized rats, and numbers and labeling indices of various cell types in liver, as a function of time after injection of labeled IDU. A Injection of [131]IDU 22 h after partial hepatectomy. Means and standard errors of radioactivity in liver DNA are indicated. B and C Injection of [125]IDU 22 h after partial hepatectomy. ○·····○ Parenchymal cells. ⊙– –⊙ Non-parenchymal cells. ● — ● Cells exhibiting nuclear pyknosis and lysis

of mitotic cell division are apparently more frequent in old than in young animals (KLINGE, 1968, 1973). In addition to mitotic abnormalities, cells exhibiting nuclear pyknosis and lysis may be detected in regenerating liver.

In order to study the relationship between kinetics of liver cells and radioactivity in DNA of regenerating liver, we injected groups of rats with [131]IDU or [125]IDU 22 h after partial hepatectomy. At different periods after administration of the radioactive precursor, animals were sacrificed, and label from [131]IDU incorporated into liver DNA was determined; in addition, liver sections of rats injected with [125]IDU were processed for autoradiography. As Fig. 9B shows, 24 h after partial hepatectomy, i.e. 2 h after precursor injection, cells with disintegrating nuclei represented a relatively large proportion of the total parenchymal cell population, whereas later on the relative number of such cells gradually decreased. It should be pointed out that these degenerative changes were observed to the same extent in the liver of partially hepatectomized rats not injected with [125]IDU.

It is of interest that the labeling index of cells exhibiting nuclear pyknosis and lysis increased by a factor of approximately 2 between 2 and 24 h after [125]IDU injection and at 48 h was again at nearly the same level as at 2 h (Fig. 9C). On the other hand, the labeling index of intact parenchymal cells underwent a pronounced decrease with time after [125]IDU injection. Even though a decrease of measured labeling indices due to dilution of label during cell multiplication cannot be excluded, these findings, taken together, suggest that a considerable fraction of parenchymal cells is lost by cell death in the course of liver regeneration. This conclusion is consistent with the observation (Fig. 9A) that radioactivity in liver DNA decreased between 2 and 24 h after [131]IDU injection to approximately 65% of its original value. This decrease was found to be statistically significant ($P < 0.05$).

With respect to non-parenchymal cells in liver, a different pattern was observed. The labeling index increased between 2 and 24 h after [125]IDU injection and remained at this level up to 48 h after administration of the labeled precursor. In addition, the total number of these cell types per cross-sectioned area underwent an increase during the second 24 h interval. Also during this period, radioactivity in total liver DNA tended to increase, despite the loss of labeled parenchymal cells. This suggests that at this stage of regeneration, labeled monocytes (macrophages) may immigrate into the liver to become Kupffer and/or littoral cells. An extrahepatic origin of at least some Kupffer cells has been reported previously (EDWARDS and KOCH, 1964; BOAK *et al.*, 1968; FABRIKANT, 1968). In addition, thoracic duct cells may become hepatic macrophages, at least under certain conditions (BOAK *et al.*, 1968). An extrahepatic origin of Kupffer cells was also demonstrated by estrogenic stimulation of parabiotic mice (KINSKY *et al.*, 1969). Among cellular events taking place during experimental liver regeneration, immigration of cells from extrahepatic sites into the growing liver should, therefore, be considered in addition to locally occurring cell proliferation and cell death.

G. Conclusions

The specificity of labeled IDU as a DNA precursor is limited (a) by metabolic degradation of this unnatural nucleoside to products that are incorporated into DNA poorly or not at all, and (b) by incorporation of label from these products into lipids and macromolecules other than DNA. In comparison with labeled thymidine, the relative extent of catabolic reactions is larger, and only 5 to 10% of injected labeled IDU is usually incorporated into DNA. On the other hand, label contained in low-molecular-weight products of iodine-labeled IDU is eliminated more rapidly than tritium from ^{3}H-thymidine. Nevertheless, at short periods after injection of labeled IDU, label in the acid-soluble fraction represented a considerable part of the total radioactivity of normal and regenerating liver. Under these conditions, total liver radioactivity was thus not representative of IDU incorporated into DNA.

In addition, elimination of label from the acid-soluble fraction of liver after injection of ^{131}IDU differed in partially hepatectomized and control animals. Differences were also observed in the distribution of radioactivity between the acid-soluble fraction and DNA after i.p. and i.m. injection of ^{131}IDU. Under all the conditions tested, a major part of the radioactivity in liver tissue was in the acid-soluble fraction 2 h after injection of labeled IDU.

Label in this fraction may, however, be removed by the simple procedure of extracting the tissue with formalin, as used in our studies, or with other solutions, such as 5 to 10% trichloroacetic acid (HUGHES *et al.*, 1964). Of the radioactivity retained in the tissue, the major portion was shown to be in the DNA fraction. When this experimental procedure is used, it seems that the specificity of incorporation of labeled IDU into DNA depends to some extent on the rate of DNA synthesis in the tissue at the time of injection of the labeled precursor. Even under the most unfavorable conditions, however, almost half of the radioactivity present in liver tissue after formalin extraction was in the DNA fraction.

If labeled IDU is to be used for studies of proliferating cell systems, the possibility of artifacts due to toxic effects of this unnatural nucleoside and/or the radiation emitted should be carefully considered. With respect to toxic effects of unlabeled IDU in cell culture, concentrations of this analog as low as 0.01 to 0.1 µmole/ml had an inhibitory effect on cell multiplication (MATHIAS *et al.*, 1959; CHEONG *et al.*, 1960). The toxic effects of IDU appear to result primarily from its incorporation into DNA, as shown in cultures of murine neoplastic mast cells (MORRIS and CRAMER, 1966, 1968). In the intact animal, however, the toxicity of IDU may be limited by its rapid degradation and the low extent of incorporation into DNA during the short time the precursor is available.

Changes in the kinetics of replication of ileal and spleen cells have been reported after injection into rats of 1.3 nmole of IDU per g of body weight (POST and HOFFMAN, 1969), i.e. at a level approximately 2.5 times higher than that used for labeling with ^{125}IDU in our studies. The toxicity of IDU was also evaluated by measuring incorporation of ^{3}H-IDU as a function of the dose of unlabeled IDU. In this assay system, IDU was inhibitory in mice at doses as low as 0.5 nmole per g of body weight (DETHLEFSEN, 1974). The effects of varying doses of IDU on incorporation of labeled IDU may, however, be misleading because the incorporation of this precursor is not necessarily proportional to the dose.

With respect to radiotoxic effects of the isotope used for labeling IDU, it was shown that after incorporation of ^{125}IDU into DNA of L 1210 leukemia cells, a 50% reduction in the number of surviving cells was caused by approximately 4 disintegrations per cell per hour, while 47 or 62 disintegrations per cell per hour were required to produce this effect after incorporation of ^{131}IDU or ^{3}H-thymidine, respectively (HOFER and HUGHES, 1971). The radiotoxicity of ^{125}IDU incorporated into DNA thus appears to be higher than that of ^{3}H-thymidine by a factor of 10 to 15. On the other hand, the efficiency of incorporation of IDU into DNA after injection into animals is lower by a factor of approximately 10 than that of thymidine. This supports the conclusion that similar degrees of radiotoxicity will be produced by injection of equal doses (μCi per g of body weight) of ^{125}IDU or ^{3}H-thymidine, whereas the effects of ^{131}IDU will be considerably smaller. Since ^{3}H-thymidine at a dose of 1 μCi per g of body weight is commonly used in autoradiographic studies, the same dose of ^{125}IDU, as applied in our studies, should not cause any major radiotoxicity.

As reported by FEINENDEGEN *et al.* (1966a), injection into rats of 1.5 μCi of ^{125}IDU per g of body weight did not result in detectable radiotoxicity, as judged by measurements of the mitotic index of bone marrow cells. On the other hand, injection of 1 μCi of ^{3}H-thymidine into partially hepatectomized young rats was found to delay entry of hepatocytes into mitosis and to cause an increase in frequency of mitotic abnormalities (GRISHAM, 1960). In our studies, however, the time course of DNA synthesis and of mitotic activity was not significantly different in rats injected with 1 μCi of ^{125}IDU per g of body weight and those given 0.02 to 0.04 μCi of ^{131}IDU per g of body weight. In addition, the ratios between numbers of labeled cells and numbers of mitotic cells, as well as the frequency of atypic mitotic figures and of degenerative cellular and nuclear changes, did not differ significantly between the two groups of animals. This supports the assumption that toxic effects of IDU as well as radiation artifacts due to ^{125}IDU or ^{131}IDU were negligible under the conditions used in our studies.

The use of labeled IDU as DNA precursor in studies of proliferating cell systems has two main advantages as compared with ^{3}H-thymidine. First, IDU labeled with gamma-emitting iodine isotopes permits determination of total radioactivity of tissues, organs, and even small animals, thus obviating the need for such time-consuming procedures as extraction of DNA or autoradiographic analysis. Second, with respect to liver tissue, extraction with formalin represents a simple means of removing the label contained in the acid-soluble fraction. A major portion of the radioactivity retained in liver tissue after formalin extraction was shown to represent IDU incorporated into DNA. This was found to be the case even under rather unfavorable conditions, i.e. if the labeled precursor was administered at a time when the rate of DNA synthesis was minimal. DNA synthetic activity may therefore be assessed in regenerating liver by measuring radioactivity in formalin-treated tissue at short time intervals after injection of labeled IDU.

Determination of radioactivity in formalin-treated liver tissue after injection of labeled IDU appears especially useful for studying variations in DNA synthetic activity as a function of time after partial hepatectomy. In particular, the time lag between the operation and onset of increased DNA synthesis may be conveniently determined. Changes in IDU incorporation occurring after this lag period probably do not exclusively reflect the corresponding changes in rate of overall DNA synthesis, since the extent of incorporation of injected IDU is also affected by vascularization, diffusion of the precursor within the tissue, activity of enzymes involved in anabolic and catabolic reactions, as well as pool sizes of thymidine and its nucleotides. Nevertheless, qualitative differences in the time course of precursor incorporation may be used to study the effects of various factors on the pattern of liver regeneration. For instance, diurnal variations in regenerative response may be analyzed, and the effects of drugs such as phenobarbital on the time course of liver regeneration may be evaluated (Bürki *et al.*, 1971 b).

Labeled IDU has another advantage over thymidine in its low extent of reutilization. It is therefore useful for analyzing cell kinetic events during prolonged periods after injection of the precursor. Heiniger *et al.* (1971 b) found that, in mice injected with ^{3}H-thymidine or ^{125}IDU before partial hepatectomy, reutilization of tritium by the regenerating liver was lower by factors of 10 to 35 than that of ^{125}iodine. In our studies, after injection of ^{131}IDU into rats 22 h after partial hepatectomy, a decrease in radioactivity of liver DNA was observed during the following 24 h. This decrease was shown to be correlated with loss of radioactivity from disintegrating parenchymal cells. In addition, migration of parenchymal cells within lobules of regenerating liver was demonstrated. During the second 24 h interval after injection of labeled IDU into partially hepatectomized rats, radioactivity in liver DNA was found to increase again. This increase may be attributable to immigration of labeled mesenchymal cells into the growing liver.

In summary, determination of radioactivity in liver DNA combined with autoradiographic analysis of liver tissue appears promising for future studies on the time course and extent of cellular events during liver regeneration. Labeled IDU is a useful DNA precursor in this type of investigation because reutilization of label from dying cells is minimal.

References

Alston, W. C., Thomson, R. Y.: Humoral and local factors in liver regeneration. Cancer Res. **23**, 901–905 (1963).

Altmann, H.-W.: Der Zellersatz, insbesondere an den parenchymatösen Organen. Verh. dtsch. Ges. Path. **50**, 15–53 (1966).

Appelgren, L.-E., Söremark, R., Ullberg, S.: Improved resolution in autoradiography with radioiodine using the extranuclear electron radiation from ^{125}I. Biochim. biophys. Acta (Amst.) **66**, 144–149 (1963).

Barbiroli, B., Potter, V. R.: DNA synthesis and interaction between controlled feeding schedules and partial hepatectomy in rats. Science **172**, 738–741 (1971).

Baugnet-Mahieu, L., Goutier, R.: Mechanisms responsible for the low incorporation into DNA of the thymidine analogue, 5-iodo-2′-deoxyuridine. Biochem. Pharmacol. **17**, 1017–1023 (1968).

Blank, H., McCarthy, P. L., de Lamater, E. D.: A non-vacuum freezing-dehydrating technic for histology, autoradiography and microbial cytology. Stain Technol. **26**, 193–197 (1951).

Boak, J. L., Christie, G. H., Ford, W. L., Howard, J. G.: Pathways in the development of liver macrophages: alternative precursors contained in populations of lymphocytes and bone-marrow cells. Proc. roy. Soc. B **169**, 307–327 (1968).

Bryant, B. J.: Reutilisation of leukocyte DNA by cells of regenerating liver. Exp. Cell Res. **27**, 70–79 (1962).

Bryant, B. J.: Reutilisation of lymphocyte DNA by cells of intestinal crypts and regenerating liver. J. Cell Biol. **18**, 515–523 (1963).

Bucher, N. L. R.: Regeneration of mammalian liver. Int. Rev. Cytol. **15**, 245–300 (1963).

Bucher, N. L. R.: Experimental aspects of hepatic regeneration. New Engl. J. Med. **277**, 686–696, 738–746 (1967).

Bucher, N. L. R., Malt, R. A.: Regeneration of liver and kidney. Boston: Little, Brown & Co. 1971.

Bucher, N. L. R., Swaffield, M. N.: The rate of incorporation of labeled thymidine into the deoxyribonucleic acid of regenerating rat liver in relation to the amount of liver excised. Cancer Res. **24**, 1611–1625 (1964).

Bucher, N. L. R., Swaffield, M. N., DiTroia, J. F.: The influence of age upon the incorporation of thymidine-2-C^{14} into the DNA of regenerating rat liver. Cancer Res. **24**, 509–512 (1964).

Bürki, K., Schaer, J. C., Grieder, A., Schindler, R., Cottier, H.: Studies on liver regeneration. I. ^{131}Iododeoxyuridine as a precursor of DNA in normal and regenerating rat liver. Cell Tiss. Kinet. **4**, 519–527 (1971a).

Bürki, K., Schindler, R., Pfenninger, M.: Studies on liver regeneration. II. Effects of phenobarbital on the onset and pattern of rat liver regeneration following partial hepatectomy. Cell Tiss. Kinet. **4**, 529–537 (1971b).

Calabresi, P., Cardoso, S. S., Finch, S. C., Kligerman, M. M., von Essen, C. F., Chu, M. Y., Welch, A. D.: Initial clinical studies with 5-iodo-2'-deoxyuridine. Cancer Res. **21**, 550–559 (1961).

Canellakis, E. S., Jaffe, J. J., Mantsavinos, R., Krakow, J. S.: Pyrimidine metabolism. IV. A comparison of normal and regenerating rat liver. J. biol. Chem. **234**, 2096–2099 (1959).

Cheong, L., Rich, M. A., Eidinoff, M. L.: Introduction of the 5-halogenated uracil moiety into deoxyribonucleic acid of mammalian cells in culture. J. biol. Chem. **235**, 1441–1447 (1960).

Clifton, K. H., Szybalski, W., Heidelberger, C., Gollin, F. F., Ansfield, F. J., Vermund, H.: Incorporation of I^{125}-labeled iododeoxyuridine into the deoxyribonucleic acid of murine and human tissues following therapeutic doses. Cancer Res. **23**, 1715–1723 (1963).

Commerford, S. L.: Biological stability of 5-iodo-2'-deoxyuridine labelled with iodine-125 after its incorporation into the deoxyribonucleic acid of the mouse. Nature (Lond.) **206**, 949–950 (1965).

Curtis, H. J.: Cellular processes involved in aging. Fed. Proc. **23**, 662–667 (1964).

Dethlefsen, L. A.: Comparison of tumor radioactivity after the administration of either ^{125}I- or ^{3}H-labeled 5-iodo-2'-deoxyuridine. Cancer Res. **29**, 1717–1720 (1969).

Dethlefsen, L. A.: Reutilization of ^{131}I-5-iodo-2'-deoxyuridine as compared to ^{3}H-thymidine in mouse duodenum and mammary tumor. J. nat. Cancer Inst. **44**, 827–840 (1970).

Dethlefsen, L. A.: An evaluation of radioiodine-labeled 5-iodo-2'-deoxyuridine as a tracer for measuring cell loss from solid tumors. Cell Tiss. Kinet. **4**, 123–138 (1971).

Dethlefsen, L. A.: ^{3}H-5-iodo-2'-deoxyuridine toxicity. Problems in cell proliferation studies. Cell Tiss. Kinet. **7**, 213–222 (1974).

Djordjevic, B., Szybalski, W.: Genetics of human cell lines. III. Incorporation of 5-bromo- and 5-iododeoxyuridine into the deoxyribonucleic acid of human cells and its effect on radiation sensitivity. J. exp. Med. **112**, 509–531 (1960).

Edwards, J. L., Koch, A.: Parenchymal and littoral cell proliferation during liver regeneration. Lab. Invest. **13**, 32–43 (1964).

Eidinoff, M. L., Cheong, L., Rich, M. A.: Incorporation of unnatural pyrimidine bases into deoxyribonucleic acid of mammalian cells. Science **129**, 1550–1551 (1959).

Erikson, R. L., Szybalski, W.: Molecular radiobiology of human cell lines. III. Radiation-sensitizing properties of 5-iodo-deoxyuridine. Cancer Res. **23**, 122–130 (1963).

Fabrikant, J. I.: The kinetics of cellular proliferation in regenerating liver. J. Cell Biol. **36**, 551–565 (1968).

Feinendegen, L. E., Bond, V. P., Hughes, W. L.: ^{125}I-DU (5-iodo-2'-deoxyuridine) in autoradiographic studies of cell proliferation. Exp. Cell Res. **43**, 107–119 (1966a).

FEINENDEGEN, L. E., BOND, V. P., HUGHES, W. L.: Physiological thymidine reutilization in rat bone marrow. Proc. Soc. exp. Biol. (N.Y.) **122**, 448–455 (1966b).

FEINENDEGEN, L. E., BOND, V. P., SHREEVE, W. W., PAINTER, R. B.: RNA and DNA metabolism in human tissue culture cells studied with tritiated cytidine. Exp. Cell Res. **19**, 443–459 (1960).

FORBERG, S., ODEBLAD, E., SÖREMARK, R., ULLBERG, S.: Autoradiography with isotopes emitting internal conversion electrons and Auger electrons. Acta radiol. (Stockh.) **2**, 241–262 (1964).

FOX, B. W., PRUSOFF, W. H.: The comparative uptake of I^{125}-labeled 5-iodo-2'-deoxyuridine and thymidine-H^3 into tissues of mice bearing hepatoma-129. Cancer Res. **25**, 234–240 (1965).

FRITZSON, P.: The relation between uracil-catabolizing enzymes and rate of rat liver regeneration. J. biol. Chem. **237**, 150–156 (1963).

FRITZSON, P.: Delayed synthesis of uracil-degrading enzymes in regenerating rat liver. Biochim. biophys. Acta (Amst.) **91**, 374–379 (1964).

GRISHAM, J. W.: Inhibitory effect of tritiated thymidine on regeneration of the liver in the young rat. Proc. Soc. exp. Biol. (N.Y.) **105**, 555–558 (1960).

GRISHAM, J. W.: A morphologic study of deoxyribonucleic acid synthesis and cell proliferation in regenerating rat liver; autoradiography with thymidine-H^3. Cancer Res. **22**, 842–849 (1962).

GRUNDMANN, E., BACH, G.: Amitosen, Endomitosen und Mitosen nach partieller Hepatektomie. Beitr. path. Anat. **123**, 144–172 (1960).

GRUNDMANN, E., SEIDEL, H. J.: Die reparative Parenchymregeneration am Beispiel der Leber nach Teilhepatektomie. In: Handbuch der allgemeinen Pathologie, Band VI/2, S. 129–243. Berlin-Heidelberg-New York: Springer 1969.

GÜNTHER, G., HÜBNER, K., PAUL, A.: Mitose-Rhythmen der Leber nach Teilhepatektomie. Virchows Arch. Abt. B **1**, 69–79 (1968).

HAMPTON, E. G., EIDINOFF, M. L.: Administration of 5-iododeoxyuridine-I^{131} in the mouse and rat. Cancer Res. **21**, 345–352 (1961).

HEINIGER, H. J., FEINENDEGEN, L. E., BÜRKI, K.: Reutilization of thymidine in various groups of rat bone marrow cells. Blood **37**, 340–348 (1971a).

HEINIGER, H. J., FRIEDRICH, G., FEINENDEGEN, L. E., CANTELMO, F.: Reutilization of 5-^{125}I-iodo-2'-deoxyuridine and ^{3}H-thymidine in regenerating liver of mice. Proc. Soc. exp. Biol. (N.Y.) **137**, 1381–1384 (1971b).

HIGGINS, G. M., ANDERSON, R. M.: Experimental pathology of the liver. I. Restoration of the liver of the white rat following partial surgical removal. Arch. Path. **12**, 186–202 (1931).

HOFER, K. G.: Radiation effects on death and migration of tumor cells in mice. Radiat. Res. **43**, 663–678 (1970).

HOFER, K. G., DIBENEDETTO, J., HUGHES, W. L.: Natural and asparaginase-induced death of L5178Y leukemia cells *in vivo*. Z. Krebsforsch. **75**, 34–44 (1970).

HOFER, K. G., HOFER, M.: Kinetics of proliferation, migration, and death of L 1210 ascites cells. Cancer Res. **31**, 402–408 (1971).

HOFER, K. G., HUGHES, W. L.: Incorporation of iododeoxyuridine-^{125}I into the DNA of L 1210 leukemia cells during tumor development. Cancer Res. **30**, 236–243 (1970).

HOFER, K. G., HUGHES, W. L.: Radiotoxicity of intranuclear tritium, ^{125}iodine and ^{131}iodine. Radiat. Res. **47**, 94–109 (1971).

HOFER, K. G., PRENSKY, W., HUGHES, W. L.: Death and metastatic distribution of tumor cells in mice monitored with ^{125}I-iododeoxyuridine. J. nat. Cancer Inst. **43**, 763–773 (1969a).

HOFER, K. G., PRENSKY, W., ROSENOFF, S., HUGHES, W. L.: Spontaneous and amethopterin-induced death of L 1210 leukaemia cells *in vivo*. Nature (Lond.) **221**, 576–577 (1969b).

HUGHES, W. L., COMMERFORD, S. L., GITLIN, D., KRUEGER, R. C., SCHULTZE, B., SHAH, V., REILLY, P.: Deoxyribonucleic acid metabolism *in vivo*. I. Cell proliferation and death as measured by incorporation and elimination of iododeoxyuridine. Fed. Proc. **23**, 640–648 (1964).

JAFFE, J. J.: Diurnal mitotic periodicity in regenerating rat liver. Anat. Rec. **120**, 935–954 (1954).

Kinsky, R. G., Christie, G. H., Elson, J., Howard, J. G.: Extrahepatic derivation of Kupffer cells during oestrogenic stimulation of parabiosed mice. Brit. J. exp. Path. **50**, 438–447 (1969).

Klinge, O.: Altersabhängige Beeinträchtigung der Zellvermehrung in der regenerierenden Rattenleber. Virchows Arch. Abt. B **1**, 342–345 (1968).

Klinge, O.: Kernveränderungen und Kernteilungsstörungen der Altersleber. Gerontologia (Basel) **19**, 314–329 (1973).

Klinge, O., Mathyl, J.: Tageszeitliche Mitose-Rhythmen in der teilektomierten Rattenleber. Virchows Arch. Abt. B **2**, 154–162 (1969).

Kopriwa, B. M., Leblond, C. P.: Improvements in the coating technique of radioautography. J. Histochem. Cytochem. **10**, 269–284 (1962).

Looney, W. B., Chang, L. O., Banghart, F. W.: The rate of DNA replication at the molecular, chromosomal, cellular, and intercellular levels in regenerating rat liver. Proc. nat. Acad. Sci. (Wash.) **57**, 972–978 (1967).

Mak, S., Till, J. E.: Use of I^{125}-labeled 5-iodo-2′-deoxyuridine for the measurement of DNA synthesis in mammalian cells *in vitro*. Canad. J. Biochem. **41**, 2343–2351 (1963).

Mathias, A. P., Fischer, G. A., Prusoff, W. H.: Inhibition of the growth of mouse leukemia cells in culture by 5-iododeoxyuridine. Biochim. biophys. Acta (Amst.) **36**, 560–561 (1959).

Morris, N. R., Cramer, J. W.: DNA synthesis by mammalian cells inhibited in culture by 5-iodo-2′-deoxyuridine. Molec. Pharmacol. **2**, 1–9 (1966).

Morris, N. R., Cramer, J. W.: 5-Iodo-2′-deoxyuridine and DNA synthesis in mammalian cells. Exp. Cell Res. **51**, 555–563 (1968).

O'Farrell, T. P., Dunaway, P. B.: Incorporation and tissue distribution of a thymidine analog in the cotton rat *Sigmodon hispidus*. Comp. Biochem. Physiol. **22**, 435–450 (1967).

O'Farrell, T. P., Dunaway, P. B.: Effects of acute ionizing radiation on incorporation of ^{131}IUDR by cotton rats, *Sigmodon hispidus*. Radiat. Res. **38**, 109–124 (1969).

Porschen, W., Feinendegen, L. E.: In-vivo-Bestimmungen der Zellverlustrate bei Experimentaltumoren mit markiertem Joddeoxyuridin. Strahlentherapie **137**, 718–723 (1969).

Post, J., Hoffman, J.: The effects of 5-iodo-2′-deoxyuridine upon the replication of ileal and spleen cells *in vivo*. Cancer Res. **29**, 1859–1865 (1969).

Potter, V. R.: Discussion of availability time of labeled DNA-precursors. In: The kinetics of cellular proliferation (F. Stohlman, ed.), p. 113–115. New York-London: Grune & Stratton 1959.

Prusoff, W. H.: Incorporation of iododeoxyuridine into the deoxyribonucleic acid of mouse Ehrlich-ascites-tumor cells *in vivo*. Biochim. biophys. Acta (Amst.) **39**, 327–331 (1960).

Prusoff, W. H., Jaffe, J. J., Günther, H.: Studies in the mouse of the pharmacology of 5-iododeoxyuridine, an analogue of thymidine. Biochem. Pharmacol. **3**, 110–121 (1960).

Rabes, H.: Untersuchungen zur humoralen Regulation bei regenerativem und malignem Wachstum. Veröffentlichungen aus der morphologischen Pathologie, Heft 73. Stuttgart: Gustav Fischer Verlag 1967.

Rabes, H., Tuczek, H. V.: Quantitative autoradiographische Untersuchung zur Heterogenität der Leberzellproliferation nach partieller Hepatektomie. Virchows Arch. Abt. B **6**, 302–312 (1970).

Rotenberg, A. D., Bruce, W. R., Baker, R. G.: Incorporation of 5-iododeoxyuridine ^{131}I in spontaneous C3H mouse mammary tumours. Brit. J. Radiol. **35**, 337–342 (1962).

Scherer, E., Friedrich-Freksa, H.: Zur Zentralvene gerichtete Wanderung von Leberzellen der Ratte nach partieller Hepatektomie und nach Verabfolgung von Diäthylnitrosamin. Z. Naturforsch. **25**b, 637–642 (1970).

Schindler, R.: Biochemie der Regeneration. In: Handbuch der allgemeinen Pathologie, Band VI/2, S. 1–128. Berlin-Heidelberg-New York: Springer 1969.

Schmidt, G., Thannhauser, S. J.: A method for the determination of desoxyribonucleic acid, ribonucleic acid, and phosphoproteins in animal tissues. J. biol. Chem. **161**, 83–89 (1945).

SCHNEIDER, G., MAURER, W.: Autoradiographische Untersuchung über den Einbau von H-3-Cytidin in die Kerne einiger Zellarten der Maus und über den Einfluß des Fixationsmittels auf die H-3-Aktivität. Acta histochem. (Jena) 15, 171–181 (1963).

SCHNEIDER, W. C.: Phosphorus compounds in animal tissues. III. A comparison of methods for the estimation of nucleic acids. J. biol. Chem. 164, 747–751 (1946).

SEEMAYER, N., HAAS, R., MAASS, G.: Vergleichende autoradiographische Untersuchungen der Generationszeit, DNS-Synthesezeit und des Einbaues in die Chromosomen nach Markierung mit ^{3}H-5-Jod-2′-desoxyuridin und ^{3}H-Thymidin an Gewebekulturzellen. Arch. ges. Virusforsch. 18, 155–162 (1966).

STEEL, G. G., LAMERTON, L. F.: The turnover of tritium from thymidine in tissues of the rat. Exp. Cell Res. 37, 117–131 (1965).

STÖCKER, E.: Der Proliferationsmodus in Niere und Leber. Verh. dtsch. Ges. Path. 50, 53–74 (1966).

STÖCKER, E.: Autoradiographische Untersuchungen zum zellulären Proliferationsstoffwechsel im Parenchym von Leber und Niere der Ratte. Acta histochem. (Jena), Suppl. 8, 205–229 (1968).

STÖCKER, E., HEINE, W. D.: Über die Proliferation von Nieren- und Leberepithel unter normalen und pathologischen Bedingungen. Autoradiographische Untersuchungen mit H^3-Thymidin an der Ratte. Beitr. path. Anat. 131, 410–434 (1965).

TAYLOR, J. H., WOODS, P. S., HUGHES, W. L.: The organization and duplication of chromosomes as revealed by autoradiographic studies using tritium-labeled thymidine. Proc. nat. Acad. Sci. (Wash.) 43, 122–128 (1957).

VERLY, W. G., HUNEBELLE, G.: Préparation de thymidine marquée avec du tritium Bull. Soc. chim. Belg. 66, 640–649 (1957).

Department of Pathology, Children's Hospital and General Hospital,
and Department of Pediatrics, University of Cincinnati Medical Center

The Human Placental Villitides:
A Review of Chronic Intrauterine Infection*

GEOFFREY ALTSHULER, M.B.B.S.
PETER RUSSELL, M.B.B.S.

With 25 Figures

Contents

* Supported in part by the Fels Division of Pediatric Research.

I. Introduction

In this era wherein we are becoming increasingly concerned about the quality of all human life, we are neglecting to pursue basic concerns of the fetus and newborn. Though many of us have developed expertise in the interpretation of various elegant biopsy preparations, relatively few of us in our study of diseases of the newborn ever bother to examine the diary of the patient's gestational life, the placenta. If it be true that the achievements of pathologists contribute to a higher standard of medical care, then it must be observed that any failure on their part to contribute towards knowledge of congenital diseases might retard the progress stimulated by contributions elsewhere.

Within the last ten years our microbiology colleagues have opened exciting vistas from which we may view the study of congenital diseases. A much deeper understanding of chronic intrauterine infections has been forthcoming from the ability of the virologist to culture rubella virus (Parkman *et al.*, 1962; Weller and Neva, 1962), cytomegalovirus (Rowe *et al.*, 1956; Smith, 1956; Weller *et al.*, 1957), and herpes simplex virus (Nahmias and Roizman, 1973).

It behooves many pathologists to have knowledge of the placenta, so that improved assessments of perinatal diseases may provide even better standards of perinatal medicine. Within this review we would like to share with our colleagues those experiences we have had and those scientific papers we have encountered, that have helped us in our understanding of human chronic intrauterine infection.

II. Normal Placental Histology

Recognition of abnormal placental histology presupposes a knowledge of the normal organ. It is perhaps a lack of confidence in the recognition of normality that causes many pathologists to avoid examining these specimens. An appreciation of placental histology can be gained from the excellent book of Boyd and Hamilton (1970) particularly with respect to the changes that constitute placental maturation.

Citing Becker (1959, 1962) they list four indices of the developing maturity of the normal human placenta: (1) decrease in the villous diameter

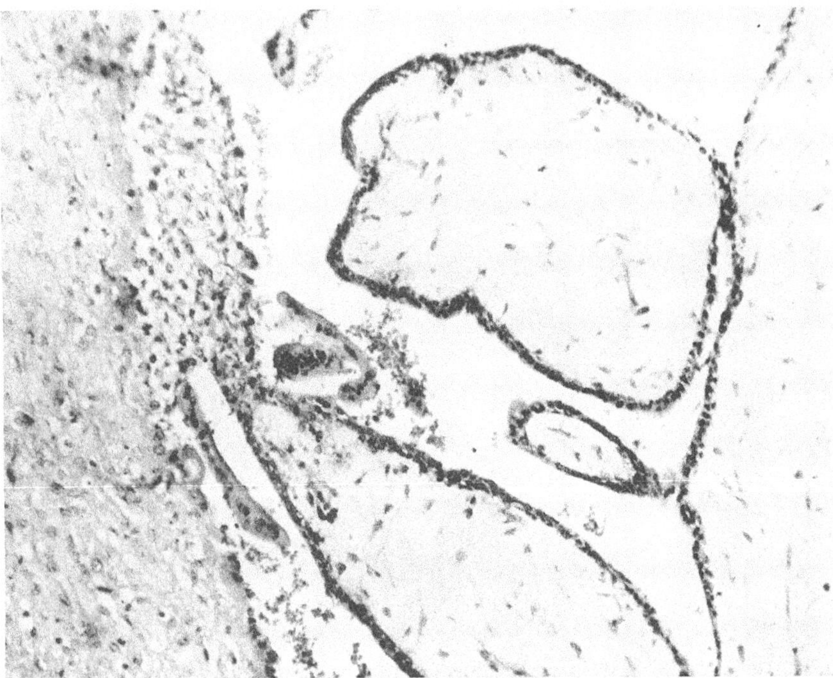

Fig. 1. Three week (post-ovulation) implantation. Note the lack of vasculogenesis of the loose-textured stroma. Original magnification × 100. Hematoxylin and Eosin

with increase in the surface of the individual villi; (2) increase in the fetal vascular spaces in the villi; (3) diminution of the peripheral intravillous connective tissue with increase in the number of syncytial bridges; and (4) marked increase in the connective tissue sheaths of the vessels in the trunci chorii. These maturational changes are illustrated in Figs. 1–4. In Fig. 1 a 2–3 weeks (post ovulation) implantation site is demonstrated. This illustration of the placental villi emphasizes the delicate immature mesenchyme, the lack of fetal vasculogenesis and the differentiation of the trophoblast into layers of syncytio- and cytotrophoblast. This differentiation is more developed by 6 to 8 weeks gestation (Fig. 2), at which time an augmented proliferation of cytotrophoblastic shell tissue is present. By 12–20 weeks there has been progressive loss of the delicate loose texture of the villous stroma and a peak in the proliferation of Hofbauer cells (Figs. 3, 4). It is likely that these cells participate in the transport of nutrients from mother to fetus and in host defence responses against foreign antigens. BENIRSCHKE and BOURNE (1958) have suggested that Hofbauer cells may transform to plasm cells during chronic placental infection. During mid-trimester, the progressive condensation of the villous stroma manifests a diminution of the size of the villi, vascularization at this time being increasingly prominent. By 20–24 weeks gestation, the villous blood vessels become more central in the villi. During mid-trimester the development of the trophoblast proceeds concomitantly with the evanes-

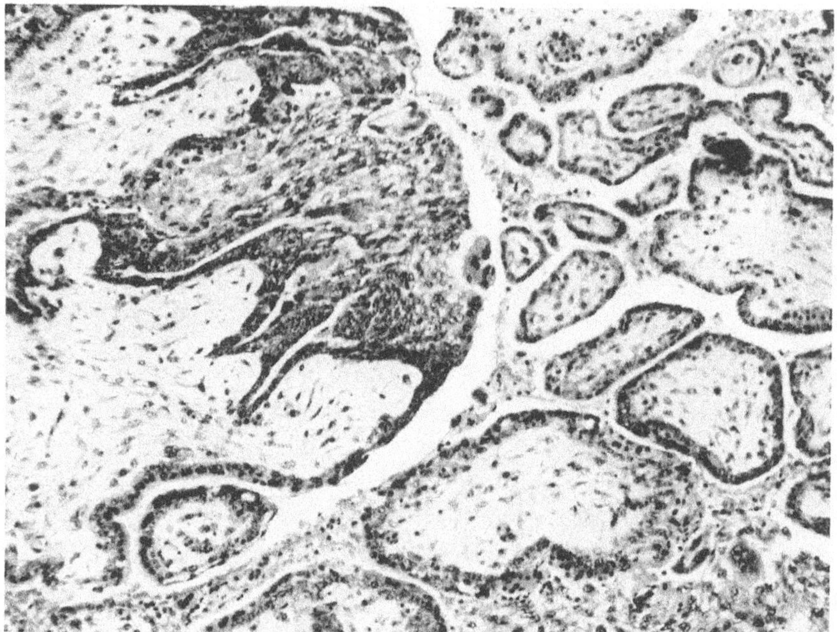

Fig. 2. A 6–8 week placenta in which proliferation and differentiation of the trophoblast
are apparent. Original magnification × 130. Hematoxylin and Eosin

cence of the cytotrophoblast and the progressive development of the syncytiotrophoblast in which knotting becomes prominent. The cytotrophoblast never
totally disappears, being recognizable at higher power light microscopy even
in term placentas. At term, the hallmarks of maturity are present, including
dense villous stroma with occasional Hofbauer cells, villous boundaries inclusive of syncytial knots and occasional deposits of maternal fibrin about the
villi (Fig. 5).

Some writers suggest that all mature placentas are "senile" or "pathologic". BOYD and HAMILTON (1970) summarize their detailed discussion
succinctly:

"Finally, though pathological changes (e.g. infarcts) and quasi-pathological
changes (e.g. increased fibrin deposits) tend to increase as pregnancy advances,
being particularly frequent in post-mature placentae . . . they are so variable
that it is dangerous to draw too firm conclusions as to placental age from
them."

III. The Concept of Villitis

Many pathologists recognize old and recent infarcts, fibrin deposits and
the severe ischemic features of the so-called "Tenney" change (Fig. 6) as
being correlates of clinically diagnosed preeclampsia, but either do not
recognize or ignore focal villitis lesions that often are additionally present.

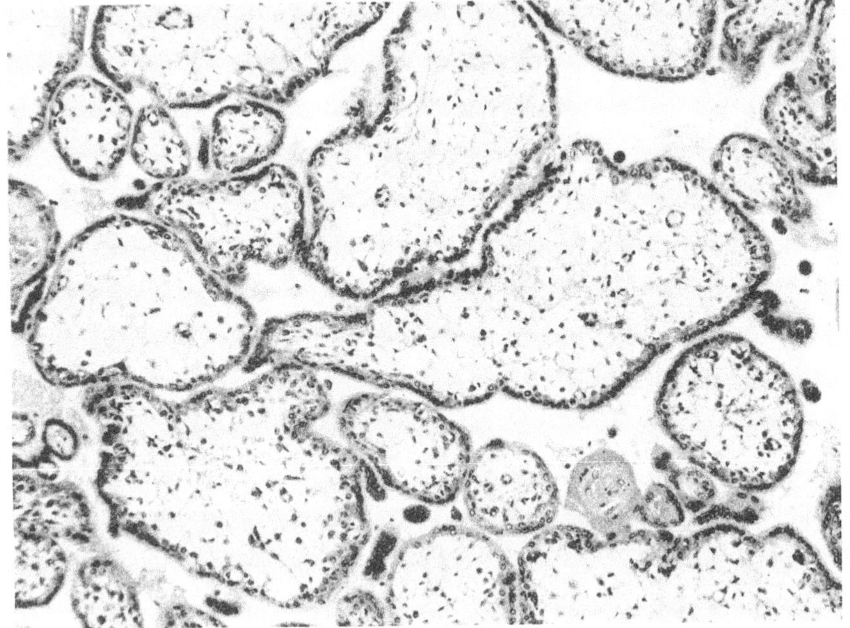

Fig. 3

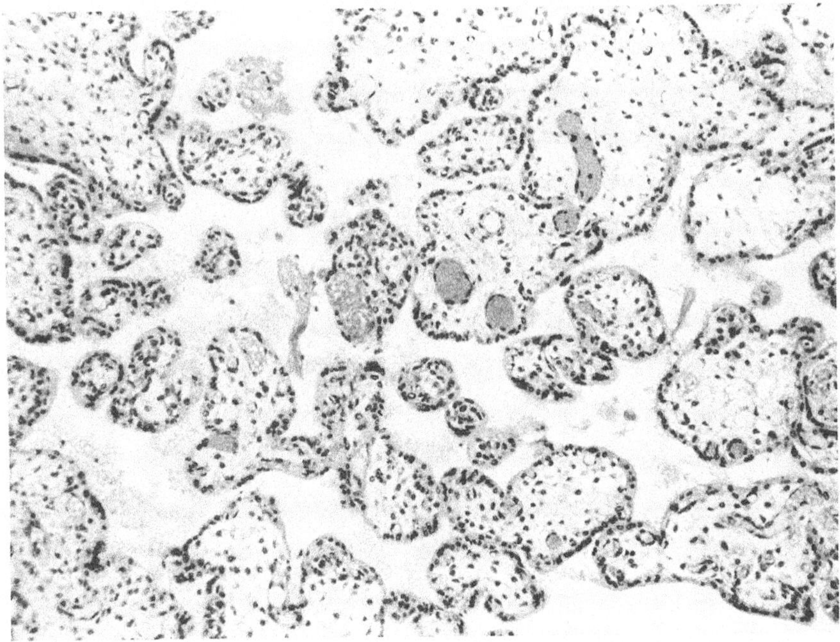

Fig. 4

Figs. 3 and 4. These placentas of 16 and 22 weeks gestation respectively show progressive increase in fetal blood vessels and stromal cells. Original magnification × 90. Hematoxylin and Eosin

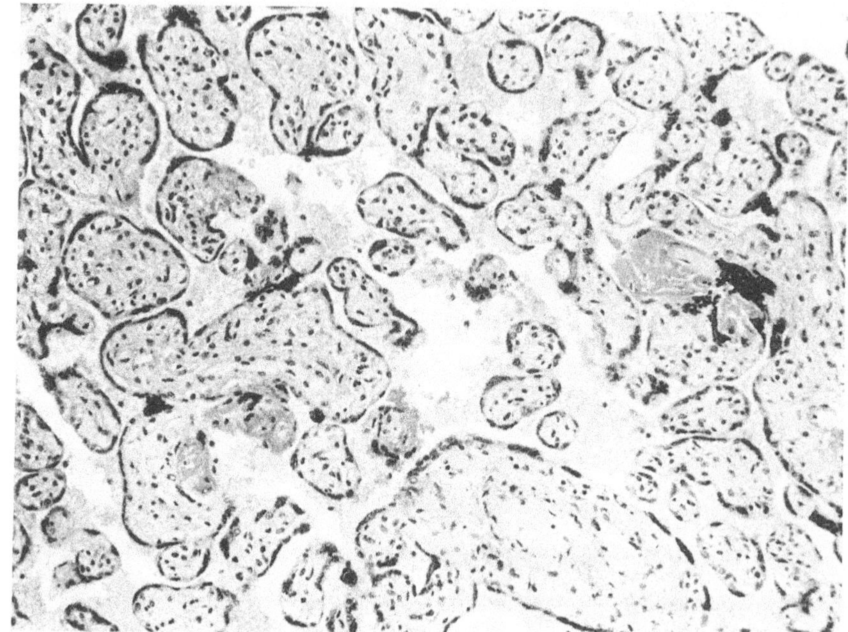

Fig. 5. Term placenta: Note the smaller size of the villi, the condensation of the stroma and prominence of syncytial knots. Original magnification × 120. Hematoxylin and Eosin

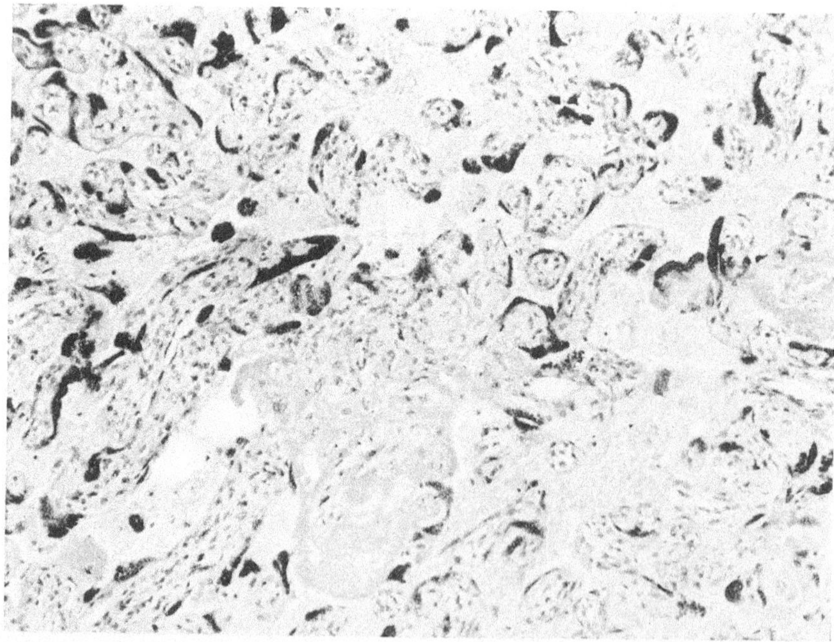

Fig. 6. Term placenta: Abundant syncytial knots and fibrin deposition characteristic of the "Tenney" effect. Original magnification × 120. Hematoxylin and Eosin

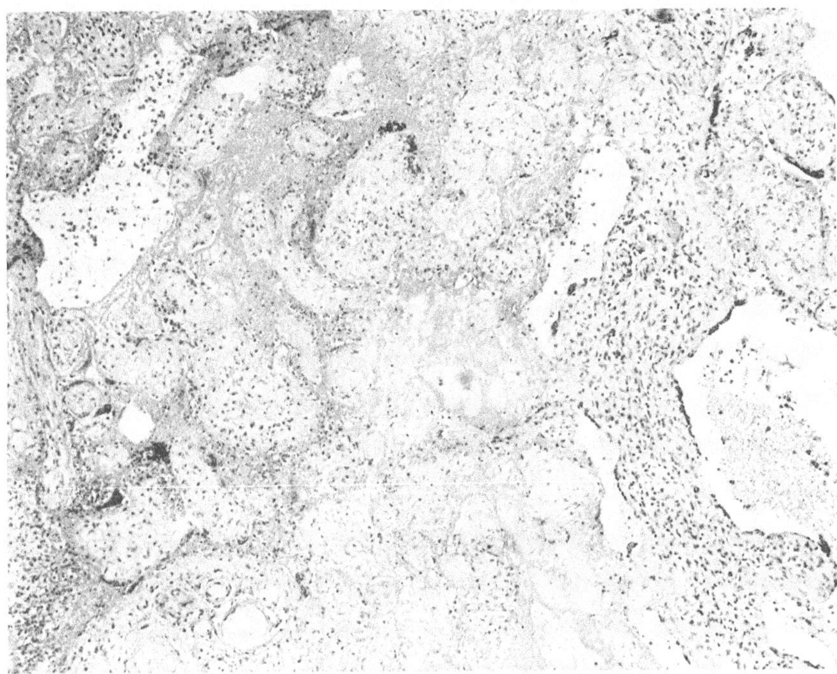

Fig. 7. Leukoerythrostasis within maternal sinusoids (left) circumscribes the central infarct, and is contrasted with villitis identified by the proliferation of inflammatory cells within the villous tissue (right). Original magnification × 60. Hematoxylin and Eosin

Thus, the significance of the lesions escapes attention. If shown similar lesions in other organs, these same pathologists certainly would recognize the inflammatory nature of the lesions and would consider the possibility of an infectious etiology. Stromal cell proliferation diffusely throughout many villi is another pathologic feature that may suggest chronic intrauterine infection. Since all chorionic tissue is fetal in origin, focal or diffuse villitis must be regarded as evidence of potential infection in the associated fetus or newborn. Although it is recognized that polymorphonuclear leukocytes of maternal origin may marginate placental infarcts of non-infectious etiology, it is emphasized that proliferation of inflammatory cells within villi (Fig. 7) should be considered as prima facie evidence of placental infection, irrespective of whether or not cultural studies lead to the isolation of an organism. Instances of chronic villitis that include plasma cell proliferation have been suggested to be of immunologic significance (HOMBERGER et al., 1971). We consider that these lesions most likely occur as a consequence of infection, even if immunologic aberrations are also present. Viruses are well known to affect the function of the immune system (SILVERSTEIN, 1964; STIEHM, 1966; ALFORD et al., 1967; DENT and RAWLS, 1971). It has been shown by immunofluorescent light microscopy that the plasma cells of chronic villitis lesions label with antibodies against the immunoglobulin IgM, the so-called "marker" of chronic intrauterine infection. Finally, in "Rh Disease", the commonly seen circumstance of feto-maternal incompatibility, in the absence of any coincidental infection, plasma cells are not present.

IV. Terms and Definitions

A. Villitis

An intrinsic inflammatory response occurring within one or more villi, the proliferating or infiltrating cells being fetal in origin. This inflammatory response is initiated by the fetus against an external antigenic stimulus. These lesions are to be differentiated from maternal sinusoidal leuko-erythrostasis about fetal villi and from maternal sinusoidal inflammatory cells chemotactically attracted to the periphery of necrotic or infarcted placental villi of non-infective origin (Fig. 7).

B. Focal Villitis

Lesions present in random, isolated villi or in small clusters of neighboring villi (Fig. 8).

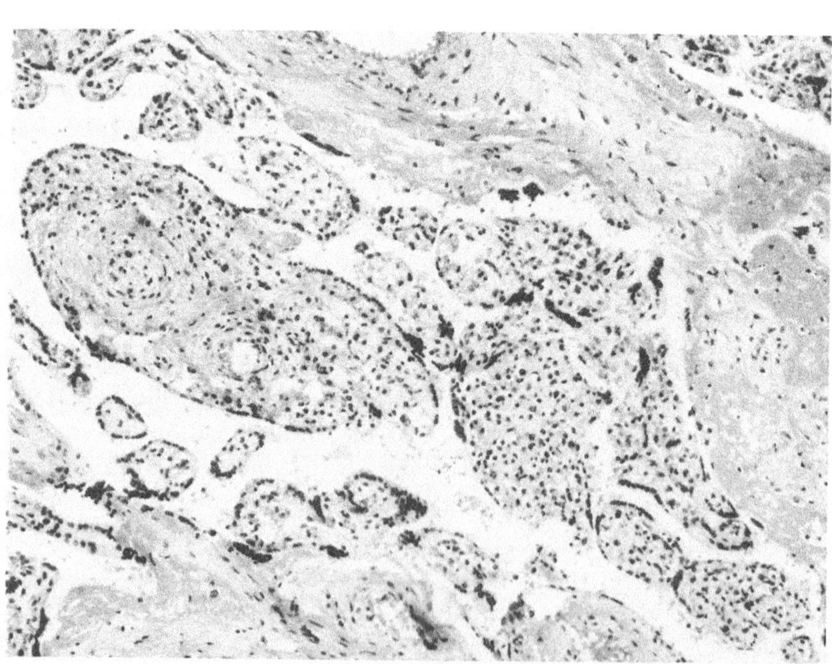

Fig. 8. In addition to proliferative villitis, there is endovascular proliferation within the villus of the left. Original magnification × 100. Hematoxylin and Eosin

C. Diffuse Villitis

Extensive involvement of contiguous villi throughout many cotyledons but not necessarily throughout the entire placenta (Fig. 9). Co-existent ischemic change may be present, for example, as a consequence of abruptio placentae or of other abnormalities of the maternal floor.

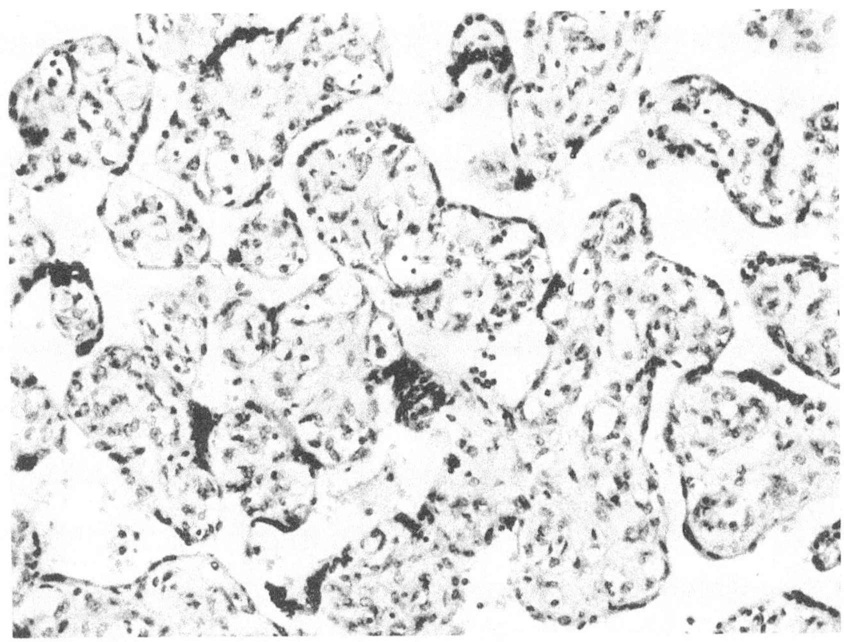

Fig. 9. Relative immaturity. This term placenta shows severe stromal cell proliferation and a retarded maturation of the trophoblast. Original magnification × 120. Hematoxylin and Eosin

D. Proliferative Villitis

A numerically increased population of chronic inflammatory cells within the affected villous tissue. (Fig. 10). If the inflammatory cells are predominantly histiocytic, a granulomatous variant may result.

E. Necrotizing Villitis

This term is used to qualify those lesions that include tissue necrosis (Fig. 11). In the context of proliferative villitis it is regarded as representing the acute stage of the spectrum of this lesion. In the context of focal lesions

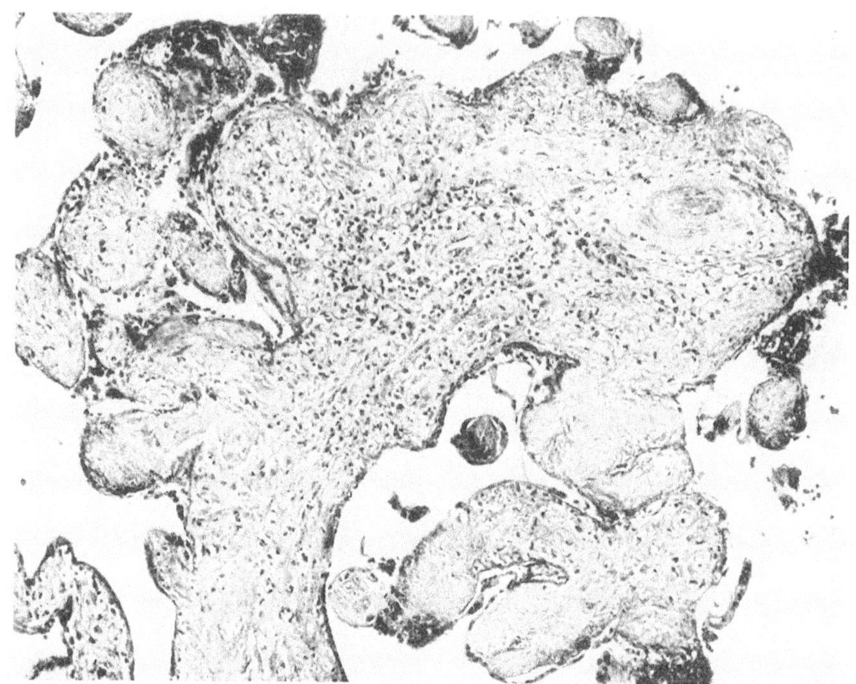

Fig. 10. Acute proliferative villitis. Note the vascular lesion at the top right aspect of the villus. Original magnification × 90. Hematoxylin and Eosin

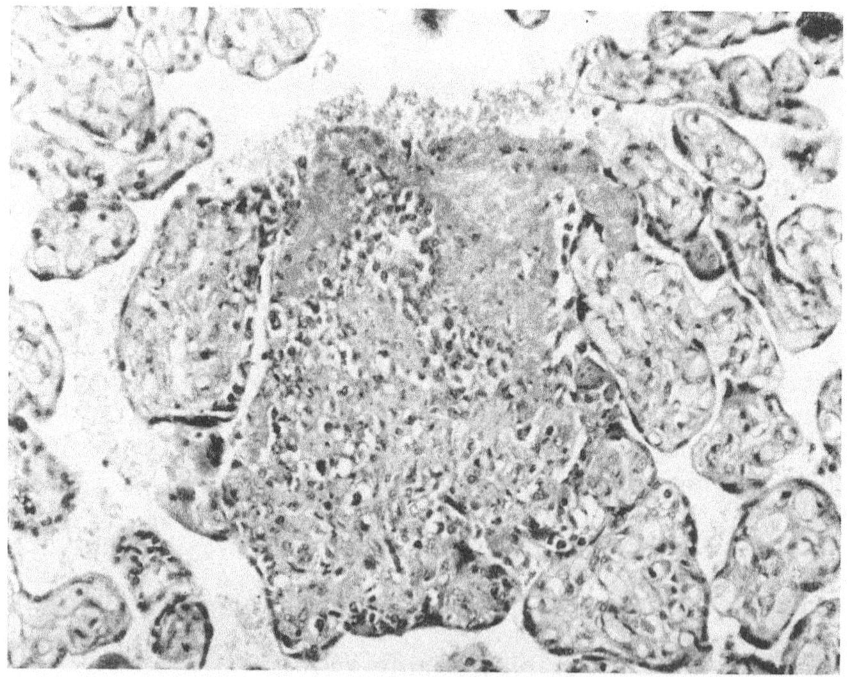

Fig. 11. Acute necrotizing villitis. Original magnification × 140. Hematoxylin and Eosin

in the decidua ("focal decidual necrosis"), these lesions should not be considered "bland" even though they often include relatively few inflammatory

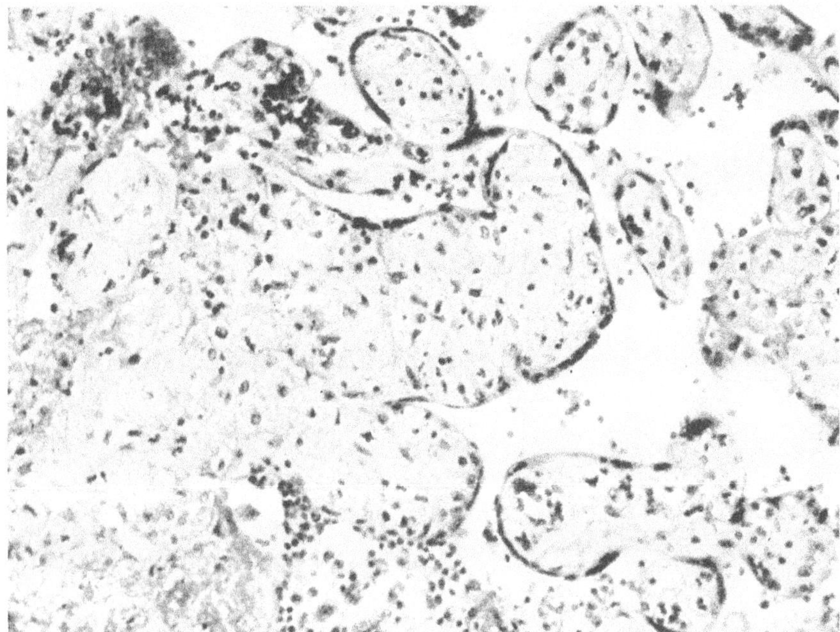

Fig. 12. Reparative villitis with cicatricial repair. Original magnification × 140.
Hematoxylin and Eosin

cells. They may be manifestations, for example, of infection with herpes simplex virus or cytomegalovirus.

F. Reparative Villitis

A later stage, characterized by cicatricial repair including the organization of histiocytes and fibroblast-like cells (Fig. 12). Vascular obliteration is a common accompaniment. Granulomatous villitis also will terminate in a reparative phase. Evanescent villitis denotes stages of repair in which occasional chronic inflammatory cells are present. The lesions (Fig. 13) typically are precursors of the entity known as avascular villi (GRUENWALD, 1961).

G. Stromal Fibrosis

Cicatricial lesions showing a condensation of connective tissue in the relative absence of inflammatory cell infiltration. This is considered the common end stage of the various forms of proliferative and reparative villitis.

H. Endovasculitis/Endovascular Sclerosis

These lesions include endovascular proliferation with intimal hyperplasia (Figs. 8, 14), acute vasculitis or concentric sclerosis of the vessel wall with ultimate luminal occlusion. Although these lesions may be seen in many of the villitides to be discussed in this review, they are particularly characteristic of placental syphilis (RUSSELL and ALTSHULER, 1974).

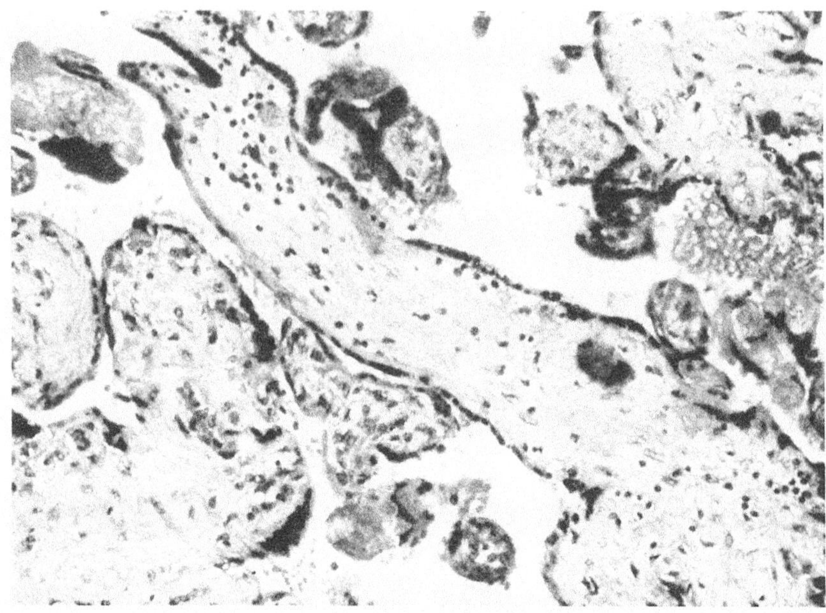

Fig. 13. Stromal fibrosis in the presence of few chronic inflammatory cells. Original magnification × 180. Hematoxylin and Eosin

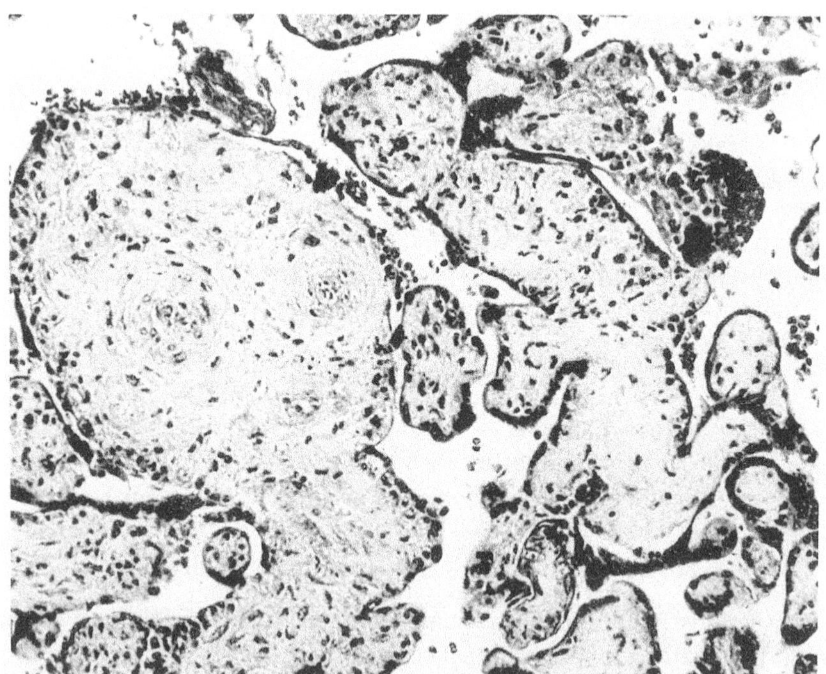

Fig. 14. This illustration shows contrasting features of intimal proliferation and endovascular sclerosis of the fetal vessels. An evanescent villitis is present in the villus to the right. Original magnification × 180. Hematoxylin and Eosin

I. Relative Immaturity

This term is one of convenience rather than of accuracy and is not meant to imply that the placenta studied is appropriate for an earlier gestational age than that stated for the associated infant. These placentas are pathologic and do not resemble normal placentas whether these be of implantation age (Fig. 1) or of any subsequent stage of normal maturation (Figs. 2–5). The characteristic features of relative immaturity are the lack of syncytiotrophoblast differentiation and knotting, persistence and proliferation of cytotrophoblast with frequently observed mitoses, and hypercellularity of the villous stroma. They are enlarged but do not have the abundant loose stroma of truly immature placental villi. It is the striking degree of stromal hypercellularity that makes this entity overtly pathologic. Normally, the most cellular villous stroma occurs between 12 and 20 weeks gestation. Comparisons between Figs. 3, 4, which represent that particular phase of development, and Fig. 9, which illustrates relative immaturity, serve to differentiate the pathologic features. The entity represents retardation of maturation of the villi. In our experience, if immunohemolytic disease and the rare occurrence of a chronic feto-maternal transfusion can be excluded, the most likely cause of relative immaturity is chronic intrauterine infection. We have not seen it in association with generalized placental ischemia due to "maternal floor infarction" (BENIRSCHKE and DRISCOLL, 1967), or with chronic abruptio placentae. Although the term implies retardation of placental maturation, only two of our 7 placentas which show severe relative immaturity (Cases 10 and 11 of Table 1) were associated with small-for-gestational-age infants.

V. Classification of the Placental Villitides

For an excellent review of the pathogenesis of fetal and neonatal infection we should like to recommend the classic paper of BLANC (1961).

DAVIES (1971), in her review of bacterial infections in the fetus and newborn, lists over 30 bacteria which may be responsible for serious perinatal infection. Within the last five years, group B streptococci have become the most frequent bacterial cause of perinatal sepsis at the University of Cincinnati Medical Center, succeeding gram-negative enteric organisms, whose incidence was predominant in the preceding 15 years. Many other medical centers in the United States have encountered a similar changing pattern of infection (FRANCIOSI et al., 1973).

Great differences exist from country to country, in the incidence of diseases caused by various pathogens. Listeriosis, for example, while not rare in Scandinavian countries or in Australia, has only occasionally been reported as a cause of recurrent reproductive failure elsewhere. Recent variola and vaccinia epidemics have occurred in Great Britain, Africa, India and South America (FOEGE and EDDINS, 1973), but in the United States there has not

Table 1. Clinicopathologic correlations

Case number	Gestation (weeks)	Birth weight (g)	Clinical correlation
1	39	2800	Cord IgM 9.6 mg% Bilirubin 14.2 mg% at one week of age (with elevated direct) despite phototherapy. No liver biopsy
2	40	4705	Sacrococcygeal teratoma
3	40	2870	Respiratory distress syndrome. Shock. Disseminated intravascular coagulation. Liver biopsy at one month = neonatal hepatitis. Repeat liver biopsy at five months = cirrhosis. Alpha-1-antitrypsin normal
4	39	3980	Maternal hepatitis at 30 weeks gestation. No problems in neonate
5	39	3140	Meconium stained. Cord IgM 7 mg%. Purpura, hepatosplenomegaly. Total bilirubin 29 mg% (direct 13 mg%)
6	34	2210	Hepatosplenomegaly with jaundice. Disseminated intravascular coagulation. Total bilirubin 16.5 mg% (direct = 2 mg%). No liver biopsy. Exchange transfusion at 3 days of age
7	39	2230	Mother a heroin addict. Child small for gestational age
8	40	2940	Hirschsprung's disease
9	39	3500	History suggestive of maternal hepatitis in first trimester. No problems in neonate
10	38	2520	Hepatosplenomegaly. Total bilirubin 18 mg% with direct 6 mg%. Liver biopsy at 3 weeks consistent with neonatal hepatitis. At 7 months of age head circumference over 98th %ile with retarded motor development
11	40	1850	Jaundice. Liver biopsy showed neonatal hepatitis and cirrhosis. At 2 years of age, follow up suggests mental retardation
12	40	3320	Myelomeningocele and hydrocephalus

[a] 0 = Test not performed.

been a death from smallpox for 25 years (Kempe, 1968). The protozoan, Toxoplasma gondii, a common neonatal pathogen in France, is a very unusual cause of destructive brain damage elsewhere (Editorial: Lancet, 1973). Although cultural mores may explain some geographic patterns of incidence of disease (e.g. the eating of raw meat by Parisians relates to toxoplasmosis), other patterns of incidence are related to ecologic factors, including the worldwide effects of malnutrition.

A. Bacterial Infections

1. Enteric and other Gram-Negative Organisms

Whereas coliforms have at various times been the most common pathogens of perinatal disease, it is rare for them to produce villitis. Placental mem-

of predominantly diffuse villitis

[cut]	Serology[a]					"Focal"						"Diffuse"		Associated lesions				
	Toxoplasma	Rubella	VDRL	Australia antigen	Herpesvirus	Severity	Proliferative	Necrotizing	Reparative	Obliterative vasculopathy	Stromal fibrosis	Relative immaturity	Fetal nucleated RBC	Chorioamnionitis	Unrelated ischemia	Maternal floor infarction	Focal decidual necrosis	Basal villitis
	0	0	0	0	0	+	+	−	−	−	+	++	−	−	+	−	+	−
	0	0	0	0	0	−	−	−	−	−	+	++	−	−	−	−	−	−
	$\frac{1}{16}$	$\frac{1}{8}$	−	−	0	−	−	−	−	−	−	++	−	−	−	−	−	−
	0	0	−	−	0	−	−	−	−	−	−	+	−	−	−	−	−	−
	$\frac{1}{16}$	$\frac{1}{64}$	−	0	$\frac{1}{16}$	−	−	−	−	−	−	++	−	−	+	±	−	−
	0	0	0	0	0	−	−	−	−	+	−	++	−	−	−	−	−	−
	0	0	−	0	0	+	±	−	±	−	−	+	−	−	−	−	−	±
	0	0	0	0	0	+	+	−	−	++	+	+	−	−	++	−	−	+
	0	0	−	0	0	−	−	−	−	−	+	+	−	−	−	+	−	±
−	−	−	−	0	0	−	−	−	±	−	−	++	−	−	++	+	−	+
−	−	−	−	−	0	−	−	−	−	++	−	++	++	−	++	−	−	−
	0	0	−	0	0	+	±	−	−	−	+	+	−	−	−	−	−	−

branitis (chorioamnionitis) is the typical lesion associated with these bacteria, infection usually occurring at 20 weeks gestation or later. In our experience the placentas of almost all spontaneous abortions occurring at 20 weeks gestation show chorioamnionitis (BENIRSCHKE and ALTSHULER, 1971). Recent studies indicate that mycoplasma organisms are frequently present (BRAUN et al., 1971; MARKHAM et al., 1972; SHURIN et al., 1974).

The ascending pathway of placental infection by enteric organisms has been described by BLANC (1961). It is appropriate to emphasize here that his term, "placentitis", refers to membranitis or chorioamnionitis, not villitis. In those rare instances wherein villitis has occurred in association with coliform infections, membranitis has been often present, supporting the concept of an ascending infection.

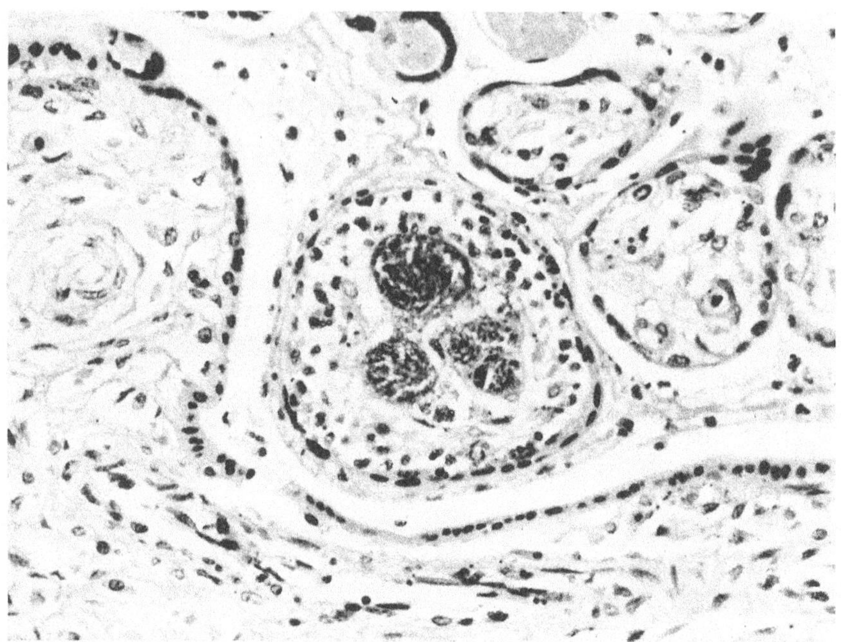

Fig. 15. Abundant intravascular organisms are seen in the central villus, which shows additional features of early suppurative villitis. Original magnification × 240. Hematoxylin and Eosin

In the past, criminal abortions or maternal septicemia in early pregnancy have been the usual cause of bacterial villitis. The increasing use of amniocenteses and intrauterine transfusions may iatrogenically produce bacterial villitis (Goodlin, 1965; Lucy, 1967; Creasman et al., 1968). Scott and Henderson (1972) reported a case of Rh incompatibility for which an intrauterine transfusion was given at 28 weeks gestation. The following morning the fetal heart sounds were inaudible and the mother had developed signs of systemic infection. As a consequence, labor wa sinduced and a 1400 g macerated fetus delivered. The transfused blood was discovered to be contaminated with the gram-negative coccus Acinetobacter calcoaceticus. This organism was also found in the blood of both mother and fetus, and from other blood supplied by the same transfusion service. Scott and Henderson emphasized that the associated placenta was free of membranitis. They suggested that the ascending route of infection, which is that typically seen to complicate intrauterine transfusion (Charles and Friedman, 1969), did not occur in their case. Maternal septicemia most likely was a consequence of fetal and therefore villous bacteremia originating from the contaminated blood in the abdomen of the fetus.

With regard to pathways of infection, it is reasonable to assume that occasional instances of bacterial villitis may follow hematogenous spread from various maternal sites. The maternal endocervical glands are the most common site in which relevant infective organisms reside. This fact is important because despite the fact that almost all mid-gestational spontaneous abortions are associated with membranitis, there has been a relative lack of study of cervical cultures of women with recurrent mid-trimester reproductive failure.

The histologic diagnosis of gram-negative villitis can be made with ease. The villitis is characterized by maternal intervillous fibrin and leukoerythrostasis prominently around villi showing various stages of evolution of microabscesses (Fig. 15). The organisms are so abundant that a gram stain is not necessary for their recognition (Fig. 15).

2. Vibrio Fetus

This organism has been well known to veterinarians as a venereally transmitted cause of abortion in sheep. EDEN (1966), in a review of human perinatal mortality caused by Vibrio fetus, indicated the need to consider the role of this organism as a cause of human reproductive failure. He cites the placental reports of HOOD and TODD (1960) and of VAN WERING and ESSEVELD (1963) and gives particular acknowledgement to VINZENT et al. (1947), who first described human infection caused by Vibrio fetus. VINZENT (1949) and VINZENT et al. (1950) have provided considerable details of the placental pathology of this infection, the classic features being widespread, acute and subacute zones of placental necrosis. An intense neutrophil response is induced, and organisms are described as being present within the lesions.

The case report of HOOD and TODD (1960) describing Vibrio fetus as a cause of human abortion is of particular interest in that the mother, who had four consecutive pregnancies each terminating either in abortion or premature delivery, denied any contact with aborting livestock or other farm animals.

The organism is a curved, gram-negative coccobacillus, fastidious in its anaerobic cultural requirements. WHEELER and BORCHERS (1961) described four cases of vibrionic enteritis in infants. In explaining the rarity of the diagnosis as a function of blood culture techniques rather than a true reflection of the incidence of the disease they state: "The unusual requirements of the organisms would almost insure that they would not be propagated and identified in most medical laboratories." WILLIS and AUSTIN (1966) reported the case of a premature infant who died at 17 hours of age, for whom neither autopsy nor placental study was available. These authors drew attention to the similarity between the epidemiology of listeriosis and of Vibrio fetus infection and explained the difference in their reported incidences as being attributable to both a lack of awareness of the latter and difficulty in its microbiologic recognition.

3. Group B Beta-Hemolytic Streptococcus

Many studies have drawn attention to the reemergence of group B betahemolytic streptococcus as the most common cause of congenital sepsis but none have included any significant information of the associated placental pathology (Eickhoff *et al.*, 1964; Franciosi *et al.*, 1973; Baker *et al.*, 1973; Baker and Barrett, 1973). An extract of a recent letter to a journal (Anthony *et al.*, 1974) highlights an urgent need for placental studies to contribute to the understanding of the pathogenesis of this disease: "The report from the Denver Study (Franciosi *et al.*, 1973) of a clear-cut separation of early and late group B streptococcal infections in the newborn infant on the basis of streptococcal serotypes and possible differences in sources of neonatal infection is intriguing and warrants additional study. However, the association of certain serotypes with early infection and of other types with later disease has not been observed by others, including Baker and her colleagues (Baker *et al.*, 1973) who found type III to be the usual organism in both early and late neonatal sepsis. Although nonmaternal sources of group B streptococci in early infancy have been suggested by several experiences (Winterbauer *et al.*, 1966; Kvittingen, 1968; Eickhoff, 1972), the only conclusively demonstrated origin is the maternal birth canal."

Grossman and Tompkins (1974) reported the simultaneous occurrence of group B beta-hemolytic streptococcus in a mother and her newborn infant. The organism was cultured from the blood of both, and each clinically manifested meningitis. The term infant was first symptomatic at 18 h of age, the mother's symptoms developing 12 h later. Unfortunately the report did not include a description of the placenta. In our experience of congenital group B beta-hemolytic streptococcus infections, approximately one third of the associated placentas feature chorioamnionitis, evidence of *in utero* infection.

4. Francisella Tularensis

This gram-negative coccobacillus is an uncommon pathogen in the United States and the Soviet Union and is stated to be geographically confined to the Northern Hemisphere (Davis *et al.*, 1973). Human tularemia is acquired by contact with infected rabbits, ticks, or flies but rarely has been reported to cause intrauterine infection.

Lide (1947) described the case of a mother who contracted tularemia at approximately 30 weeks gestation, probably as a consequence of preparing rabbits for the family dinner. One month after the development of a digital ulcer, nausea and vomiting, she spontaneously delivered a macerated 2400 g fetus. Details of the placental histopathology are described and illustrated. There were many confluent granulomatous lesions, several of which were centrally necrotic. Similar lesions were present in fetal organs. Although abundant organisms were demonstrated, Lide (1947), citing Lillie, emphasized that in many other instances of human infection with Francisella tularensis, organisms have not been found in the tissues examined.

5. Treponema Pallidum

As with beta-hemolytic streptococcal infection, several countries are experiencing a resurgence of syphilis (King, 1970). Despite its importance, there

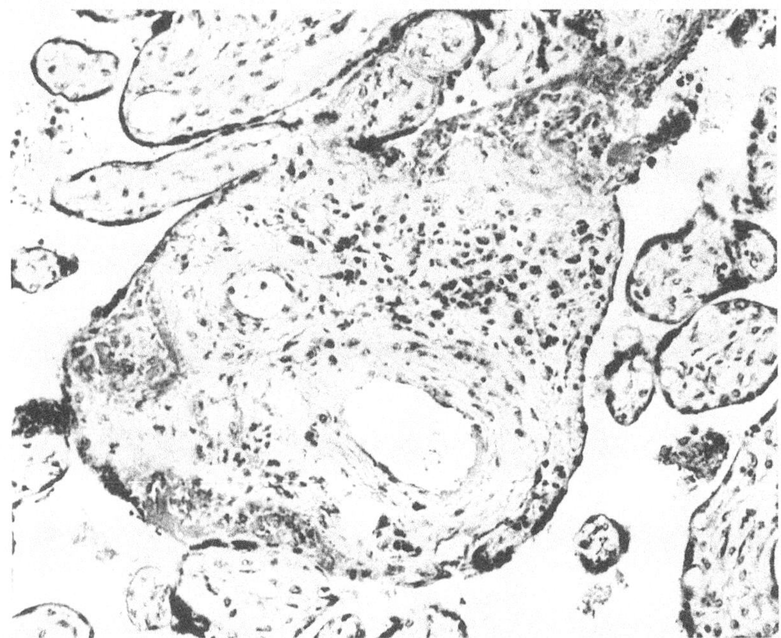

Fig. 16. Proliferative villitis in syphilis. The inflammatory cells in this illustration are lymphocytes and plasma cells. Original magnification × 180. Hematoxylin and Eosin

is a lack of knowledge of the pathologic features syphilis produces in the placenta. This is ironic when one considers the historic incidence of the disease and the fact that it was from the study of syphilis that SILVERSTEIN (1962) pioneered fundamental concepts of fetal immunologic competence.

DORMAN and SAHYUN (1937) in a study of 105 cases showed that the diagnosis of placental syphilis may be made reliably by the use of the Levaditi stain. They described histopathologic lesions briefly, and understandably their illustrations were limited. In their study they reviewed the literature of authors who had stated dogmatically that there is no placental pathology characteristic of syphilis. The error of those claims became apparent in the discussion of placental syphilis presented by BENIRSCHKE and DRISCOLL (1967), and in the excellent article of HÖRMANN (1954).

From recent experience of three cases of congenital syphilis (RUSSELL and ALTSHULER, 1974), we have indicated a triad of histopathologic placental lesions from which the diagnosis of syphilis should be strongly suspected: (1) focal villitis, (2) endovasculitis and associated endovascular sclerosis, and (3) relative immaturity of the placental villi. In each placenta of the three reported cases, this triad of changes was present, although there were differences in severity and distribution.

Proliferative necrotizing (Fig. 8), and occasionally granulomatous, villitis represent the active lesions of the disease with chronic lesions of reparative and evanescent villitis (Fig. 14) additionally being common. Plasma cells may

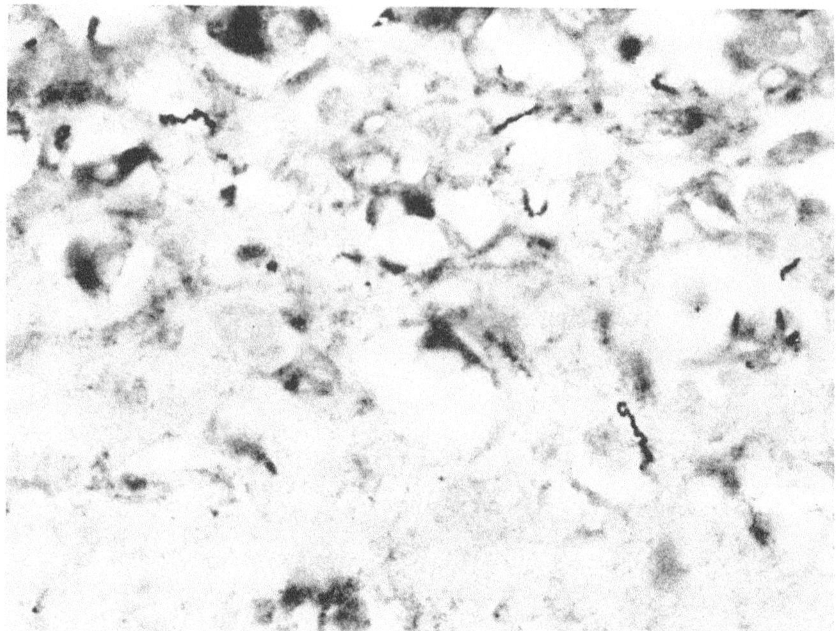

Fig. 17. Spirochetes. Original magnification × 1100. Warthin-Starry

be focally quite numerous (Fig. 16). Typically they are associated with widespread vascular changes of proliferative or sclerotic type (Fig. 14). While some of these features may occur in cytomegalovirus (CMV) placentitis, the latter is easily differentiated by the following: (1) Although CMV attacks endothelial cells and produces endovascular sclerosis (often with associated nearby hemosiderin pigment), it does not so strikingly produce the proliferative endovasculitis characteristic of syphilitic placentitis. (2) Relative immaturity is not a feature of CMV placentitis. (3) On conscientious search of appropriate material, specific diagnoses can be made by the identification of CMV inclusions or of spirochetes (Fig. 17).

Finally, it is emphasized that the Warthin-Starry method of staining spirochetes (Zugibe, 1970) is not only more reliable than the Levaditi, but also will provide a result some three days earlier.

6. Listeria Monocytogenes

Uncommon as human listeriosis is, its predilection for infecting products of conception relates it significantly to recurrent reproductive failure (Rappaport et al., 1960). In animals, listeriosis is well known to cause abortion and fetal wastage, and in humans the two largest reported series (Seeliger, 1957; Potel, 1958) indicate a combined incidence of over 50% of their cases to be in neonates and pregnant women. The reported incidence of human listeriosis is low but, as stressed by Driscoll et al. (1962), this may be due to a lack of recognition. These short gram-positive facultatively anaerobic rods may be confused with diphtheroids. They are difficult to recognize culturally unless specifically sought.

Placentitis is characteristically seen in congenital listeriosis (BRET and GREPINET, 1967). As in the infant or fetus showing "granulomatosis infantiseptica" (disseminated micro-abscesses and purpura not truly granulomatous), Listeria monocytogenes produces widespread necrotizing lesions and micro-abscesses. Neutrophil polymorphs are the predominant inflammatory cells. These lesions are seen both in membranes and cord, and in the placenta, manifesting as purulent chorioamnionitis, umbilical vasculitis, and nodular placental lesions of bland necrotic or abscess type. It is an important observation of SARRUT and ALISON (1967) that organisms are not always demonstrable in association with these lesions. In the series of SARRUT and ALISON (1967), both transplacental (hematogenous) and membranous (ascending) routes are proposed. It is likely, therefore, that local infection of the endometrium or endocervix precedes infection of the placenta and fetus. DRISCOLL *et al.* (1962) state that in a high percentage of such women the urinary tract is the primary source of infection.

7. Mycobacterium Tuberculosis

One should be mindful of the relationship of tuberculosis to congenital disease firstly because it is still a significant cause of human disease (Editorial: Lancet, 1974b) and secondly because knowledge of its pathogenesis stimulates questions as to the protective role of the placenta in chronic intrauterine fetal infection.

SIEGEL (1934) made several contributions to the understanding of congenital tuberculosis and extensively reviewed many earlier studies (SIEGEL and SINGER, 1935). Even before the turn of the century, SCHMORL (SCHMORL and BIRCH-HIRSCHFELD, 1891; SCHMORL and KOCKEL, 1894) had presented an illustrated description of the placental pathology of tuberculosis and in one of their cases included details of a fetus in whom transplacental passage of acid-fast bacilli had occurred. Some years later SCHMORL and GEIPL (1904), from an examination of 2000 serial sections, demonstrated characteristic tuberculous infection in nine of 20 placentas studied. Details of their observations and of those of WARTHIN and COWIE (1904), who studied a single specimen with thousands of sections, are summarized by BENIRSCHKE and DRISCOLL (1967). Neither in these Herculean studies nor in any subsequent investigation, has tuberculous amnionitis, inclusive of acid-fast bacilli, been demonstrated. Although it is certainly possible that the pathogenesis of congenital tuberculous pneumonia may involve aspiration, whether that occurs before or after rupture of the placental membranes, this pneumonia might equally result from intrauterine hematogenous passage of bacilli via the umbilical vein (RICH, 1950). The placental lesions of tuberculosis are essentially the same as the tubercular lesions of other organs.

The transmission of tuberculosis from mother to fetus is rare. Review of pathology literature indicates that in the presence of severe and extensive tuberculous placentitis, with a multitude of tubercle bacilli, there are typically no lesions or bacilli in the associated fetus or newborn (Rich, 1950). It has been suggested that this may result from the inhibition of mycobacterial growth by the low oxygen tension of fetal blood (Rich and Follis, 1942).

Many additional important studies of congenital tuberculosis, for example, may be found in the reports of Nokes et al. (1957), Boesaart (1959), Blackall (1969), and Ramos et al. (1974).

8. Mycoplasma Hominis

Within the last 10 years, in many articles, there has been discussion of the role of T-strain mycoplasma infection as a cause of reproductive failure (Kundsin et al., 1967; Gnarpe and Friberg, 1972, 1973; di Musto et al., 1973). Many of these articles have been reviewed by McCormack et al. (1973). Cervical infection with these T-strain mycoplasmas occurs frequently, these organisms having been isolated from the cervix of as many as 58% of 199 women cultured during their first trimester (Foy et al., 1970).

Kundsin et al. (1967) were the first to emphasize the association of this infection with human reproductive failure. A relationship between genital mycoplasmas and chorioamnionitis has been demonstrated (Shurin et al., 1974) but insufficient investigations have been performed to assess any association between mycoplasma infection and villitis. The organism has been shown to be acquired venereally (Gregory and Payne, 1970). Because T-strain mycoplasma infection occurs so commonly in the genital tract and because of its association with reproductive failure, it is mandatory that morphologic studies of pathogenesis be performed. From endometrial biopsy study of women who have genital mycoplasma infection and a history of reproductive failure, Horne et al. (1973) have recently demonstrated a presence of focal granulomatous endometrial lesions. Morphologically these lesions have a similar granulomatous appearance to some of the focal reparative villitis lesions of unknown etiology that we have encountered. In the same manner that we advocate conscientious examination of placentas, Horne et al. emphasize that lesions in endometrial biopsy specimens can easily be missed if the latter are not examined carefully.

9. Chlamydia Psittaci

The recent observations of Page and Smith (1974) that Chlamydia psittaci, isolated from human aborted placenta, can cause abortion with placentitis in cattle, appear to be of great significance. Although no placental lesions have to date been attributed to this organism in humans, one should be mindful that it is a common inhabitant of the female genital tract and that it may have abortifacient potential.

B. Fungal Infections

Histoplasmosis is the most common fungus infection capable of causing serious disease that we have seen in the Midwestern United States. There has never been a reported case of placental infection with this organism (JAN SCHWARZ, pers. comm.). Coccidioidomycosis, endemic elsewhere in the United States, has been reported to produce placental lesions variously of necrotic, caseous and purulent types. It would appear, however, that even in the presence of severe placental infection, passage of the organism to the fetus does not occur (VAUGHAN and RAMIREZ, 1951; BAKER, 1955). Although Candida albicans may be associated with chorioamnionitis, it has not been reported to produce villitis. We are not aware of any other fungal organisms, encountered by other investigators, that cause placental villitis.

C. Parasitic and Protozoan Infections

1. Toxoplasma Gondii

Of the various diseases encountered world-wide, toxoplasmosis has one of the more interesting histories. A period of over 30 years elapsed between its original description as a disease of rabbits (SPLENDORE, 1908) and its documentation as a fatal disease of newborn humans (WOLF et al., 1939).

Several excellent reviews (FRENKEL, 1967; FELDMAN, 1968; REMINGTON, 1970; WORK, 1971; HUME, 1972) and fascinating studies of the ecology of this disease have been forthcoming (FRENKEL and DUBEY, 1972; PETERSON et al., 1972; WALLACE et al., 1972; WATSON, 1972; KROGSTAD et al., 1972). The infective organism, Toxoplasma gondii, is an obligate intracellular parasite, the mechanism of its entry into mammalian cells and its fate therein, being only recently established (JONES et al., 1972). The life cycle of the infective agent has now been delineated. HUTCHISON (1965) demonstrated that Toxoplasma gondii could be spread by the feces of cats fed on toxoplasma-infected mice. He initially considered that the nematode Toxocara cati was a vector that spread the disease. Later, however, in association with several colleagues he established that transmission could occur in the absence of this nematode (WORK and HUTCHISON, 1969; SIIM et al., 1969; HUTCHISON et al., 1970). Studies performed simultaneously across the Atlantic confirmed these findings (FRENKEL et al., 1970; DUBEY et al., 1970).

Persistent enigmas of toxoplasmosis include its striking geographic pattern of incidence and its pathogenetic significance. The latter aspect is well reviewed by SHARF et al. (1973) in their recent study of latent toxoplasmosis and pregnancy. So many investigators have studied the relationship of toxoplasmosis to reproductive failure that we would like to offer four observations, rather than attempt to summarize all the relevant literature.

1. We stress the opinion of FRENKEL (1967):

"To prove that a syndrome is associated with toxoplasmosis, it is important to establish the incidence of latent infection, which needs to be

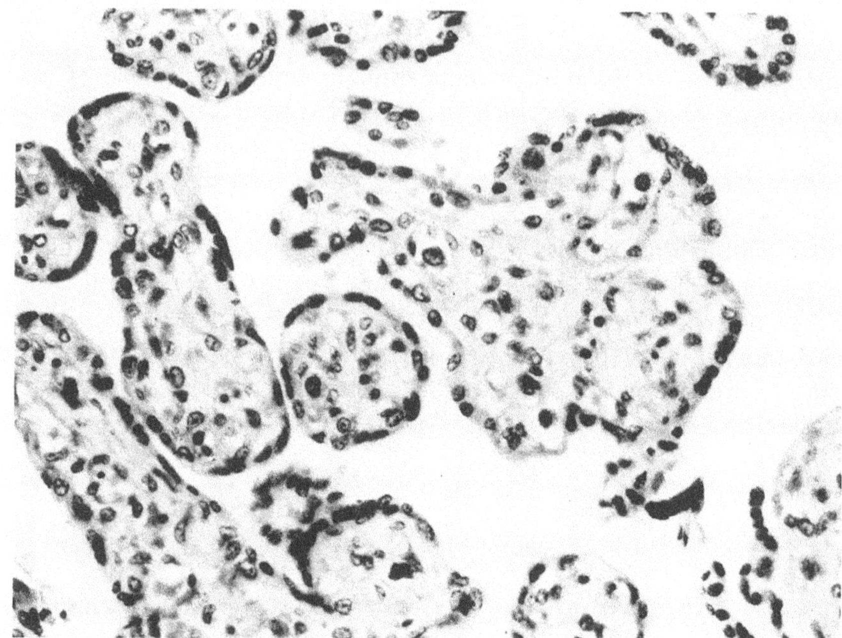

Fig. 18. Toxoplasmosis in a full-term placenta. Note severe stromal hypercellularity and retarded maturation of the trophoblast and erythtoblasts in the terminal villous vessels. Compare with Fig. 9. Original magnification × 120. Hematoxylin and Eosin

determined simultaneously from the exact area where the survey is made using comparable age groups and similar selection factors. The antibody titers must be consistent with the diagnosis to be related. If in a certain region 20% of the adults had antibodies, and positive dye tests for toxoplasmosis were found in 70% of patients with retinochoroiditis, then approximately 70 minus 20 = 50% of the patients with retinochorioditis can be concluded to have lesions as a result of toxoplasmosis. The same type of proof would have to be brought forth for patients with habitual abortions if this is to be established as a frequent event. Subgroups of patients and control groups differing in age should show a consistent pattern."

2. In over 2000 fetal and perinatal autopsies in Cincinnati we have encountered only two cases proven to be toxoplasmosis.

3. Desmonts and Couvreur (1974), from large prospective studies in an endemic area, state: "... the great majority of babies born to women who acquire toxoplasma during pregnancy are uninfected or minimally so."

4. In regarding subclinical rather than overt toxoplasmosis as being more often hazardous to man, it is well to consider the work of Alford's group (Saxon et al., 1973), which has shown intellectual deficits in children born with subclinical congenital toxoplasmosis. Toxoplasmosis may escape detection in newborns. This is particularly tragic since spiramycin has been established to be very effective in the control of toxoplasmosa infection (Beverley et al., 1973; Desmonts and Couvreur, 1974).

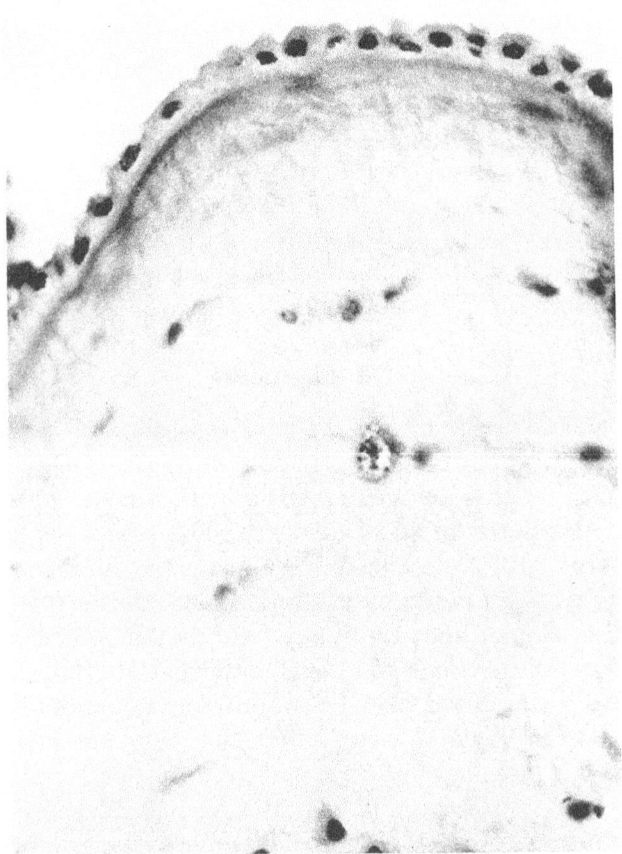

Fig. 19. Toxoplasma cyst. Pathognomonic of placental toxoplasmosis. Original magnification × 240. Hematoxylin and Eosin

There have been difficulties in diagnosing cases of congenital toxoplasmosis not only because the disease may be clinically silent but also because some of these newborn infants have been shown to lack elevated IgM-immunofluorescent antibody titers (REMINGTON and DESMONTS, 1973). Histopathologic assessment of the placenta thus may be even more significantly contributory to diagnosis since the placental pathology of this disease is characteristic (ALTSHULER, 1973b). Various reports of placental toxoplasmosis that are available in the literature have been mentioned by ELLIOTT (1970). Excellent descriptions have been presented by BENIRSCHKE and DRISCOLL (1967), who list the abnormalities of 5 placentas they studied, according to involvement of the decidua, the membranes, the umbilical cord and the villi. Placental toxoplasmosis resembles placental erythroblastosis fetalis in that relative immaturity is extensive in both entities. In placentas of chronic intrauterine infection with toxoplasmosa that we have had the opportunity to review, we have been impressed that villous stromal hypercellularity is much more severe (Fig. 18) than in erythroblastosis fetalis. Pari passu with this hypercellularity there is less villous hydrops than occurs in erythroblastosis. The presence of focal villitis further differentiates toxoplasmosis and finally, the observation of a toxoplasma cyst (Fig. 19) in the placental membranes, decidua, or villi enables a specific diagnosis to be made.

A rare case of congenital toxoplasmosis whose placenta lacks pathologic features other than the presence of toxoplasma cysts has been cited (Benirschke, 1967). Serious perinatal toxoplasmosis has its origin in second trimester maternal infection (Desmonts and Couvreur, 1974). Relative immaturity and focal villitis might thus be considered as possible morphologic indices of the prognosis of the associated newborn.

2. Plasmodia

Although still common in several countries, malaria is a disease that has not stimulated much study of its effects upon the fetus and newborn. Occasional discussions and reports of congenital malaria (Eckstein and Nixon, 1946; Potter, 1961; Benirschke and Driscoll, 1967) have been published since Wickramasuriya (1935) described his experiences in Colombo, but they have not provided significantly more information. Prior to 1935 many authors were of the firm opinion that transplacental infection with malaria does not occur. Wickramasuriya, however, explained that the inability to demonstrate parasites in the blood of the newborn does not negate a diagnosis of congenital malaria. He established "that not only are malarial parasites transmitted to the fetus but also that such transmission is not an uncommon cause of death of the fetus in utero." Potter (1961) described villous inflammatory infiltrates of macrophages and lymphocytes in addition to changes in the maternal sinusoids, which Wickramasuriya (1935) referred to as a storehouse of parasites. It may be, therefore, that the diagnosis of congenital malaria could be confirmed more easily by a smear and light microscopy examination of the placenta than of the blood of the fetus or newborn.

3. Schistosoma

Schistosomiasis (Bilharziasis) is endemic in Africa, South America, the West Indies and the Far East. Cort (1921) cites as the earliest observation of congenital Bilharziasis that of Fujinama and Nakamura (1911), who described the infection in the fetus of a dog. Awareness of the disease in humans has largely resulted from the contributions of Sutherland, who first described placental bilharziasis (Sutherland et al., 1965). Although schistosoma ova in the liver stimulate the production of giant-celled granulomas, consequent repair being manifested by so-called "pipe-stem fibrosis" (Symmers, 1904), there is a lack of inflammatory reaction to these ova in the placenta. Sumherland recommends that in areas where schistosomiasis is endemic, the placentas of eclamptic women be thoroughly studied to exclude the presence of ova, suggesting that the patient's seizures may be due to the presence of even a single ovum or adult worm in the brain, rather than

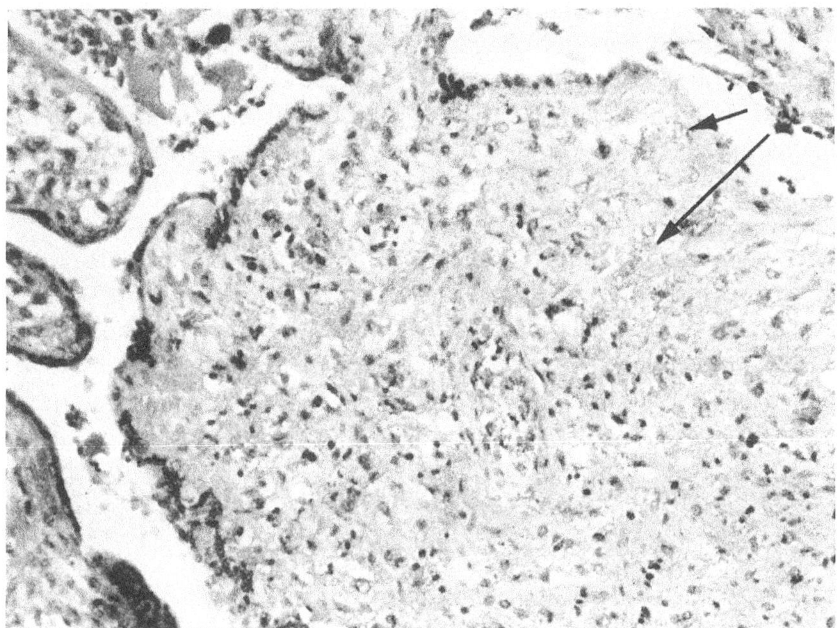

Fig. 20. Placental trypanosomias. Leishmanial forms appear like fine granules in the area of the arrows. Also not the proliferative villitis. Original magnification × 240. Hematoxylin and Eosin

eclampsia of pregnancy. The method SUTHERLAND describes for the detection of placental ova is digestion of segments of placenta in sodium hydroxide, and light microscopy examination of the sediment.

4. Trypanosoma Cruzi

Through the kindness of colleagues, Drs. KURT BENIRSCHKE, JACK FRENKEL and KARL SALFELDER, we have been informed of not only of the particularly high incidence of congenital Chagas' disease in South and Central America but also of the numerous publications on that subject, excellently bibliographed by OLIVIER et al. (1972).

The disease is essentially confined to South America and Mexico, being spread by the reduvid bug to the final host, man. Armadillos, opposums and bats act as animal reservoirs. The lesions produced by trypanosomal infection are characteristically granulomatous but may also be exudative. Leishmanial infection of the sarcoplasm of heart muscle with associated myocarditis is a hallmark of the disease. Leptomeningitis and liver lesions, both of necrotic and reparative types, are additionally characteristic. Vasculitis is common. Chagas' disease in infants and young children typically pursues a fulminant and fatal course, the symptoms being those of acute meningoencephalitis. In children who survive and in adults, the disease manifests an insidiously chronic course.

The first documentation of transplacental Chagas' disease was in the study of Bittencourt (1960), who reported the histopathology of 6 cases. Details of the placentas of 9 cases of Chagas' disease were later described, tabulated, and well illustrated (Bittencourt, 1963). Severe villitis was typical. Bittencourt *et al.* (1972) emphasized that occasionally it may be difficult to find leishmania forms (Fig. 20) in placentas and fetal organs, even in the presence of severe inflammatory lesions; this recent study indicates the rate of transplacental transmission of infection by chagasic mothers to be 10.5%.

With regard to the high incidence of Chagas' disease in South America, it will be important to learn the precise role of this infection as a possible cause of recurrent reproductive failure, an association suggested by the report of a mother who apparently transmitted this disease transplacentally, on two occasions (Bittencourt and Gomes, 1967).

D. Viral Infections

1. Cytomegalovirus

Since the first isolation of cytomegalovirus from a living infant (Weller *et al.*, 1957), a great number of investigations have been made to elucidate the role of this infection in the production of congenital disease. These have been well reviewed (Hanshaw, 1971; Weller, 1971), many of the problems having been summarized editorially: "Cytomegalovirus (CMV) is the commonest known microbiological cause of brain damage in infancy. Infection by CMV is particularly common during pregnancy, for 3 to 6% of pregnant women excrete virus in their urine and an even greater proportion via the cervix. The incidence of viruria and cervical excretion increases progressively from trimester to trimester. In patients of different ethnic groups in Pittsburgh, the overall incidence of viruria was similar (about 4%), but cervical excretion was much more common among Navajo Indians (14%) than among Blacks (5%) or Whites (4%). Pregnant Japanese women had even higher rates of cervical CMV excretion—10% and 28% during the second trimester and at term, respectively. CMV may also be excreted in breast milk: Australian workers have shown that 27% of apparently healthy recently delivered, seropositive women have virolactia. Nevertheless, although intrauterine CMV infection may damage the fetus, there is no evidence as yet to suggest that infection acquired during birth or in the immediate postnatal period is harmful" (Editorial: Lancet, 1974a).

Occasional reports have described CMV villitis in placentas of immature fetuses (Strauss and Seki, 1962; Rosenstein and Navarrete-Reyna, 1964; Altshuler and McAdams, 1971; Altshuler, 1974a). In a case of chronic intrauterine infection with CMV, occurring at the thirteenth week of gestational life, the observation of severe villitis including plasma cells has been suggested as evidence that the fetus is at this stage immunologically competent (Altshuler, 1974a).

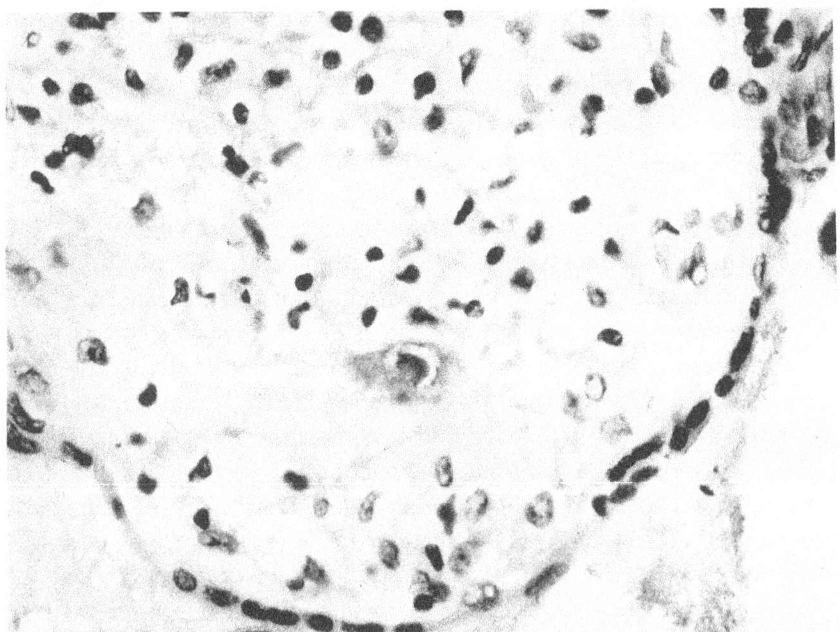

Fig. 21. Centrally, a typical intranuclear inclusion is shown. Original magnification × 400. Hematoxylin and Eosin

BENIRSCHKE *et al.* (1974) recently reported 5 cases of fetal CMV infection, with descriptions of the placentas and a review of earlier publications of the placental pathology of CMV infection. MONIF and DISCHE (1972) tabulated a summary of the histopathologic findings in two of their cases in addition to four cases previously reported by other authors (LEPAGE and SCHRAMM, 1958; LELONG *et al.*, 1960; BLANC, 1961; QUAN and STRAUSS, 1962). Almost all of these placentas were stated to be edematous. Of the 10 specimens that we have studied in Cincinnati, however, only three have featured edema. The most characteristic appearance of CMV placentitis that we have encountered has been a focal proliferative villitis with lymphocytes and plasma cells and when conscientiously sought, pathognomonic inclusions (Fig. 21). Focal evanescent villitis and villous stromal fibrosis have been additionally characteristic and within all of these lesions, in hematoxylin and eosin sections, we have found an apparent severe presence of hemosiderin pigment to be a valuable clue to the presence of cytomegalovirus. Although deposits of hemosiderin in the villi occur with other chronic intrauterine infections, they are often especially severe with CMV villitis.

Within our own material and that of other investigators, in which CMV inclusions have been seen, we have observed four different patterns of CMV placentitis:

1. Normal placental parenchyma showing random, necrotizing, proliferative or evanescent villitis and also random foci of villous stromal fibrosis.

A variant of this pattern shows these lesions in a placenta with ischemia or infarction due to unrelated causes.

2. Edematous placental parenchyma showing similar random focal lesions.

3. Placental parenchyma with severe extensive focal villitis.

In our experience the presence of each of these three patterns has correlated with clinical cytomegalovirus disease in the associated neonate. By cultural studies, Hayes and Gibas (1971) documented a case of placental CMV infection in which the associated full-term infant was free of this infection. They state that a light microscopic examination of the placenta did not reveal inflammatory changes or CMV inclusions in several sections.

4. Focal necrotizing deciduitis, which is present subjacent to the placenta or placental membranes. It may be that such placental lesions, together with those of CMV in the cervix, decidua and endometrium (Goranov and Gancev, 1963; Jundrak, 1964; Diosi et al., 1967; Goldman et al., 1969; McCracken et al., 1974; Benirschke et al., 1974), correlate with the 1% of asymptomatic newborns observed to excrete CMV in their urine (Stern, 1968; Starr et al., 1970; Hanshaw, 1971; Kumar et al., 1973).

While it is impractical to culture the urine of all newborns for the purpose of retrieval of this 1% excretors, it is reasonable to screen with placental examination all premature infants, not only to seek treatable pathology in such infants, but also to select those infants whose urines should be cultured for the possible presence of this virus. The importance of inapparent congenital CMV infection has recently been demonstrated. Reynolds et al. (1974) detected newborns with inapparent congenital CMV infection by means of umbilical cord serum IgM studies. From longitudinal studies of these infants, these investigators have demonstrated an association between inapparent congenital CMV infection and a tendency to the development of hearing deficits and subnormal intelligence.

In studies of an asymptomatic man 14 months after his initial clinical illness, Lang et al. (1974) demonstrated the presence of persistent CMV in his semen. Such evidence of venereal spread of CMV adds greatly to the understanding of the pathogenesis of congenital CMV infection. It may help also to explain the role of CMV as a cause of spontaneous abortion (Kriel et al., 1970), recurrent abortion, as convincingly demonstrated by Berenberg and Nankervis (1970), and recurrent congenital infection (Embil et al., 1970; Krech et al., 1971; Stagno et al., 1973). The role of CMV as a cause of congenital malformations (McCracken et al., 1969; Oppenheimer and Esterly, 1973) is also to be further evaluated.

2. Rubella

Although over 20000 infants born in the United States were afflicted by the 1964 rubella epidemic, only one study provides detailed information of the placental pathology of that epidemic (Driscoll, 1969). Recently, Ornoy et al. (1973) reported their findings of the fetal and placental pathology associated with the 1972 rubella epidemic in Israel. As a consequence of this lack of

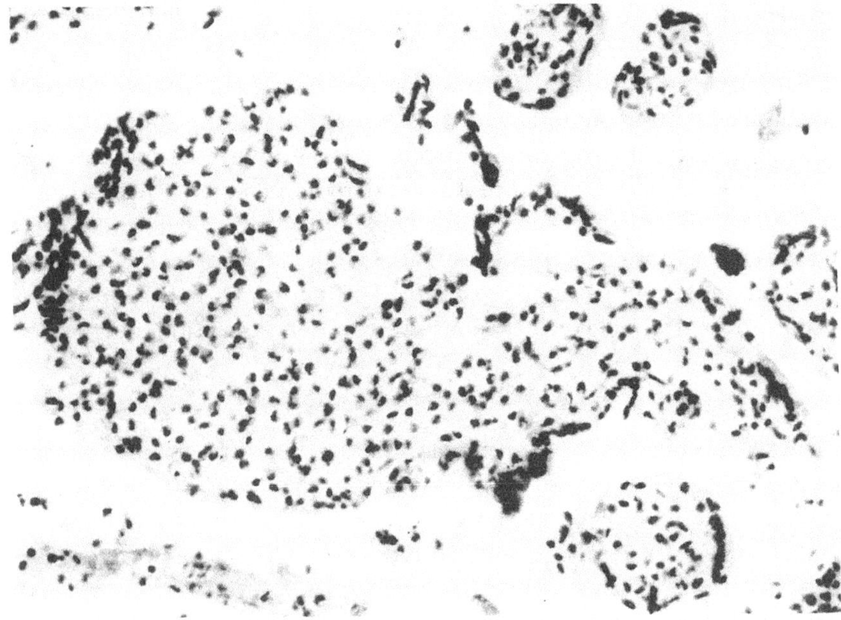

Fig. 22. Severe rubella villitis from a therapeutic abortion performed at 20 weeks gestation. Original magnification × 180. Hematoxylin and Eosin.
(Courtesy of ASHER ORNOY M.D.)

studies, our understanding of the pathogenesis of congenital rubella has been significantly limited. Only recently has it been shown by microbiologists that reinfection with rubella virus is not uncommon and that, rarely, reinfection of pregnant women may produce viral infection of the fetus (NORTHROP et al., 1972; EILARD and STRANNEGARD, 1974). Mention of the placental findings was included in the comprehensive review of fetal rubella pathology of TÖNDURY and SMITH (1966). They stated that the probable route of fetal infection is maternal viremia with subsequent embolization of infected endothelial cells of the villous fetal blood vessels. It has been emphasized that, in addition to villous fibrosis and atrophy, vascular damage within the villous blood vessels, villous infiltrates (Fig. 22) with lymphocytes, histiocytes, polymorphonuclear leukocytes and occasional plasma cells, chronic deciduitis is present in specimens with rubella placentitis (BENIRSCHKE and DRISCOLL, 1967). This described histopathology in conjunction with the evidence of SEPPALA and VAHERI (1974) that rubella virus may be excreted from the human cervix raises the possibility that fetal infection with rubella may occur as a consequence of an ascending infection from the cervix directly to the decidua and fetal tissues, in the absence of maternal viremia.

3. Varicella

Congenital chicken pox was first described by HUBBARD (1878) and since that time has been a rare cause of intrauterine fetal infection. Most of the cases reviewed by Keutel (1968) occurred following maternal infection late in pregnancy. More recently, however, cases of infants with multiple congenital anomalies following maternal infection early in pregnancy have attested to the rubella-like teratogenic effects of this virus (Srabstein *et al.*, 1974). The placental pathology of congenital varicella can be inferred from the description of the single reported instance (Garcia, 1963) in which a necrotizing and granulomatous villitis was seen. Epithelioid and giant cell granulomas were widespread throughout the placenta with prominence of associated villous necrosis and maternal fibrin deposition. The maternal floor showed acute deciduitis, and intranuclear inclusions were observed within decidual cells.

4. Vaccinia and Variola

Prenatal vaccinia as a complication of vaccination in pregnancy has appeared as sporadic reports in the literature (MacArthur, 1952; MacDonald and MacArthur, 1953; Wielenga *et al.*, 1961; Tucker and Gibson, 1962; Entwistle *et al.*, 1962; Hood and McKinnon, 1963; Naidoo and Hirsch, 1963). Apart from causing generalized vaccinia in the infant, it has been suggested that first trimester vaccination may be a cause of stillbirth (Dixon, 1962). The placental lesions described in congenital vaccinia (Wielenga *et al.*, 1961; Entwistle *et al.*, 1962; Hood and McKinnon, 1963) are essentially focal villous necrosis and acute villitis with deposition of maternal fibrin. Entwistle *et al.* (1962) found typical eosinophilic cytoplasmic inclusions.

"Intra-uterine smallpox, too, is not unknown, and it is said that Mauriceau, one of the world's greatest obstetricians, came into the world, pock-marked" (Wickramasuriya, 1935). The villitis of congenital smallpox would appear to be similar to that of the other pox viruses, varicella and vaccinia. The two cases of congenital alastrim (variola minor) of Garcia (1963) are, to our knowledge, the only histological documentation of placental variola, both featuring necrotizing and granulomatous villitis with deposition of maternal fibrin and infiltration by neutrophils. Nuclear and cytoplasmic inclusions within decidual cells were prominent.

5. Herpes Simplex Virus

A veritable explosion of information has occurred in recent years regarding the role of herpes simplex virus in the causation of human disease. Notable in this regard is the reported ability of herpes simplex virus-2 to produce a spectrum of infections in the newborn. Evidence now points clearly to the mother's infected genital tract as being the major source of this virus' transmission to the infant, at or around the time of delivery (Nahmias *et al.*, 1970). Less commonly, herpesvirus may be transmitted to the fetus *in utero*, occasionally with teratogenic effects (South *et al.*, 1969). Although it is true that maternal viremia is a mode of transplacental transmission (Hanshaw, 1973), it is logical to emphasize local ascending spread of the virus from the cervix to the placental bed and membranes. The observation of herpetic lesions (including intranuclear inclusions) in the endometrium (GOLDMAN, 1970) and herpetic chorioamnionitis (ALTSHULER, 1974b) support this concept. The single report in the literature of herpesvirus placental villitis (WITZLEBEN and DRISCOLL, 1965) describes small but widespread, focal, necrotizing lesions which interestingly enough are relatively lacking in inflammatory response by the fetus. They are thus of similar appearance to herpesvirus lesions in other fetal organs.

6. Other Viruses (C-type Virus, Influenza, Coxsackie, Polio, Mumps)

The observation has been made of C-type viral particles within normal human placentas (VERNON et al., 1974) and normal baboon placentas (KALTER et al., 1973), but its significance is unknown. Transplacental transfer of influenza virus has been documented (YAWN et al., 1971). Although the placenta was stated to be normal in this case, one should observe that the clinical course was extremely rapid (four days), possibly too rapid to allow morphologically identifiable lesions in the placenta to evolve.

Although known to cause intrauterine fetal infections, coxsackie, polio and mumps viruses have not been observed to cause placental lesions.

E. Villitis of unknown Etiology

Recognition of this entity has evolved from an intention to compare inflammatory placental lesions of unknown etiology with histologically similar lesions of known infective etiology. Demonstration of known placental pathogens, histologically, culturally or serologically has not been forthcoming, and therefore, clinicopathological studies have been used to correlate the presence of these lesions with pathology in the fetus and neonate.

Tables 1–3 (see p. 76ff.) indicate clinicopathological correlates of 63 cases of villitis of unknown etiology between 1972 and 1974. In a contemporary series of 100 random third trimester placentas, we found villitis of unknown etiology in 6%.

1. Focal

These villitis lesions are not newly observed but, until recently, their significance has escaped clarification. GRUENWALD (1961), in placentas of small-for-gestational-age infants, observed inflammatory villous infiltrates adjacent to villi showing fibrosis and vascular obliteration. He observed several such lesions but did not interpret their significance. In the same year, GERSHON and STRAUSS (1961) described a chronic inflammatory infiltrate associated with ischemic placentas of small-for-gestational-age infants. More recently, HOMBERGER et al. (1971) presented a series of cases of "lymphoplasmacytic placentitis" in which intrinsic chronic inflammatory infiltrates were found within the placental villi. Known pathogens were excluded in almost all of

 G. Altshuler and P. Russell:

Table 2. Clinicopathologic correlations

Case number	Gestation (weeks)	Birth weight (g)	Clinical correlation
13	38	3040	Cord IgM 17 mg-%
14	33	1105	Maternal jaundice in 1st trimester. Neonate small for gestational age (S.G.A.). Meconium stained. Seizures
15	36	2260	Recurrent reproductive failure. Stillborn. Autopsy showed no gross abnormality
16	41	3260	Respiratory distress syndrome. Signs of sepsis. No organism grown
17	30	1500	Cord IgM—"absent"
18	37	1570	S.G.A.
19	40	3000	Cord IgM 15.7 mg-%
20	40	3110	Mild jaundice ?physiological
21	39	1500	S.G.A. Disseminated intravascular coagulation, polycythemia, thrombocytopenia, petechiae. IgM 16 mg-%
22	42	2340	Cord IgM 12 mg-%. Vesicular rash on face. Cytomegalovirus cultured from urine
23	39	2400	Head circumference 50th percentile despite S.G.A.
24	41	3700	Polycythemia, tachypnoea, pneumomediastinum
25	42	1540	S.G.A. patent ductus arteriosus with aneurysmal dilatation and thrombosis. Neonatal death
26	37	2120	S.G.A. Neonatal death. Autopsy showed cataracts and massive diaphragmatic hernia. Viral cultures negative for virus
27	39	3020	Tachypnoea, cyanosis. Viral cultures negative
28	39	2410	S.G.A. meconium stained. Cord IgM 8.4 mg-% Fissure in ano at 3 days of age
29	40	2320	Cord IgM 8.6 mg-%. S.G.A.
30	40	3700	Neonatal seizures
31	40	3260	Pneumomediastinum. Bilateral pneumothorax
32	43	3590	Fever, cultures negative for viruses and bacteria
33	35	2120	Respiratory distress syndrome. Cord IgM 17 mg-%. Positive viral culture but not identification of virus
34	40	2475	S.G.A. Meconium stained. Maternal toxemia
35	40	3880	Beckwith's syndrome
36	40	3500	Hypoglycemia
37	34	940	Severely macerated stillbirth. Head enlargement observed by X-ray at 24 weeks geststation

[a] 0 = Test not performed.

: predominantly focal villitis

	Serology[a]				"Focal"						"Diffuse"		Associated lesions				
	Toxoplasma	Rubella	VDRL	Herpesvirus	Severity	Proliferative	Necrotizing	Reparative	Obliterative vasculopathy	Stromal fibrosis	Relative immaturity	Fetal nucleated RBC	Chorioamnionitis	Unrelated ischemia	Maternal floor infarction	Focal decidual necrosis	Basal villitis
-	—	—	—	0	±	±	—	—	—	—	—	—	—	—	—	—	—
	0	0	0	0	±	±	—	—	++	—	—	—	—	+++	—	—	—
	0	0	0	0	±	±	—	—	—	—	—	—	—	±	—	—	—
	0	0	0	0	±	±	—	—	—	—	—	—	—	—	—	—	—
	0	—	0	0	±	±	—	—	—	—	—	—	—	+++	—	—	—
	0	0	—	0	±	±	—	±	—	—	—	—	—	±	±	—	—
	0	0	—	0	+	—	—	+	—	—	—	—	—	—	±	—	—
	0	0	0	0	+	+	—	—	—	—	—	—	—	—	—	—	—
-	0	—	—	0	+	+	—	—	+	—	—	—	—	++	+	—	—
	0	0	0	0	+	+	—	—	—	—	—	—	—	+	+	—	—
	0	0	—	0	+	+	—	—	—	—	—	—	—	+	—	—	—
;	$\frac{1}{16}$	$\frac{1}{16}$	—	0	+	+	—	—	—	—	±	—	—	+	—	—	—
	0	—	—	0	+	+	—	—	++	—	+	—	+	++	+	—	—
-	—	$\frac{1}{1024}$	—	0	+	+	—	+	+	—	—	—	—	—	—	—	—
	0	0	—	0	+	+	—	—	—	—	—	—	—	+	—	—	—
	0	0	—	0	+	+	—	+	++	+	—	—	—	+	—	—	—
	0	0	0	0	+	+	—	+	+	—	—	—	+	—	—	—	+
	0	0	—	0	+	+	—	±	—	—	—	—	—	—	—	—	—
	0	0	—	0	+	—	++	±	++	—	—	—	+	—	—	—	—
	0	0	—	0	+	+	—	—	—	—	—	—	—	—	—	—	—
	0	0	—	0	+	+	—	+	—	—	±	—	—	+	—	—	+
	0	0	0	0	+	+	—	—	+	±	+	—	—	+	—	—	—
	0	0	0	0	+	+	—	—	++	—	+	—	—	—	±	—	—
	0	0	—	0	+	+	—	—	—	—	±	—	—	+	±	—	—
	0	0	—	0	+	+	—	—	—	—	—	—	+	—	—	+	+

Table 2.

Case number	Gestation (weeks)	Birth weight (g)	Clinical correlation
38	37	1 520	S.G.A. Hypoglycemia. IgM 43 mg-% at 1 week age
39	39	3 680	Cord IgM 8.9 mg-%
40	38	1 900	Recurrent reproductive failure. S.G.A. Maternal pre-eclampsia
41	36	2 115	"Low cord IgM". Head circumference 90th percentile (weight at 25th percentile). Normal skull X-ray
42	30	1 580	Renal dysplasia. Cord IgM 4.8 mg-%. Neonatal death
43	40	2 650	Facial palsy. "Abormal looking child"
44	40	2 780	Stillborn. Autopsy showed no gross abnormality
45	43	2 280	S.G.A. Chromosomally confirmed Down's syndrome. Cord IgM 11 mg-%
46	36	2 800	Hypoglycemia
47	41	4 140	Well neonate
48	29	720	S.G.A. Stillborn. Autopsy showed no gross anomaly
49	40	3 500	Ventricular septal defect with transposition of great vessels. Post-operative death at 10 weeks
50	38	3 400	Mother on dexamethazone at time of conception. Cord IgM 6.6 mg-%
51	40	2 025	S.G.A. Cord IgM 20 mg-%
52	39	2 100	S.G.A. Cord IgM 5.8 mg-%. Idiopathic seizures at five months of age. Skull X-ray normal
53	39	2 630	Meconium stained. Cord IgM 4.2 mg-%. Head circumference at 8 months of age below 10th percentile (weight at 70th percentile)
54	40	2 460	S.G.A. Cord IgM 5 mg-%
55	38	3 970	Hepatosplenomegaly. "Low IgM" at 4 days of age
56	40	3 760	Hyperbilirubinemia
57	40	1 860	Recurrent reproductive failure. S.G.A. Stillborn. Autopsy not done

[a] 0 = Test not performed.

their cases but they did infer that this villitis of unknown etiology was infectious in origin.

As can be seen from Table 2, the most significant clinical correlate of this lesion is intrauterine growth retardation, 17 out of 45 associated infants being small for gestational age. This association of villitis to intrauterine growth retardation has been documented elsewhere (Benirschke and Altshuler, 1971; Laga *et al.*, 1972; Altshuler, 1973a; Altshuler *et al.*, 1974). It is our contention that villitis is in fact of etiologic importance in the genesis of

Continued)

| Serology[a] | | | | | "Focal" | | | | | | "Diffuse" | | Associated lesions | | | | |
Cytomegalovirus	Toxoplasma	Rubella	VDRL	Herpesvirus	Severity	Proliferative	Necrotizing	Reparative	Obliterative vasculopathy	Stromal fibrosis	Relative immaturity	Fetal nucleated RBC	Chorioamnionitis	Unrelated ischemia	Maternal floor infarction	Focal decidual necrosis	Basal villitis
)	$\frac{1}{16}$	$\frac{1}{8}$	—	0	+	+	—	—	+++	—	—	—	—	++	+	—	—
)	0	0	—	0	+	+	—	—	—	—	+	—	—	+	+	—	—
;	0	$\frac{1}{32}$	—	$\frac{1}{8}$	+	+	—	—	—	—	—	—	—	++	+	—	+
—	—	$\frac{1}{128}$	—	0	++	+	—	+	++	—	—	—	—	—	+	—	+
$\frac{1}{2}$	—	—	—	0	+	+	—	++	—	+	—	—	—	+	—	—	—
)	0	0	—	0	++	++	—	+	—	—	—	—	—	+	—	—	+
)	0	0	0	0	++	++	—	—	+++	—	—	—	—	±	+	—	—
)	0	0	0	0	++	++	—	—	±	—	—	—	—	++	—	+	—
)	0	0	—	0	++	+	—	—	+	—	—	—	+	—	+	—	+
)	0	0	—	0	++	+	—	—	++	—	—	—	—	—	—	—	—
)	0	0	—	0	++	—	+++	—	—	—	—	—	—	—	—	—	—
$\frac{1}{4}$	$\frac{1}{16}$	$\frac{1}{8}$	—	0	+++	++	—	+	+	+	+	—	—	—	—	—	+
)	0	0	0	0	+++	+++	±	+	—	—	—	—	—	—	—	+	—
—	$\frac{1}{16}$	$\frac{1}{8}$	—	$\frac{1}{8}$	+++	++	—	++	+	—	—	—	—	+	—	—
)	0	—	0	0	+++	++	—	++	—	—	—	—	—	—	—	—	—
·	0	$\frac{1}{8}$	—	0	+++	+	—	++	++	+	—	—	+	—	—	—	—
)	0	0	—	0	+++	+	—	+	++	—	—	—	—	—	—	—	+
)	0	0	—	0	+++	+	—	+	++	+	—	—	—	++	+	—	++
)	0	0	0	0	+++	++	+	—	—	—	—	—	+	—	—	—	+
:	$\frac{1}{8}$	$\frac{1}{32}$	—	$\frac{1}{8}$	+++	+++	—	++	+	—	—	—	+	++	—	—	+

a significant percentage of small-for-gestational-age infants. It has been suggested that fetal growth retardation may result from the direct effects of viral infection in addition to those effects of severe and chronic placental ischemia (BLANC, 1969). This speculation is reasonable in the light of recent investigations. NAEYE has shown that viruses can cause growth retardation by means of inhibition of cellular proliferation (NAEYE and BLANC, 1965; NAEYE, 1967). More recently, COID and RAMSDEN (1973) demonstrated that inapparent Coxsackie B3 virus infection can produce growth retardation in mice.

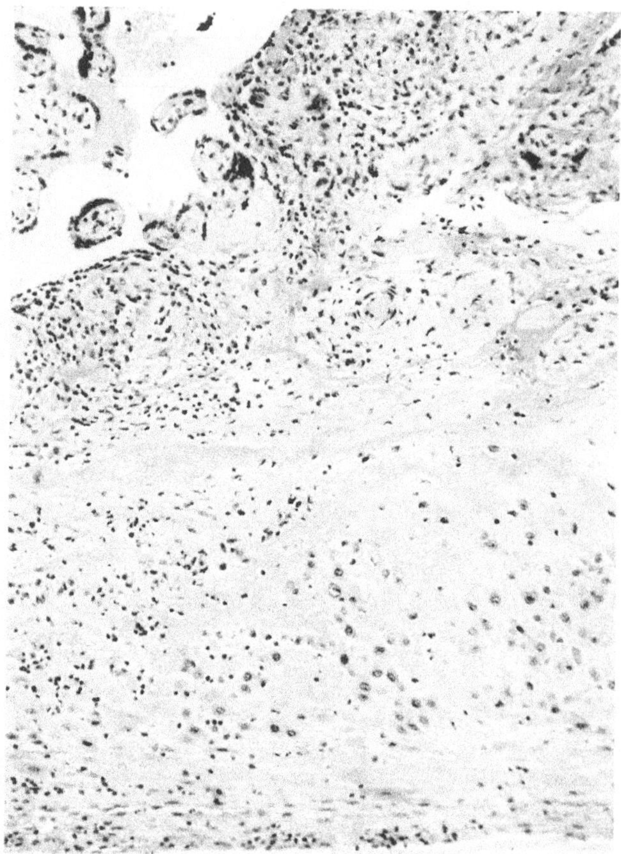

Fig. 23. Although a common feature of villitis of unknown etiology, the inflammatory infiltrates of this basal villitis are non-specific. Original magnification × 120. Hematoxylin and Eosin

Two instances of recurrent reproductive failure are included in Table 2 (Case 15 and Cases 40 and 57; the latter two represent successive pregnancies in the same woman). As with the case presented by Dollmann and Schmitz-Moormann (1972), known pathogens were excluded by either negative serology or cultures. Two cases of biopsy-proven neonatal hepatitis showed focal villitis, in addition to diffuse relative immaturity (Cases 10 and 11 in Table 1, p. 16). Other examples of symptomatic neonatal disease suggestive of an infective etiology are cases 25, 26, 38, 49 and 53. Cases 25 and 49 are both instances of congenital heart disease. In case 38, although the only abnormality found in the infant at birth was low birth weight (1520 g for 37 weeks gestation), the serum IgM at one week of age was 43 mg%. Case 53 showed progressively decreasing percentile of head circumference so that at eight months of age, despite the child's weight being at the 70th percentile, head circumference was below the 10th percentile. Case 26 may have been one of congenital rubella infection, but extensive efforts to isolate and grow the

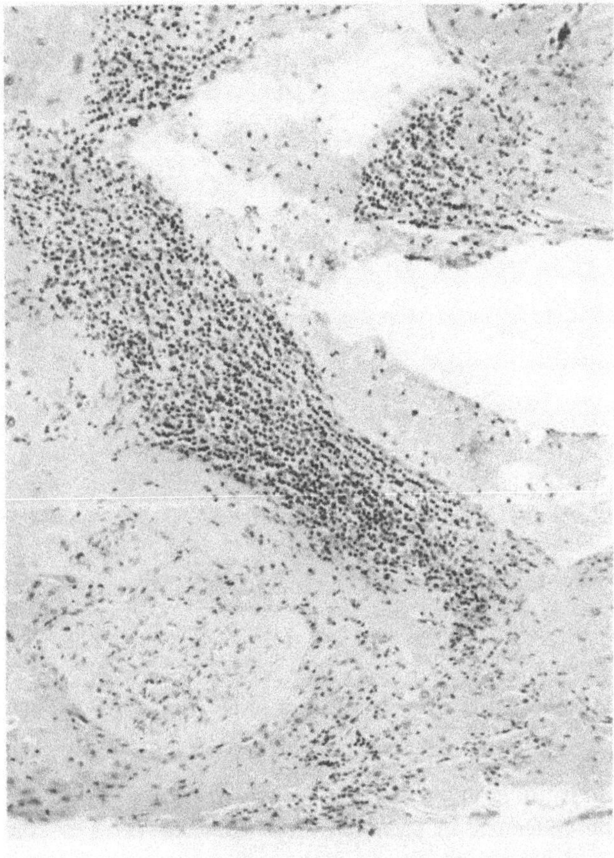

Fig. 24. Basal lymphoplasmacytic villitis. Compare with Fig. 23. Original magnification
× 90. Hematoxylin and Eosin

virus were unsuccessful. Case 22 (Table 2, p. 96), where CMV was isolated
from the urine, is not considered to represent intrauterine CMV infection.
The placental lesions were not those of CMV villitis. It is likely that the virus
was acquired by the infant either during delivery or postnatally.

The histology of almost all of our focal villitis lesions of unknown etiology
is indistinguishable from that of rubella villitis. There is an intrinsic infiltrate
of chronic inflammatory cells, usually lymphocytes, within the villous stroma.
Occasionally these cells are localized beneath the trophoblast but more commonly their distribution is random. Proliferation of stromal mesenchymal
cells is also often a feature. The trophoblast may be damaged in association
with local fibrin deposition. Tissue necrosis associated with the villitis may
be confined to small groups of villi or may extend to large areas of confluent
necrosis (Fig. 7) (seen grossly as white infarcts). Vascular abnormalities may
also be prominent (Fig. 10). An endovasculitis is sometimes seen that is
analogous to the virus-induced endothelial necrosis of rubella or CMV infection.
Secondary changes such as fibrin thrombi are occasionally seen in nearby

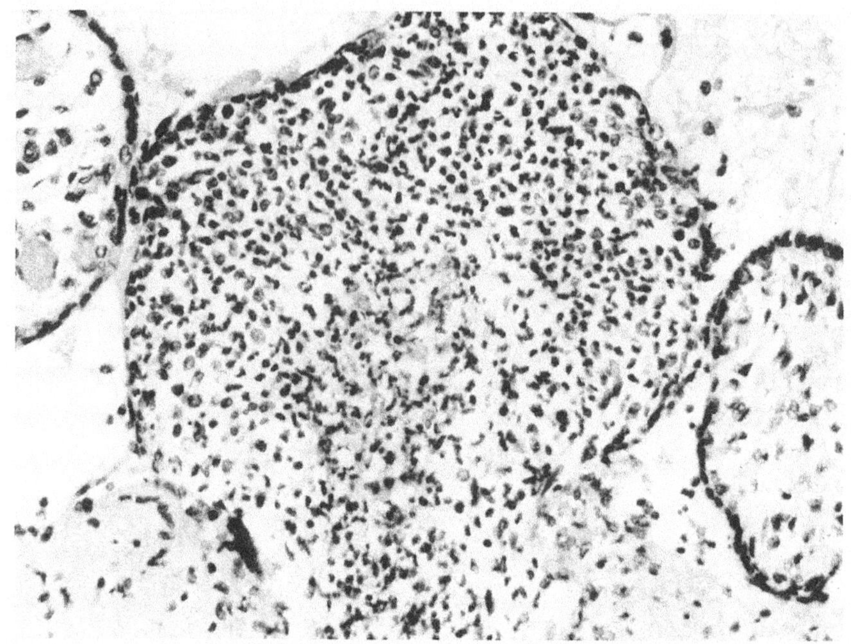

Fig. 25. In this suppurative villitis no organisms were identifiable even with use of special stains. Original magnification × 240. Hematoxylin and Eosin

vessels, although in some instances fibrin thrombi have been widespread throughout the placenta in cases of disseminated intravascular coagulation in the associated infant. Maternal floor inflammatory lesions including focal

Table 3. Clinicopathologic corrrelation

Case number	Gestation (weeks)	Birth weight (g)	Clinical correlation
58	40	3 540	Neonatal seizures. Cord IgM 25 mg-% and reported as suggestive of intrauterine infection
59	24	640	Stillborn. Autopsy showed no gross abnormality
60	40	4 100	Acrocyanosis. Cord IgM 28 mg-%
61	40	3 900	IgM 7.4 mg-%. Beta-hemolytic streptococcus isolated from ear
62	32	2 000	Rh incompatability. Intrauterine transfusion. Antepartum betamethazone
63	35	2 000	Hypocalcemic seizures. IgM 5 mg-%. Respiratory distress syndrome

[a] 0 = Test not performed.

decidual necrosis and chronic non-specific (Fig. 23) or lymphoplasmacytic deciduitis (Fig. 24) were commonly observed. The lesions of focal villitis show a spectrum of change, dependent on both severity and duration. We have not observed any pattern which would indicate that gestational age significantly modifies the histologic appearance of these lesions. The mildest changes (evanescent villitis, Fig. 13) usually involve a few lymphocytes in villi showing reparative features. More severe changes are marked by a more intense inflammatory infiltrate, more numerous lesions in the placenta, and individual lesions involving not single villi but groups of adjacent villi or even large zones of placental tissue. Early lesions show lymphocytic infiltration and early vascular changes. Later lesions show scarring of the affected villi, vascular sclerosis and obliteration. Rarely, we have encountered focal villitis of unknown etiology which was morphologically similar to that of listeriosis, vaccinia and variola (Fig. 25). We have not seen any positive correlation between the severity of focal villitis of unknown etiology and the presence of fetal or neonatal abnormalities.

2. Diffuse Villitis (with Particular Reference to Neonatal Hepatitis)

Of the 63 cases of villitis of unknown etiology (Tables 1–3), 12 were associated with a predominantly diffuse pattern of relative immaturity (Table 1). The reason we subtype this villitis is the observation that four of twelve instances of this lesion were associated with infants having biopsy-proven neonatal hepatitis and two other infants had severe jaundice clinically resembling neonatal hepatitis (although biopsy was not done). Of perhaps more significance is that in an additional two cases there were maternal

f predominantly basal lymphoplasmacytic villitis

Serology[a]					"Focal"						"Diffuse"		Associated lesions				
	Toxoplasma	Rubella	VDRL	Herpesvirus	Severity	Proliferative	Necrotizing	Reparative	Obliterative vasculopathy	Stromal fibrosis	Relative immaturity	Fetal nucleated RBC	Chorioamnionitis	Unrelated ischemia	Maternal floor infarction	Focal decidual necrosis	Basal villitis
	0	0	−	0	−	+	−	−	−	−	−	−	−	−	−	−	+
	0	0	0	0	−	+	−	−	−	−	−	−	−	−	−	−	+ +
−	−	$\frac{1}{30}$	0	0	+	+	−	−	+	−	−	−	−	−	−	−	+ +
	0	0	−	0	±	±	−	−	−	−	±	−	−	+	−	−	+
	0	0	0	0	−	+	−	−	+ +	−	+	−	−	+ +	+	−	+ +
	0	0	−	0	−	+	−	−	−	−	−	−	−	−	−	−	+

symptoms of hepatitis during pregnancy and in a third instance the mother was a known heroin addict.

The transmission of Australia antigen (H.A.A.) and epidemic-hepatitis-associated antigen (E.H.A.A.) from mother to infant may occur in any of four ways of which one is the transplacental transmission of the antigens *in utero* (Schweitzer *et al.*, 1973). Considerable controversy surrounds the question of whether these antigens actually cross the intact placenta (Moroni *et al.*, 1971; Garty *et al.*, 1971; Schweitzer *et al.*, 1973; Krech *et al.*, 1973; Aziz *et al.*, 1973). In the absence of postnatal antigenemia, no circumstantial evidence is, to date, available to support the hypothesis of their transplacental transmission. Although Australia antigen was sought in the infant's serum of only three of our cases and in each instance not found, the placental changes observed here are morphologic support for transplacental transmission of a hepatitis-associated antigen. Histologically the features of this lesion are essentially those of relative immaturity (Fig. 9). Erythroblastosis was present in some but not all cases. It was a feature of the placentas of the clinically hepatitic infants and thus may be a marker of the severity of the infection.

3. Basal Lymphoplasmacytic Villitis

Basal lymphoplasmacytic villitis (Fig. 24) was seen in many of the placentas with villitis of unknown etiology but was predominant in only six out of 63 (Table 3). Our cases showed essentially the same features as those described by Homberger *et al.* (1971). In no case was there a significant clinical correlate in the associated fetus or infant.

VI. Reprise

This review has focused attention upon those human diseases caused by chronic intrauterine infection. Just as we have emphasized the value of placental examinations to the elucidation of such problems, so it is appropriate for us additionally to emphasize the importance of these examinations to the understanding of the majority of afflictions of the fetus and newborn. To this end we cite the words of those whose contributions continuously stimulate our concern for the welfare of the developing fetus and newborn. Benirschke and Driscoll (1967): "With burgeoning interest in fetal and infant welfare, more and more attention is being focused on pregnancy failure, whether the latter includes only fetal wastage or extends to the handicaps of damaged surviving progeny. Systematic reviews of these problems usually disregard the placenta as a source of valid data relevant to the pathophysiology of gestation and its outcome. Adequate placental function is paramount to fetal survival, and the placenta is the co-victim with the fetus in many antenatal disorders. Surely, the study of the placenta, as a maternal and fetal biopsy, is often rewarding in terms of specific disease, both diagnostically and pathogenetically."

Acknowledgements

Virologic studies performed for patients discussed in this Review were kindly provided by JOHN L. SEVER, M.D. and DAVID FUCILLO, Ph.D., National Institute of Neurological Diseases and Stroke, and by the laboratories of GILBERT SCHIFF, M.D., Division of Infectious Diseases, University of Cincinnati Medical Center.

References

ALFORD, C. A., SCHAEFFER, J., BLANKENSHIP, W. J., STRAUMFÇORD, J. V., CASSIDY, G.: A correlative immunologic, microbiologic and clinical approach to the diagnosis of acute and chronic infections in newborn infants. New Engl. J. Med. **277**, 437–449 (1967).

ALTSHULER, G.: Placental villitis of unknown etiology: harbinger of serious disease. J. Reprod. Med. **11**, 215–222 (1973a).

ALTSHULER, G.: Toxoplasmosis as a cause of hydranencephaly. Amer. J. Dis. Child. **125**, 251–252 (1973b).

ALTSHULER, G.: Immunologic competence of the immature human fetus. Morphologic evidence from intrauterine cytomegalovirus infection. Obstet. and Gynec. **43**, 811–816 (1974a).

ALTSHULER, G.: Pathogenesis of congenital herpesvirus infection. Amer. J. Dis. Child. **127**, 427–429 (1974b).

ALTSHULER, G., MCADAMS, A. J.: Cytomegalic inclusion disease of a nineteen-week fetus. Amer. J. Obstet. Gynec. **111**, 295–298 (1971).

ALTSHULER, G., RUSSELL, P., ERMOCILLA, R.: The placental pathology of small for gestational age infants. Amer. J. Obstet. Gynec. Accepted for publication (1974).

ANTHONY, F., HOBEL, C. J., OH, W., OKADA, D.: Group B streptococcal infections in neonates. J. Pediat. **84**, 609–610 (1974).

AZIZ, M. A., KHAN, G., KHANUM, T., SIDDIQUI, A.-R.: Transplacental and postnatal transmission of the hepatitis-associated antigen. J. infect. Dis. **127**, 110–112 (1973).

BAKER, C. J., BARRETT, F. F.: Transmission of group B streptococci among parturient women and their neonates. J. Pediat. **83**, 919–925 (1973).

BAKER, C. J., BARRETT, F. F., GORDON, R. C., YOW, M. D.: Suppurative meningitis due to streptococci of Lancefield group B: a study of 33 infants. J. Pediat. **82**, 724–729 (1973).

BAKER, R. L.: Pregnancy complicated by coccidioidomycosis: report of two cases. Amer. J. Obstet. Gynec. **70**, 1033–1038 (1955).

BECKER, V.: Über die Reifung der plazentaren Zotten. Klin. Wschr. **37**, 1204 (1959).

BECKER, V.: Mechanismus der Reifung fetaler Organe. Verh. dtsch. path. Ges. **46**, 309–314 (1962).

BENIRSCHKE, K.: Viral infection of the placenta. In: Viral etiology of congenital malformations. Bethesda: The National Heart Institute and the National Institute of Child Health and Human Development 1967.

BENIRSCHKE, K., ALTSHULER, G.: Symposium on the functional physiopathology of the fetus and neonate. St. Louis: C.V. Mosby Co. 1971.

BENIRSCHKE, K., BOURNE, G. L.: Plasma cells in an immature human placenta. Obstet. and Gynec. **12**, 495–503 (1958).

BENIRSCHKE, K., DRISCOLL, S. G.: The pathology of the human placenta. Berlin-Heidelberg-New York: Springer 1967.

BENIRSCHKE, K., MENDOZA, G. R., BAZELEY, P. L.: Placental and fetal manifestations of cytomegalovirus infection. Virchows Arch. Abt. B, Sept. 1974.

BERENBERG, W., NANKERVIS, G.: Long-term follow-up of cytomegalic inclusion disease of infancy. Pediatrics **46**, 403–410 (1970).

BEVERLEY, J. K. A., FREEMAN, A. P., HENRY, L., WHELAN, J. P. F.: Prevention of pathological changes in experimental congenital toxoplasma infections. Lyon méd. **230**, 491–498 (1973).

BITTENCOURT, A. C.: Sobre a forma congenita da doenca de Chagas. Rev. Inst. Med. trop. S. Paulo **2**, 319–334 (1960).

BITTENCOURT, A. C.: Placentite chagasica e transmissao congenita da doenca de Chagas. Rev. Inst. Med. trop. S. Paulo **5**, 62–67 (1963).

Bittencourt, A. C., Barbosa, H. S., Rocha, T., Sodre, I., Sodre, A.: Incidencia da transmissao congenita da doenca de Chagas em partos prematuros na maternidade tsylla balbino (Salvador, Bahia). Rev. Inst. Med. trop. S. Paulo 14, 131–134 (1972).

Bittencourt, A. C., Gomes, M. C.: Gestacoes successivas de uma paciente chagasica com ocorrencia de casos de transmissao congenita de doenca. Gaz. Med. Bahia 67, 166–172 (1967).

Blackall, P. B.: Tuberculosis: maternal infection of the newborn. Med. J. Aust. 2, 1055–1058 (1969).

Blanc, W. A.: Pathways of fetal and early neonatal infection: viral placentitis, bacterial and fungal chorioamnionitis. J. Pediat. 59, 473–496 (1961).

Blanc, W. A.: The future of antepartum morphological studies. In: Diagnosis and treatment of fetal disorders (ed. Adamson, K.), p. 15–49. Berlin-Heidelberg-New York: Springer 1969.

Boesaart, J. W.: Case of tuberculosis of the placenta. Ned. T. Geneesk. 103, 1849–1852 (1959).

Boyd, J. D., Hamilton, W. J.: The human placenta. Cambridge: Heffer & Sons 1970.

Braun, P., Lee, Y.-H., Klein, J. O., Marcy, S. M., Klein, T. A., Charles, D., Levy, P., Kass, E. H.: Birth weight and genital mycoplasmas in pregnancy. New Engl. J. Med. 284, 167–171 (1971).

Bret, A.-J., Grepinet, J.: Placentites et avortements d'origine infectieuse. Incidence des endometrites et de certains germes tels que le pyocyanique. Rev. franç. Gynéc. 62, 417–430 (1967).

Charles, A. G., Friedman, E. A.: Rhesus iso-immunization and erythroblastosis foetalis. London: Butterworth 1969.

Coid, C. R., Ramsden, D. B.: Retardation of fetal growth and plasma protein development in fetuses from mice injected with Coxsackie B 3 virus. Nature (Lond.) 243, 460–461 (1973).

Cort, W. W.: Prenatal infestation with parasitic worms. J. Amer. med. Ass. 76, 170–171 (1921).

Creasman, W. T., Lawrence, R. A., Thiede, H. A.: Fetal complications of amniocentesis. J. Amer. med. Ass. 204, 91–94 (1968).

Davis, B. D., Dulbecco, R., Eisen, H. N., Ginsberg, H. S., Wood, H. B., Jr., McCarty, M.: Microbiology (2nd ed.). Hagerstown: Harper & Row 1973.

Davies, P. A.: Bacterial infection in the fetus and newborn. Arch. Dis. Childh. 46, 1–25 (1971).

Dent, P. B., Rawls, W. E.: Human congenital rubella: the relationship of immunologic aberration to viral persistence. Ann. N.Y. Acad. Sci. 181, 209–222 (1971).

Desmonts, G., Couvreur, J.: Congenital toxoplasmosis: a prospective study of 378 pregnancies. New Engl. J. Med. 290, 1110–1116 (1974).

Diosi, P., Babusceac, L., Nevinglovschi, O., Kun-Stoicu, G.: Cytomegalovirus infection associated with pregnancy. Lancet 1967 II, 1063–1066.

Dixon, C. W.: Vaccination against smallpox. Brit. med. J. 1962 I, 1262–1266.

Dollmann, A., Schmitz-Moormann, P.: Rekurrierende Plazentainsuffizienz durch villöse Plazentitis mit extremer fetaler Hypotrophie. Geburtsh. u. Frauenheilk. 32, 795–801 (1972).

Dorman, H. G., Sahyun, P. F.: Identification and significance of spirochetes in the placenta. Amer. J. Obstet. Gynec. 33, 954–967 (1937).

Driscoll, S. G.: Histopathology of gestational rubella. Amer. J. Dis. Child. 118, 49–53 (1969).

Driscoll, S. G., Gorbach, A., Feldman, D.: Congenital listeriosis: diagnosis from placental studies. Obstet. and Gynec. 20, 216–220 (1962).

Dubey, J. P., Miller, N. L., Frenkel, J. K.: The toxoplasma gondii oocyst from cat feces. J. exp. Med. 132, 636–662 (1970).

Eckstein, A., Nixon, W. C. W.: Congenital malaria. Brit. med. J. 1946 I, 432–433.

Eden, A. N.: Perinatal mortality caused by Vibrio fetus. J. Pediat. 68, 297–304 (1966).

Editorial: Intrauterine infections: problems and prevention. Lancet 1973 I, 868.

Editorial: Congenital cytomegalovirus infection—more problems. Lancet 1974 I, (a) 845.

Editorial: Tuberculosis retreats-slowly. Lancet 1974 I, (b) 1087.

Eickhoff, T. C.: Group B streptococci in human infection. In: Streptococci and streptococcal diseases (eds. Wannamaker, Matsen). New York: Acad. Press 1972.

EICKHOFF, T. C., KLEIN, J. O., DALY, K. A., INGALL, D., FINLAND, M.: Neonatal sepsis and other infections due to group B beta-hemolytic streptococci. New Engl. J. Med. **271**, 1221–1228 (1964).

EILARD, T., STRANNEGARD, O.: Rubella reinfection in pregnancy followed by transmission to the fetus. J. infect. Dis. **129**, 594–596 (1974).

ELLIOTT, W. G.: Placental toxoplasmosis. Amer. J. clin. Path. **53**, 413–417 (1970).

EMBIL, J. A., OZERE, R. L., HALDANE, E. V.: Congenital cytomegalovirus infection in two siblings from consecutive pregnancies. J. Pediat. **77**, 417–421 (1970).

ENTWISTLE, D. M., BRAY, P. T., LAURENCE, K. M.: Prenatal infection with vaccinia virus: report of a case. Brit. med. J. **1962I**, 238–239.

FELDMAN, H. A.: Toxoplasmosis. New Engl. J. Med. **279**, 1370–1375, 1431–1436 (1968).

FOEGE, W. H., EDDINS, D. L.: Mass vaccination programs in developing countries. In: Progress in medical virology, vol. 15 (ed. MELNICK, J. L.), p. 205–243. Basel: S. Karger 1973.

FOY, H. M., KENNY, G. E., WENTWORTH, B. B., JOHNSON, W. L., GRAYSTON, J. T.: Isolation of mycoplasma hominis, T-strains, and cytomegalovirus from the cervix of pregnant women. Amer. J. Obstet. Gynec. **106**, 635–643 (1970).

FRANCIOSI, R. A., KNOSTMAN, J. D., ZIMMERMAN, R. A.: Group B streptococcal neonatal and infant infections. J. Pediat. **82**, 707–718 (1973).

FRENKEL, J. K.: Toxoplasmosis. In: Comparative aspects of reproductive failure (ed. BENIRSCHKE, K.), p. 296–321. Berlin-Heidelberg-New York: Springer 1967.

FRENKEL, J. K., DUBEY, J. P.: Toxoplasmosis and its prevention in cats and man. J. infect. Dis. **126**, 664–673 (1972).

FRENKEL, J. K., DUBEY, J. P., MILLER, N. L.: Toxoplasma gondii in cats: fecal stages identified as coccidian oocysts. Science **167**, 893–896 (1970).

FUJINAMI, A., NAKAMURA, H.: On the prophylaxis of shistosomiasis and some investigations on infection with this disease. Chugi Iji Shimpo. **753** (1911).

GARCIA, A. G. P.: Fetal infection in chickenpox and alastrim with histopathologic study of the placenta. Pediatrics **32**, 895–901 (1963).

GARTY, R., BAR-SCHANY, S., GORDIN, A.: Possible transplacental transmission of serum hepatitis. Lancet **1971II**, 434.

GERSHON, R., STRAUSS, L.: Structural changes in human placentas associated with fetal inanition or growth arrest ("placental insufficiency syndrome"). Amer. J. Dis. Child. **102**, 645–646 (1961).

GNARPE, H., FRIBERG, J.: Mycoplasma and human reproductive failure. I: The occurrences of different mycoplasmas in couples with reproductive failure. Amer. J. Obstet. Gynec. **114**, 727–731 (1972).

GNARPE, H., FRIBERG, J.: T-mycoplasmas as a possible cause for reproductive failure. Nature (Lond.) **242**, 210–212 (1973).

GOLDMAN, R. L.: Herpetic inclusions in the endometrium. Obstet. and Gynec. **36**, 603–605 (1970).

GOLDMAN, R. L., BANK, R. W., WARNER, N. E.: Cytomegalovirus infection of the cervix: an "incidental" finding of possible clinical significance. Obstet. and Gynec. **34**, 326–329 (1969).

GOODLIN, R. C.: Intrauterine transfusion complicated by amnionitis and maternal peritonitis. Obstet. and Gynec. **26**, 803 (1965).

GORANOV, I., GANCEV, S.: Fehlgeburt bei Zytomegalie. Zbl. Gynäk. **85**, 1037–1040 (1963).

GREGORY, J. E., PAYNE, F. E.: Mycoplasma in the uterine cervix. Amer. J. Obstet. Gynec. **107**, 220–226 (1970).

GROSSMAN, J., TOMPKINS, R. L.: Group B beta-hemolytic streptococcal meningitis in mother and infant. New Engl. J. Med. **290**, 387 (1974).

GRUENWALD, P.: Abnormalities of placental vascularity in relation to intrauterine deprivation and retardation of fetal growth. N. Y. St. J. Med. **61**, 1508–1517 (1961).

HANSHAW, J. B.: Congenital cytomegalovirus infection: a fifteen year perspective. J. infect. Dis. **123**, 555–561 (1971).

HANSHAW, J. B.: Herpesvirus hominis infections in the fetus and the newborn. Amer. J. Dis. Child. **126**, 546–555 (1973).

HAYES, K., GIBAS, H.: Placental cytomegalovirus infection without fetal involvement following primary infection in pregnancy. J. Pediat. **79**, 401–405 (1971).

Hörmann, G.: Placenta und Lues. Ein Beitrag zur Diagnose und Prognose konnataler Syphilis. Arch. Gynäk. **184**, 481–521 (1954).

Homberger, C., Chauhan, P., Blanc, W. A.: Lymphoplasmacytic placentitis, fetal infection and placental immunoglobulin synthesis. Abstract, Pediatric Pathology Meeting, International Academy of Pathology, Montreal, March, 1971.

Hood, C. K., McKinnon, G. E.: Prenatal vaccinia. Amer. J. Obstet. Gynec. **85**, 238–240 (1963).

Hood, M., Todd, J. M.: Vibrio fetus—a cause of human abortion. Amer. J. Obstet. Gynec. **80**, 506–511 (1960).

Horne, H. W., Hertig, A. T., Kundsin, R. B., Kosasa, T. S.: Sub-clinical endometrial inflammation and T-mycoplasma. A possible cause of human reproductive failure. Int. J. Fertil. **18**, 226–231 (1973).

Hubbard, T. W.: Varicella occurring in an infant twenty-four hours after birth. Brit. med. J. **1878I**, 822.

Hume, O. S.: Toxoplasmosis and pregnancy. Amer. J. Obstet. Gynec. **114**, 703–715 (1972).

Hutchinson, W. M.: Experimental transmission of Toxoplasma gondii. Nature (Lond.) **206**, 961–962 (1965).

Hutchinson, W. M., Dunachie, J. F., Siim, J. C.: Coccidian-like nature of Toxoplasma gondii. Brit. med. J. **1970I**, 142–144.

Jones, T. C., Yeh, S., Hirsch, J. G.: The interaction between Toxoplasma gondii and mammalian cells. I. Mechanism of entry and intracellular fate of the parasite. J. exp. Med. **136**, 1157–1172 (1972).

Jundrak, K.: Die Zytomegalie in der Zervixschleimhaut einer Wöchnerin. Zbl. allg. Path. path. Anat. **106**, 255–258 (1964).

Kalter, S. S., Helmke, R. J., Panigel, M., Heberling, R. L., Felsberg, P. J., Axelrod, L. R.: Observation of apparent C-type particles in baboon (*Papio cynocephalus*) placentas. Science **179**, 1332–1333 (1973).

Kempe, C. H.: To vaccinate or not? Hosp. Pract. **3**, No 9, 28–33 (1968).

Keutel, J.: Angeborene Varicellen. Bericht über einen Fall. Literaturübersicht — immunologische Gesichtspunkte. Arch. Kinderheilk. **102**, 266–274 (1968).

King, A.: Failure to control venereal disease. Brit. med. J. **1970I**, 451–457.

Krech, U., Konjajev, Z., Jung, M.: Congenital cytomegalovirus infection in siblings from consecutive pregnancies. Helv. paediat. Acta **26**, 355–362 (1971).

Krech, U., Sonnabend, W., Kistler, G., Mäder, A.: Australia antigen in cord blood. Vox Sang. (Basel), Suppl. **24**, 55–60 (1973).

Kriel, R. L., Gates, G. A., Wulff, H., Powell, N., Poland, J. D., Chin, T. D. Y.: Cytomegalovirus isolations associated with pregnancy wastage. Amer. J. Obstet. Gynec. **106**, 885–892 (1970).

Krogstad, D. J., Juranek, D. D., Walls, K. W.: Toxoplasmosis: with comments on risk of infection from cats. Ann. intern. Med. **77**, 773–778 (1972).

Kumar, M. L., Nankervis, G. A., Gold, E.: Inapparent congenital cytomegalovirus infection. New Engl. J. Med. **288**, 1370–1372 (1973).

Kundsin, R. B., Driscoll, S. G.: Mycoplasmas and human reproductive failure. Surg. Gynec. Obstet. **131**, 89–92 (1970).

Kundsin, R. B., Driscoll, S. G., Ming, P.-M. L.: Strain of mycoplasma associated with human reproductive failure. Science **157**, 1573–1574 (1967).

Kvittingen, J.: Beta-hemolytic streptococcus group B causing neonatal meningitis. Acta path. microbiol. scand. **74**, 143–144 (1968).

Laga, E. M., Driscoll, S. G., Munro, H. N.: Comparison of placentas from two socioeconomic groups. I. Morphometry. Pediatrics **50**, 24–32 (1972).

Lang, D. J., Kummer, J. F., Hartley, D. P.: Cytomegalovirus in semen: persistence and demonstration in extracellular fluids. New Engl. J. Med. **291**, 121–123 (1974).

Lelong, M., Lepage, F., Le Tan, V.: Le virus de la maladie d'inclusions cytomegaliques. Arch. franç. Pédiat. **17**, 437–450 (1960).

Lepage, F., Schramm: Aspects histologiques du placenta et des membranes dans la maladie d'inclusions cytomegaliques. Gynéc. et Obstét. **57**, 273–279 (1958).

Lide, T. N.: Congenital tularemia. Arch. Path. **43**, 165–169 (1947).

Louvris, J. de, Blades, M., Harrison, R. F., Hurley, R., Stanley, V. C.: Frequency of mycoplasma in fertile and infertile couples. Lancet **1974I**, 1073–1075.

Lucy, J. F.: Intrauterine transfusion and erythroblastosis fetalis. In: Report of 53rd Conference on pediatric research, p. 14–15. Columbus: Ross Laboratories 1967.

MacArthur, P.: Congenital vaccinia and vaccinia gravidarum. Lancet 1952II, 1104–1106.

MacDonald, A. M., MacArthur, P.: Foetal vaccinia. Arch. Dis. Childh. 28, 311–315 (1953).

Markham, N. P., Markham, J. G., Smith, E. R.: Incidence of T-strain mycoplasmas in male and female subjects attending a venereal diseases clinic. Brit. J. vener. Dis. 48, 200–204 (1972).

McCormack, W. M., Braun, P., Lee, Y.-H., Klein, J. O., Kass, E. H.: The genital mycoplasmas. New Engl. J. Med. 288, 78–89 (1973).

McCracken, A. W., D'Agostino, A. N., Brucks, A. B., Kingsley, W. B.: Acquired cytomegalovirus infection presenting as viral endometritis. Amer. J. clin. Path. 61, 556–560 (1974).

McCracken, G. H., Jr., Shinefield, H. R., Cobb, K., Rausen, A. R., Dische, R., Eichenwald, H. F.: Congenital cytomegalic inclusion disease; a longitudinal study of 20 patients. Amer. J. Dis. Child. 117, 522–539 (1969).

Monif, G. R. G., Dische, R. M.: Viral placentitis in congenital cytomegalovirus infection. Amer. J. clin. Path. 58, 445–449 (1972).

Moroni, G. A., Constantino, D., Zampieri, G., Gianotti, G. A., Doglia, M., Del Prete, S.: Do the hepatitis antigens cross the placenta? Lancet 1971II, 376.

Musto, J. C. di, Bohjalian, O., Millar, M.: Mycoplasma hominis type I infection and pregnancy. Obstet. and Gynec. 41, 33–37 (1973).

Naeye, R. L.: Cytomegalic inclusion disease: the fetal disorder. Amer. J. clin. Path. 47, 738–744 (1967).

Naeye, R. L., Blanc, W. A.: Pathogenesis of congenital rubella. J. Amer. med. Ass. 194, 1277–1283 (1965).

Nahmias, A. J., Alford, C. A., Korones, S. B.: Infection of the newborn with herpes-virus hominis. In: Advances in pediatrics, p. 185–226. Chicago: Year Book Med. 1970.

Nahmias, A. J., Roizman, B.: Infection with herpes-simplex viruses 1 and 2. New Engl. J. Med. 15, 781–789 (1973).

Naidoo, P., Hirsch, H.: Prenatal vaccinia. Lancet 1963I, 196–197.

Nokes, J. M., Claiborne, H. A., Jr., Thornton, W. N., Jr., Yiu-Tang, H.: Extrauterine pregnancy associated with tuberculous salpingitis and congenital tuberculosis in the fetus. Obstet. and Gynec. 9, 206–211 (1957).

Northrop, R. L., Gardner, W. M., Geittmann, W. F.: Rubella reinfection during early pregnancy. Obstet. and Gynec. 39, 524–526 (1972).

Olivier, Olivier, Segal: A bibliography on Chagas disease, 1909–1969. Washington: U.S.D.A. and University of Maryland 1972.

Oppenheimer, E. H., Esterly, J. R.: Cytomegalovirus infection: a possible cause of biliary atresia (abstr.). Amer. J. Path. 71, 2a (1973).

Ornoy, A., Segal, S., Nishmi, M., Simcha, A., Polishuk, W. Z.: Fetal and placental pathology in gestational rubella. Amer. J. Obstet. Gynec. 116, 949–956 (1973).

Page, L. A., Smith, P. C.: Placentitis and abortion in cattle inoculated with chlamydiae isolated from aborted human placental tissue. Proc. Soc. exp. Biol. (N.Y.) 146, 269–275 (1974).

Parkman, P. D., Buescher, E. L., Artenstein, M. S.: Recovery of rubella virus from army recruits. Proc. Soc. exp. Biol. (N.Y.) 111, 225–230 (1962).

Peterson, D. R., Trouca, E., Bouin, P.: Human toxoplasmosis prevalence and exposure to cats. Amer. J. Epid. 96, 215–219 (1972).

Potel, J.: Die Listeriose beim Menschen. In: Listeriosen-Symposion (Hrsg. Roots, E., Strauch, D.). Veterinärmedizin March, p. 70 (1958).

Potter, E.: Pathology of the Fetus and Infant. Chicago: Year Book Med. 1961.

Quan, A., Strauss, L.: Congenital cytomegalic inclusion disease: observations in a macerated fetus with congenital defect, including study of the placenta. Amer. J. Obstet. Gynec. 83, 1240–1247 (1962).

Ramos, A. D., Hibbard, L. T., Craig, J. R.: Congenital tuberculosis. Obstet. and Gynec. 43, 61–64 (1974).

Rappaport, F., Rabinovitz, M., Toaff, R., Krochik, N.: Genital listeriosis as a cause of repeated abortion. Lancet 1960I, 1273–1275.

Remington, J. S.: Toxoplasmosis: recent developments. Ann. Rev. Med. **21**, 201–218 (1970).

Remington, J. S., Desmonts, G.: Congenital toxoplasmosis: variability in the IgM-fluorescent antibody response and some pitfalls in diagnosis. J. Pediat. **83**, 27–30 (1973).

Reynolds, D. W., Stagno, S., Stubbs, K. G., Dahle, A. J., Livingston, M. M., Saxon, S. S., Alford, C. A.: Inapparent congenital cytomegalovirus infection with elevated cord IgM levels. New Engl. J. Med. **290**, 291–296 (1974).

Rich, A. R.: The pathogenesis of tuberculosis (2nd ed.). Springfield: C. C. Thomas 1950.

Rich, A. R., Follis, R. H., Jr.: The effects of low oxygen tension upon the development of experimental tuberculosis. Bull. Johns Hopk. Hosp. **71**, 345–363 (1942).

Rosenstein, D. L., Navarrek-Reyna, A.: Cytomegalic inclusion disease. Amer. J. Obstet. Gynec. **89**, 220–224 (1964).

Rowe, W. P., Hartley, J. W., Waterman, S., Turner, H. C., Huebner, R. J.: Cytopathogenic agent resembling human salivary gland virus recovered from tissue cultures of human adenoids. Proc. Soc. exp. Biol. (N.Y.) **92**, 418–424 (1956).

Russell, P., Altshuler, G.: The placental abnormalities of congenital syphilis. Amer. J. Dis. Child. **128**, 160–163 (1974).

Sarrut, S., Alison, F.: Etude du placenta dans 21 cas de listeriose congenitale. Arch. franç. Pédiat. **24**, 285–302 (1967).

Saxon, S. A., Knight, W., Reynolds, D. W., Stagno, S., Alford, C. A.: Intellectual deficits in children born with subclinical congenital toxoplasmosis: a preliminary report. Pediatrics **82**, 792–797 (1973).

Schmorl, G., Birch-Hirschfeld: Übergang von Tuberkel-Bacillen aus dem mütterlichen Blut auf die Frucht. Beitr. path. Anat. **9**, 428–439 (1891).

Schmorl, G., Geipl, L.: Über die Tuberkulose der menschlichen Plazenta. Münch. med. Wschr. **51**, 1676–1679 (1904).

Schmorl, G., Kockel, K. V.: Die Tuberkulose der menschlichen Placenta und ihre Beziehung zur kongenitalen Infection mit Tuberkulose. Beitr. path. Anat. **16**, 313–339 (1894).

Schweitzer, I. L., Dunn, A. E. G., Peters, R. L., Spears, R. L.: Viral hepatitis B in neonates and infants. Amer. J. Med. **55**, 762–771 (1973).

Scott, J. M., Henderson, A.: Acute villous inflammation in the placenta following intrauterine transfusion. J. clin. Path. **25**, 872–875 (1972).

Seeliger, H. P. R.: Some new aspects of human listeriosis. In: Human listeriosis: its nature and diagnosis. Atlanta: U.S. Dept. of Health, Education, and Welfare. Public Health Serice Communicable Disease Center 1957.

Seppala, M., Vaheri, A.: Natural rubella infection of the female genital tract. Lancet **1974I**, 46–47.

Sharf, M., Eibschitz, I., Eylan, E.: Latent toxoplasmosis and pregnancy. Obstet. and Gynec. **42**, 349–354 (1973).

Shurin, P. A., Alpert, S., Rosner, B., Driscoll, S. G., Kass, E. H.: Genital mycoplasmas—association with chorioamnionitis. Pediat. Res. **8**, 428 (1974).

Siegel, M.: Pathological findings and pathogenesis of congenital tuberculosis. Amer. Rev. Tuberc. **29**, 297–309 (1934).

Siegel, M., Singer, B.: Occurrence of tubercle bacilli in the blood of the umbilical cord and in the newborn infants of tuberculous mothers. Amer. J. Dis. Child. **50**, 636–641 (1935).

Siim, J. C., Hutchinson, W. M., Work, K.: Transmission of Toxoplasma gondii. Acta path. microbiol. scand. **77**, 756–757 (1969).

Silverstein, A. M.: Congenital syphilis and the timing of immunogenesis in the human fetus. Nature (Lond.) **194**, 196–197 (1962).

Silverstein, A. M.: Ontogeny of the immune response. Science **144**, 1423–1428 (1964).

Smith, M. G.: Propagation in tissue cultures of a cytopathogenic virus from human salivary gland (SGC) disease. Proc. Soc. exp. Biol. (N.Y.) **92**, 424–430 (1956).

South, M. A., Tompkins, W. A. F., Morris, C. R., Rawls, W. E.: Congenital malformation of the central nervous system associated with genital type (type 2) herpes virus. J. Pediat. **75**, 13–18 (1969).

SPLENDORE, A.: Un nuovo protozoa parassita dei conigli: incontrato nelle lesioni anatomiche d'una malattia che ricorda in molti punti il Kala-azar dell'uomo. Rev. Soc. Sc. S. Paulo 3, 109–112 (1908).

SRABSTEIN, J. C., MORRIS, N., LARKE, R. P. B., SA, D. J. DE, CASTELINO, B. B., SUM, E.: Is there a congenital varicella syndrome? J. Pediat. 84, 239–243 (1974).

STAGNO, S., REYNOLDS, D. W., LAKEMAN, A., CHARAMIELLO, L. J., ALFORD, C. A.: Congenital cytomegalovirus infection: consecutive occurrence due to viruses with similar antigenic compositions. Pediatrics 52, 788–794 (1973).

STARR, J. G., BART, R. D., JR., GOLD, E.: Inapparent congenital cytomegalovirus infection: clinical and epidemiologic characteristics in early infancy. New Engl. J. Med. 282, 1075–1078 (1970).

STERN, H.: Isolation of cytomegalovirus and clinical manifestations of infection at different ages. Brit. med. J. 1968I, 665–669.

STIEHM, E. R., AMMANN, A. J., CHERRY, J. D.: Elavated cord macroglobulins in the diagnosis of intrauterine infections. New Engl. J. Med. 275, 971–977 (1966).

STRAUSS, L., SEKI, M.: Plasma cells in the fetal part of the human placenta. Abstract of presentation to 59th Annual Meeting of the American Association of Pathologists and Bacteriologists. Montreal, May, 1962.

SUTHERLAND, J. C., BERRY, A., HYND, M., PROCTOR, N. S. F.: S. Afr. J. Obstet. Gynaec. 3, 76–80 (1965).

SYMMERS, WM. ST. C.: Note on a new form of liver cirrhosis due to the presence of the ova of Bilharzia haematobia. J. Path. Bact. 9, 237–239 (1904).

TÖNDURY, G. T., SMITH, D. W.: Fetal rubella pathology. J. Ped. 68, 867–879 (1966).

TUCKER, S. M., GIBSON, D. E.: Foetal complication of vaccination in pregnancy. Brit. med. J. 1962I, 237–238.

VAUGHAN, J. E., RAMIREZ, H.: Coccidioidomycosis as a complication of pregnancy. Calif. Med. 74, 121–125 (1951).

VERNON, M. L., MCMAHON, J. M., HACKETT, J. J.: Additional evidence of type-C particles in human placentas. J. nat. Cancer Inst. 52, 987–989 (1974).

VINZENT, R.: Une affection mecomme de la grossesse. L'infection placentaire a vibrio foetus. Presse méd. 57, 1230–1232 (1949).

VINZENT, R., DELARUE, J., HEBERT, H.: L'infection placentaire a vibrio foetus. Ann. Méd. 51, 23–68 (1950).

VINZENT, R., DUMAS, J., PICARD, N.: Septicemie grave au cours de la grossesse due a un vibrion. Avortement consecutif. Bull. Acad. nat. Méd. (Paris) 131, 90–92 (1947).

WALLACE, G. D., MARSHALL, L., MARSHALL, M.: Cats, rats, and toxoplasmosis on a small Pacific island. Amer. J. Epid. 95, 475–482 (1972).

WARTHIN, A. S., COWIE, D. M.: A contribution to the casuistry of placental and congenital tuberculosis. J. infect. Dis. 1, 140–169 (1904).

WATSON, W. A.: Toxoplasmosis in human and veterinary medicine. Vet. Rec. 91, 254–258 (1972).

WELLER, T. H.: The cytomegaloviruses: ubiquitous agents with protean clinical manifestations. New Engl. J. Med. 285, 203–214, 267–274 (1971).

WELLER, T. H., MACAULEY, J. C., CRAIG, J. M., WIRTH, P.: Isolation of intranuclear inclusion producing agents from infants with illnesses resembling cytomegalic inclusion disease. Proc. Soc. exp. Biol. (N.Y.) 94, 4–12 (1957).

WELLER, T. H., NEVA, F. A.: Propagation in tissue culture of cytopathic agents from patients with rubella-like illness. Proc. Soc. exp. Biol. (N.Y.) 111, 215–225 (1962).

WERING, R. F. VAN, ESSEVELD, H.: Vibrio fetus. Ned. T., Geneesk. 107, 119–121 (1963).

WHEELER, W. E., BORCHERS, J.: Vibrionic enteritis in infants. Amer. J. Dis. Child. 101, 86–92 (1961).

WICKRAMASURIYA, G. A. W.: Some observations on malaria occurring in association with pregnancy. J. Obstet. Gynaec. Brit. Emp. 42, 816–834 (1935).

WIELENGA, G., TONGEREN, H. A. E. VAN, FERGUSON, A. H., RIJSSEL, T. G. VAN: Prenatal infection with vaccinia virus. Lancet 1961I, 258–260.

WILLIS, M. D., AUSTIN, W. J.: Human Vibrio fetus infection. Amer. J. Dis. Child. 112, 459–462 (1966).

WINTERBAUER, R. H., FORTUINE, R., EICKHOFF, T. C.: Unusual occurrence of neonatal meningitis due to group B beta-hemolytic streptococci. Pediatrics 38, 661–662 (1966).

Witzleben, C. L., Driscoll, S. G.: Possible transplacental transmission of herpes simplex infection. Pediatrics **36**, 192–199 (1965).
Wolf, A., Cowen, D., Paige, B.: Human toxoplasmosis: occurrence in infants as encephalomyelitis: verification by transmission to animals. Science **89**, 226–227 (1939).
Work, K.: Toxoplasmosis: with special reference to transmission and life cycle of Toxoplasma gondii. Acta path. microbiol. scand., Suppl. **221**, Section B (1971).
Work, K., Hutchinson, W. M.: The new cyst of Toxoplasma gondii. Acta path. microbiol. scand. **77**, 414–424 (1969).
Yawn, D. H., Pyeatte, J. C., Joseph, J. M., Eichler, S. L., Garcia-Bunnel, R.: Transplacental transfer of influenza virus. J. Amer. med. Ass. **216**, 1022–1023 (1971).
Zugibe, F. T.: Diagnostic histochemistry. St. Louis: C. V. Mosby Co. 1970.

Institute of Pathology, University of Hamburg
(Director: Prof. Dr. G. Seifert)

Ultrastructural Pathology of the Adrenal Glands in Cushing's Syndrome*

H. Mitschke and W. Saeger**

With 17 Figures

Contents

I. Introduction

According to Tannenbaum (1973), the ultrastructural pathology of the adrenal cortex in man is a relatively unexplored area. The first ultrastructural examinations of human adrenal cortices were done by Carr (1958, 1961) and Ross *et al.* (1958). Before these examinations and particularly following them, adrenal cortices of numerous animal species were examined under various experimental conditions by electron microscopy (Idelman, 1970; Saeger and Mitschke, 1973 b).

These studies showed that the typical division of the adrenal cortex into zones was characterized by a specific varying structure and distribution of cell organelles (Brenner, 1966; Kawaoi, 1969; Long and Jones, 1967a,

---

* Dedicated to Prof. Dr. med. h. c. Carl Krauspe on his 80th birthday.
** Supported by the Deutsche Forschungsgemeinschaft SFB 34.

1967b; Luse, 1967; Mackay, 1969; Rhodin, 1971; Tannenbaum, 1973). By means of manifold inhibitory and stimulatory techniques, the cortical cells could be more exactly described as being in a state of hyper- and hypofunction. In animal, as well as in human studies, the significance of the smooth endoplasmic reticulum and the mitochondria for the synthesis of steroid hormones from precursors stored in the lipid vacuoles, was observed. This effected a change in the understanding of the functional activity manifested in the cortex cells. Earlier views (Liebegott, 1952; Tonutti, 1952) had presumed a progressive and regressive transformation of the adrenal cortex. The electron-microscopic examination was able to identify the compact cell as an especially active cell form (Carr, 1961; Tsuchiyama, 1967).

The ultrastructure of the adrenal glands was used in attempts to gain information not only for estimating the activity of the normal or hyperplastic cortex but also for registering the steroidogenic activity of adrenal tumors. Explanations were also sought for a differentiated morphological evidence of a varying steroid hormone production. There was also interest in establishing criteria for differentiating benign from malignant tumors. Investigations of this subject have been hitherto relatively infrequent (Mackay, 1969; Mitschke *et al.*, 1973; Neville and Mackay, 1972; Tannenbaum, 1973).

In interpreting the actual findings, the following points must be considered: the problem of taking specimens from patients with already pre-operative initiated steroid hormone medication; the phase of hypoxia following ligature of the blood vessels which can lead to especially pronounced changes of the sinusoidal endothelium but also to focal membrane changes particularly of the mitochondria in cortical cells (Horvath and Kovacs, 1973); the limited possibilities of obtaining evidence from the small particles (Mackay, 1969) with the result that representative evidence can only be obtained after examination of tissue taken from various areas.

The Cushing's syndrome offers a good example for study of the regulative and autonomous hyperfunction of the adrenal cortex. It is a disease caused by hypersecretion of cortisol or by an excessive supply of exogenous gluco-corticoid hormones (Besser and Edwards, 1972; Labhart, 1971). This hypercortisolism results in a characteristic clinical picture common to all the various forms of this syndrome.

Table 1. Pathogenetic forms of Cushing's syndrome

I. Primary extraadrenal forms	*Morphology of adrenal cortex*
1. Hypothalamic-hypophyseal causes with ACTH stimulation	diffuse or nodular hyperplasia
2. Ectopic ACTH-syndrome	diffuse or nodular (?) hyperplasia
3. ACTH therapy	diffuse or nodular (?) hyperplasia
4. Corticosteroid therapy	atrophy
II. Primary adrenal forms	
1. Adenoma a) clear cell adenoma b) compact cell adenoma	
2. Carcinoma	

According to the pathogenesis one can differentiate between 1. primary extraadrenal and 2. primary adrenal forms (SAEGER and MITSCHKE, 1973 a) (Table 1).

II. Macroscopic Changes of the Adrenal Gland in Cushing's Syndrome

The weight of hyperplastic adrenal glands is often only moderately increased above the norm weight of approximately 6–10 g. They rarely reach a weight of 25 g (SYMINGTON, 1969). Particularly high weights can be found in the ectopic ACTH-syndrome (NEVILLE and MACKAY, 1972). With regard to structure, one differentiates between *diffuse and nodular hyperplasia.*

In the diffuse form the adrenal gland has rounded contours with a lipid-rich, yellow outer zone and a varying wide brown inner layer. Small cortical nodules may also be found. These can increase in number and size and lead to compression and atrophy—due to pressure—of the bordering cortical sections. In the case of pronounced nodular changes one can also speak of *adenomatous or nodular cortical hyperplasia.* According to SYMINGTON (1969), this nodular hyperplasia accounts for approximately 17% of all cortical hyperplasias. He does not regard the multiple nodules, located on one side or bilaterally, as being autonomous as do other authors (BIERICH, 1971; KRACHT and TAMM, 1960).

The macroscopic sign of a functional active adenoma or carcinoma is the atrophy of the ipsi- and contralateral adrenal cortex due to suppression of ACTH-secretion. Tumors of the adrenal cortex occur in approximately 15–20% of all cases of Cushing's syndrome (SYMINGTON, 1969). The *adenomas* usually weigh less than 100 g and have an obvious capsule. By contrast, the *carcinomas* usually weigh more than 100 g. Furthermore, they are marked by an infiltration of the capsule and often extensive tumor necrosis.

III. Histological Findings of the Adrenal Cortex in Cushing's Syndrome

In the zona fasciculata and reticularis of the normal adrenal cortex—which can be viewed as a functional unit with regard to glucocorticoid and androgen hormone secretion—large, lipid-rich clear cells can be distinguished from compact eosinophilic cortical cells containing few lipids by light microscopy. In cases of adrenal hyperplasia the clear cells are found primarily in the outer zone in fascicular cell formations (Fig. 1 a), whereas the darker inner zone is composed of compact cells which, in part, contain a great deal of lipofuscin pigment (Fig. 1 b). The cortical noduli, which may also show a division into zones, are separated by considerable collagenous and reticular tissue (NEVILLE and SYMINGTON, 1967).

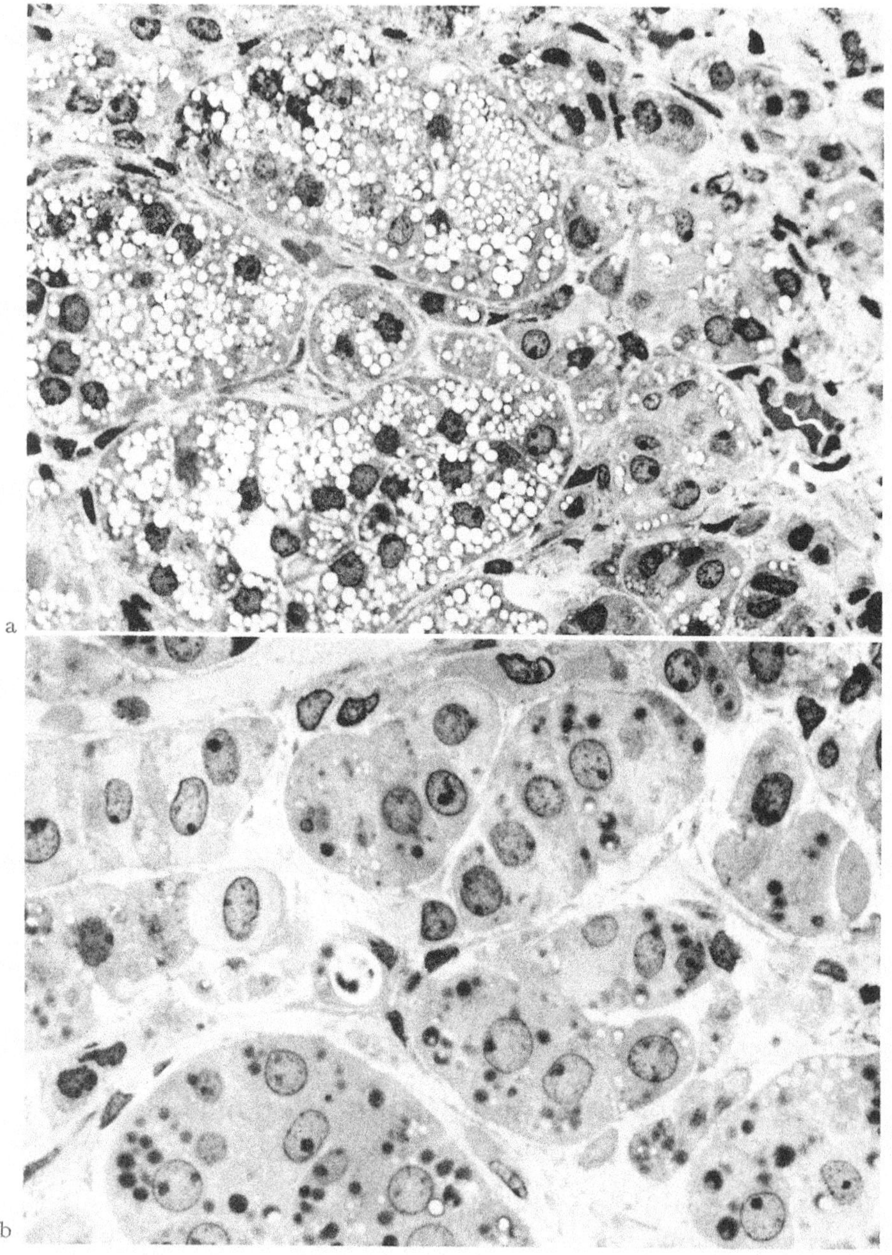

Fig. 1a. Subcapsular zone of hyperplastic adrenal cortex with regular zona glomerulosa and lipid-rich cells of the zona fasciculata. 1 μ thick section, Toluidine-blue staining, ×630

Fig. 1b. Compact cells of the inner zona fasciculata with very few lipid vacuoles and a large number of pigment bodies. 1 μ thick section, Toluidine-blue staining, ×630

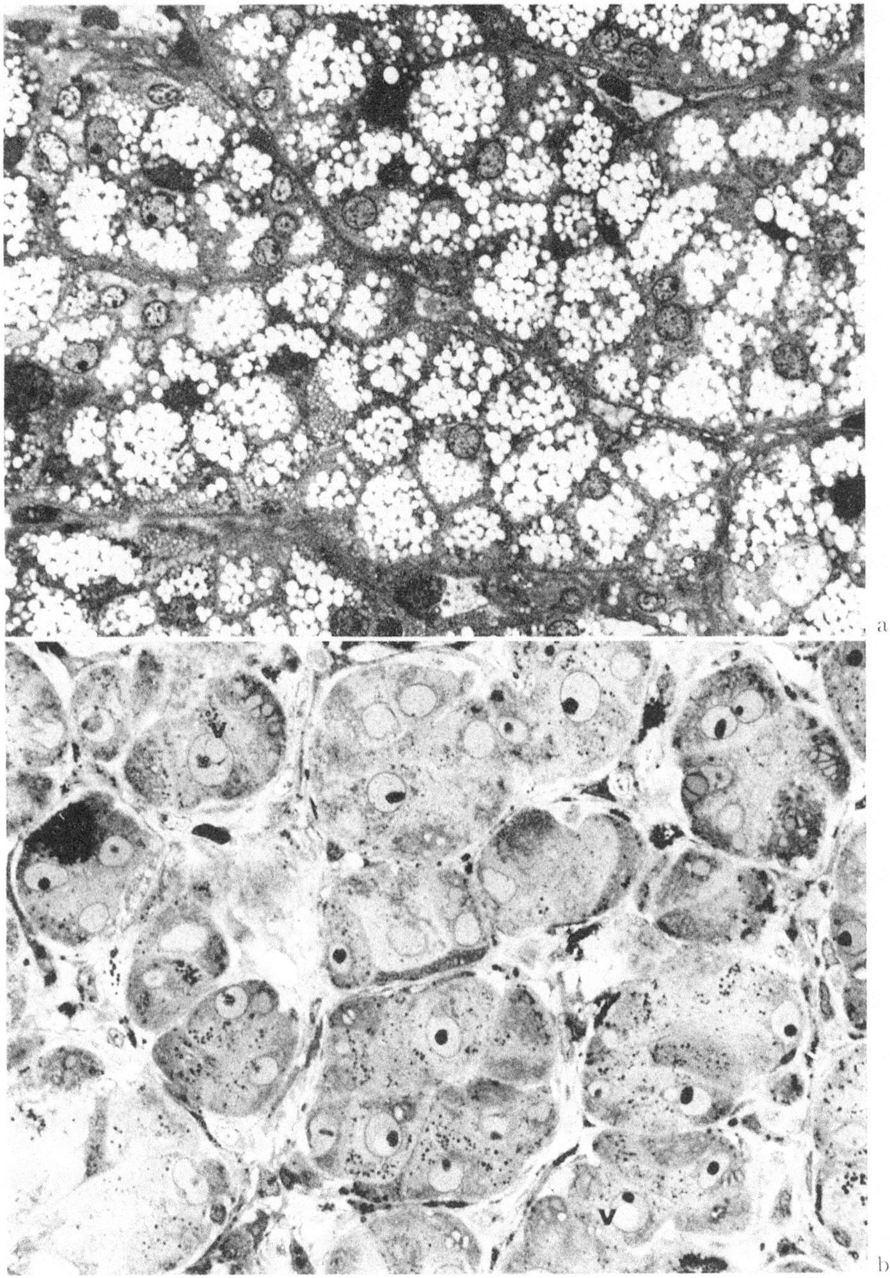

Fig. 2a. Clear cell adenoma with lipid-rich tumor cells and scanty interstitial fibrous tissue with capillaries. 1 μ thick section, Toluidin-blue staining, × 630

Fig. 2b. Compact cell adenoma with alveolar arrangement of the tumor cells. They contain only very few liposomes in contrast to a large number of pigment bodies. Nuclei with prominent nucleoli and occasionally with nuclear vacuoles (*V*). 1 μ thick section, Toluidin-blue staining, × 630

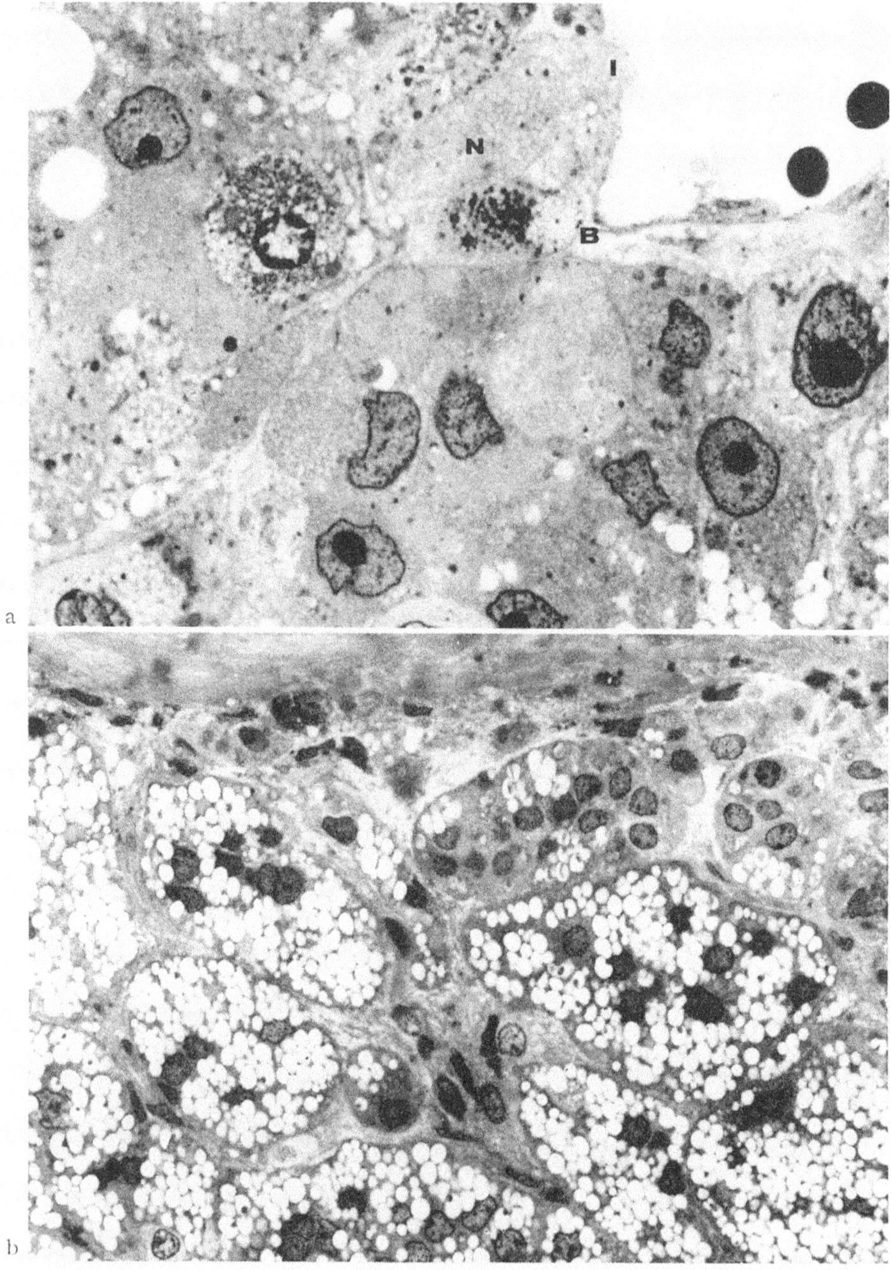

Fig. 3a. Carcinoma of the adrenal cortex with predominating pleomorphic compact tumor cells and focal necrosis (*N*). Interruption of the basement membrane (*B*) with invasion (*I*) of a sinusoidal-like capillary. Pleomorphism of nuclei with giant nucleoli. 1 µ thick section, Toluidine-blue staining, × 630

Fig. 3b. Atrophic adrenal cortex, attached to a hormonal-active adrenal adenoma. Glomerular formation of subcapsular cells with disarrangement of the zona fasciculata, composed of lipid-rich cells. Increase of interstitial collagen fibers. 1 µ thick section, Toluidine-blue staining, × 630

Both cell types may also be found in *adenomas* where the macroscopic darker areas consist of compact cells (Figs. 2a, 2b) with a high lipofuscin content. Anisocytosis as well as nuclear pleomorphism and hyperchromasia may also be found in compact and particularly in focal cell structure in clear cell adenomas. These structures do not yet justify the assumption of a malignant tumor, however.

The *carcinoma* often shows medullary structures. Numerous sinusoidal vessels may establish pseudopapillary formations. The basement membranes are often interrupted (Fig. 3a) and tumor invasion into vessels can be observed. Extensive necroses can be found in the center of the tumor. The nuclei of the carcinoma cells may appear vesicular and exhibit polymorphism right up to giant nuclear formations with large nucleoli. Mitoses are found to be rare.

IV. Ultrastructural Pathology of the Adrenal Cortex in Cushing's Syndrome

A. Adrenocortical Hyperplasia

In deviation from normal findings more pronounced changes of the *interstitium* occur primarily in cases of nodular hyperplasia (NEVILLE and MACKAY, 1972). TANNENBAUM, (1973) described as well, however, that in cases of diffuse hyperplasia an increase of collagen with extracellular microfibrils as well as substantial amounts of ground substance in the interstitium occurred. In the hyperplastic cortex the cells—as in the normal adrenal gland—are separated by basement membranes from the endothelial cells of the capillaries. The endothelium has numerous pores (MACKAY, 1969).

A surface enlargement of the *cell membranes* can be observed in the form of numerous microvilli which spread out finger-like into the intercellular space (LONG and JONES, 1967b). Such interdigitations of cell membranes also occur in the normal adrenal cortex, particularly in the zona fasciculata and reticularis (LONG and JONES, 1967a, 1967b; MACKAY, 1969).

Numerous vesicles with a fine granular electron-dense membrane (so-called *coated vesicles*) often lie in the cytoplasm adjacent to these cell membrane folds. Such vesicles can also be found near the Golgi complex (LONG and JONES, 1967a, 1967b; MACKAY, 1969). These structures are supposed to be a gauge for an increased micropinocytosis. We also saw these granular vesicles in part as seclusion of the granular endoplasmic reticulum which, in addition to an increased pinocytosis, may perhaps also serve as an increased extrusion of cellular products into the extracellular space (MITSCHKE *et al.*, 1971). Similar findings with multiplication of the microvilli as well as a substantial increase of pinocytose processes were also shown in animal experiments following ACTH stimulation.

A substantial variability of *mitochondrial structure* in Cushing's syndrome is repeatedly reported (MACKAY, 1969; MITSCHKE *et al.*, 1971; REIDBORD and

Fisher, 1968; Tannenbaum, 1973). The mitochondria have increased in number and size (Fig. 4) and the inner structures also appear to increase. Tannenbaum (1973) often found giant mitochondria in cases of diffuse and particularly in cases of nodular hyperplasia. Tubular and occasional lamellar cristae may be observed in addition to the typical vesicular cristae. The matrix is more electron-dense and may contain dense intramitochondrial bodies (Hashida et al., 1970). The outer mitochondrial membrane may display bulges (Hashida et al., 1970) with whorl-like arrangement of the bordering membrane systems (Fig. 7b) which appear in direct continuity with formations of the endoplasmic reticulum (Mitschke et al., 1971).

Kadioglu and Harrison (1972) described these in similar form as polylaminary membranous mitochondria in the rat adrenal cortex. Volk (1971b) similarly demonstrated mitochondrial tubular membrane connections in the rat adrenal cortex.

In animal experiments, as well, ACTH leads to an increase of mitochondria (Sekiyama and Yago, 1972), whereby first an increase in the volume of the individual mitochondria, then an increase in the number of mitochondria concomitant with a decrease of the individual volume, and finally an increase in mitochondrial number and volume occurs (Nussdorfer et al., 1974). After ACTH as well as after cAMP and cGMP, this trophic and steroidogenic effect can be observed not only on the mitochondria but on the nuclei, lipid vacuoles and Golgi complexes (Nussdorfer and Mazzocchi, 1972, 1973) as well.

According to Kahri (1973), the preservation of the internal structures of the mitochondria is dependent upon ACTH. The functional relationship between mitochondrial structure and steroid biosynthesis was also emphasized by Milner (1971).

Defects occur in the mitochondrial membranes in rats after treatment with ACTH with the result that the mitochondrial interior communicates with the cytoplasm (Carr, 1961; Luse, 1967) and that the outer membrane of the mitochondria cannot be clearly defined (Ashworth et al., 1959). It is possible that such apertures of the mitochondrial membranes correlate with the degree of ACTH stimulation and cortisol production. An equal explanation is ascribed to the vesicular protrusions of the outer mitochondrial membrane (Idelman, 1970; Sabatini et al., 1962).

Long and Jones (1967a, 1967b), however, viewed such findings as fixation artifacts or as tangential sections. Using morphometrical methods, Nussdorfer and Mazzocchi (1972) were able to show that the intramitochondrial membranes multiply according to the dose of ACTH given.

In the hyperplastic adrenal cortex close *relations* exist *between the mitochondria and the lipid vacuoles*, the membranes of which appear to be dented by mitochondrial protrusions. Occasionally, the passage of lipid into the mitochondrial interior accompanied by disintegration of the outer membranes can be observed (Mitschke et al., 1971). Such close relationships were also described by Mackay (1969) who, however, viewed the lipid transition as an artifact.

The disintegration of mitochondrial membranes with vesicular storage of lipids could be induced by aminoglutethimide in rats (KADIOGLU and HARRISON, 1971; MAREK et al., 1970).

In cortical hyperplasia the *lipid globules* appear as large membrane-bound vacuoles which sometimes contain a sickle or ring–shaped, slightly osmiophilic margin. Usually they appear empty due to the removal of lipids during preparation of the tissue particles and sections. Depending upon the kind of tissue preparation, an extremely varied liposomal structure could be shown in the rat adrenal (NAKAMURA, 1973). In small lipid vacuoles with an osmiophilic content a membrane could not always be observed.

A decrease of lipid vacuoles in rats was accompanied by an increased regeneration of mitochondria after ACTH stimulation (ASHWORTH et al., 1959; LUSE, 1967; MÄUSLE, 1971; RHODIN, 1971).

Close *relations* also exist *between the lipid vacuoles and the agranular endoplasmic reticulum* (Figs. 4, 5). The direct passage of lipid into the smooth endoplasmic reticulum as was shown in an adenoma in one case of Conn-syndrome (PROPST, 1965) has not, however, been demonstrated in Cushing's syndrome. The *smooth endoplasmic reticulum* in the cortical cells is conspicuously developed in cases of hyperplasia, especially in compact cells, and composed of dilated vesicular and tubular systems (HARTEMANN et al., 1971; HASHIDA et al., 1970; MACKAY, 1969; MITSCHKE et al., 1971; REIDBORD and FISHER, 1968). In human (CARR, 1961) as well as in animal experiments an increase and vesicular transformation of the smooth endoplasmic reticulum could be achieved by means of ACTH stimulation (ASHWORTH et al., 1959; IDELMAN, 1970; SEKIYAMA and YAGO, 1972) (Fig. 8). This was morphometrically quantified in animal experiments (NUSSDORFER et al., 1971). According to these findings the agranular endoplasmic reticulum is the most important parameter for judging the steroidegenic activity of the adrenal cortex cells (NUSSDORFER and MAZZOCCHI, 1970).

The close *relationship between the endoplasmic reticulum and mitochondria* is expressed by whorl-like membrane systems (Fig. 7b) with circumscribed transition into the outer mitochondrial membrane. These membrane systems are even more pronounced in the Leydig cells of the mouse (CHRISTENSEN and FAWCETT, 1966). After stimulation with ACTH or gonadotropins, a proliferation of these membrane systems was also observed in adrenal cortical cells (GIACOMELLI et al., 1965) and interpreted as hypertrophy of the smooth endoplasmic reticulum.

Whereas in normal human cortical cells the *granular endoplasmic reticulum* is only moderately pronounced, a variable increase can be observed in cases of hyperplasia and also in tumors (MACKAY, 1969). In the organogenesis of the adrenal cortex, close correlations exist between the appearance of the granular endoplasmic reticulum and the development of the smooth endoplasmic reticulum (McNUTT and JONES, 1970). In connection with the similarly increased free *ribosomes* in cortical cells in cases of hyperplasia, such changes are probably an expression of an increased structural protein synthesis.

H. Mitschke and W. Saeger:

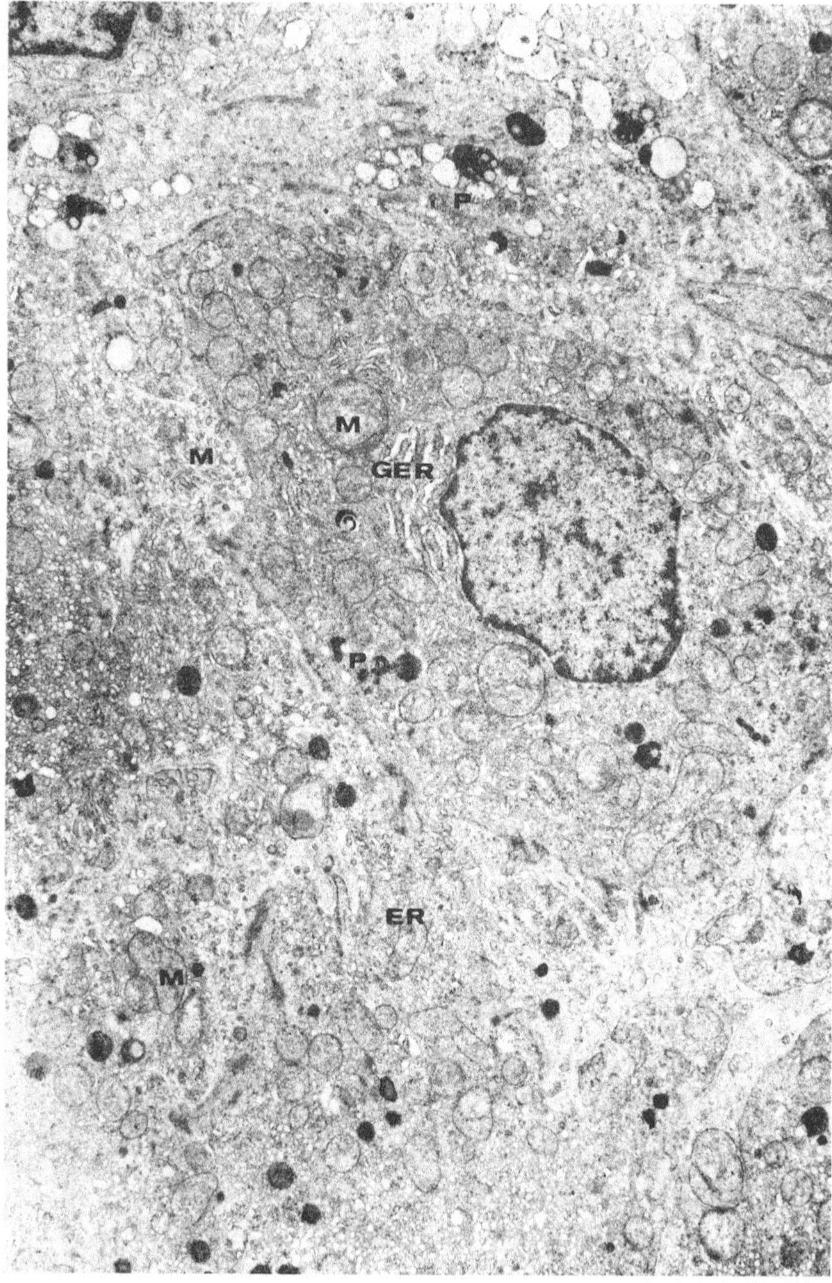

Fig. 4. Compact cells from the zona reticularis of a hyperplastic adrenal cortex. They illustrate an increase of the tubulo-vesicular smooth endoplasmic reticulum (*ER*), numerous pleomorphic mitochondria (*M*), multiple lipid-pigment complexes (*P*) and stacks of granular endoplasmic reticulum (*GER*). Microvillous projections of the cell membrane (*M*) can also be seen. × 8090

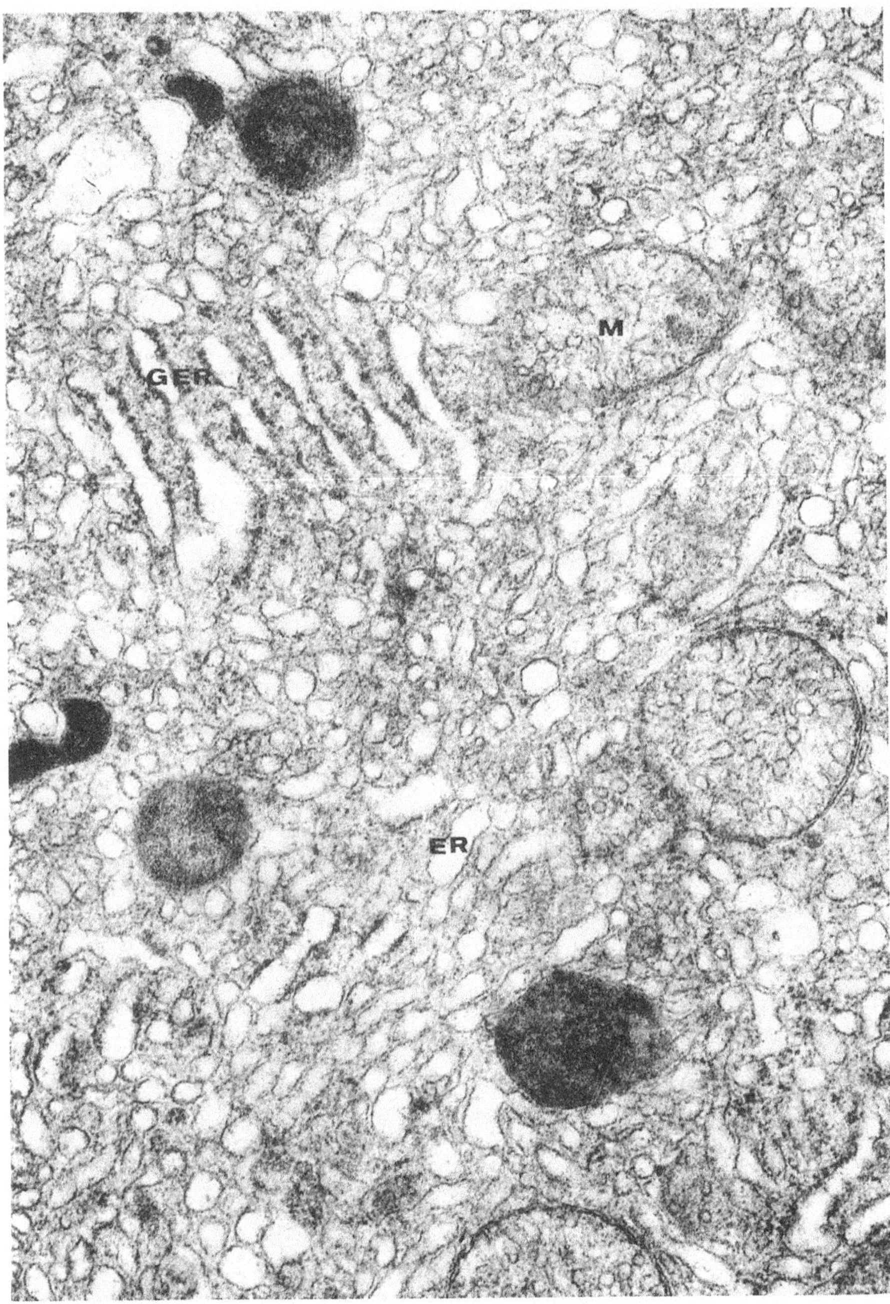

Fig. 5. Compact cell of a diffuse hyperplastic adrenal cortex with variable dilated, partially vesicular agranular endoplasmic reticulum (*ER*) which shows a direct continuity and transition into the granular endoplasmic reticulum (*GER*). The mitochondria (*M*) contain tubulo-vesicular internal structures; in addition a few dense bodies × 27 480

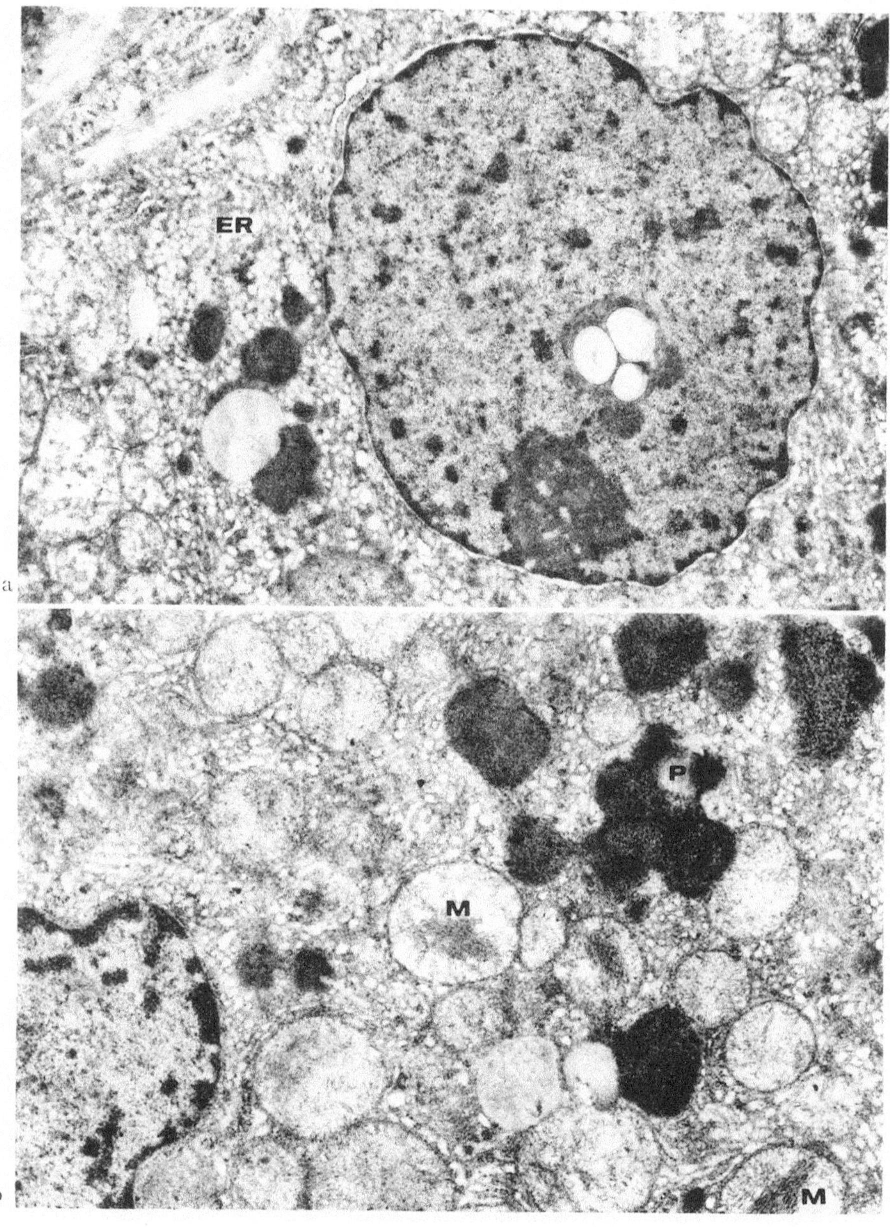

Fig. 6a and b. Nodular hyperplasia of the adrenal cortex. a Compact cell showing dense and dilated agranular endoplasmic reticulum (ER) and a multivesicular nuclear inclusion. $\times 6320$. b Part of compact cell. The mitochondria contain dense tubular internal structures (M) and an electron-lucent matrix. In addition the cytoplasm shows pigment bodies (P) and dilated smooth endoplasmic reticulum. $\times 10115$

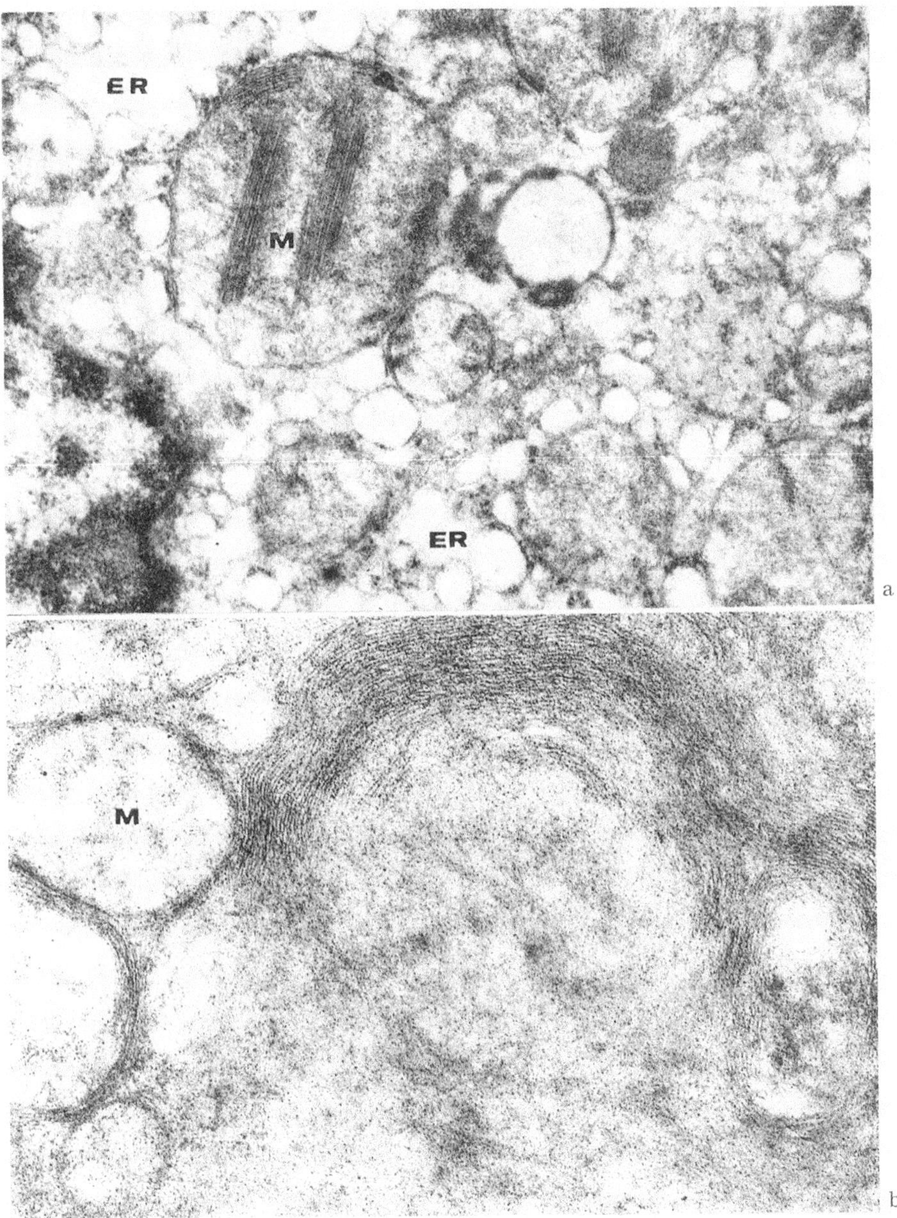

Fig. 7a and b. Nodular hyperplasia of the adrenal cortex with increased production of cortisol, aldosterone and androgens. a Compact cell with crystalline-like mitochondrial inclusion (*M*) and dilatation of the agranular endoplasmic reticulum (*ER*). × 19110. b Part of a compact cell demonstrating whorled membranes of the smooth endoplasmic reticulum in continuity with the outer mitochondrial membrane. × 15700

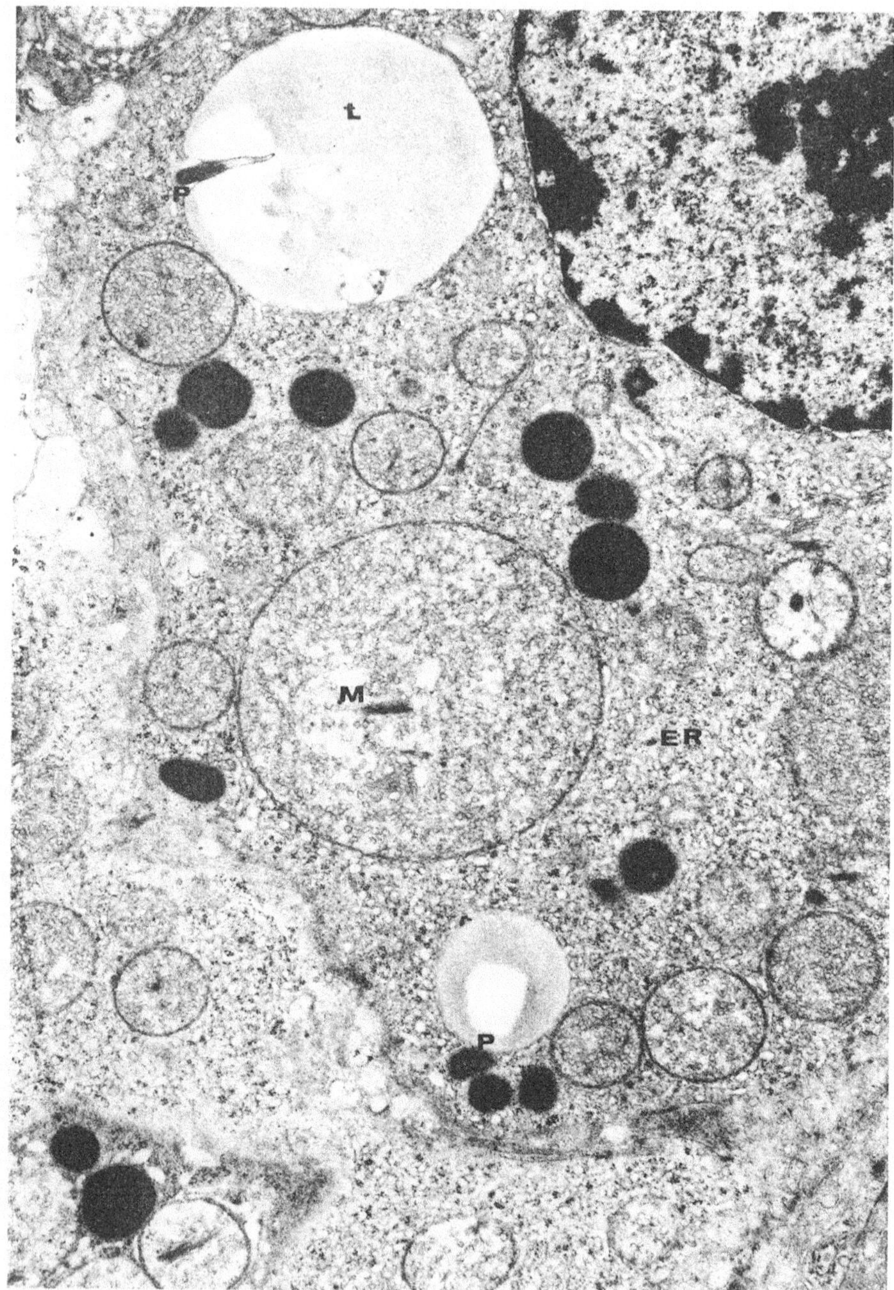

Fig. 8. Zona fasciculata cell of the rat adrenal cortex after stimulation with ACTH. The cell shows a depletion of lipid vacuoles (*L*) with beginning formation of lipid-pigment-complexes (*P*). Numerous pleomorphic mitochondria with occasionally giant mitochondria (*M*) can be seen in addition to an increase of smooth endoplasmic reticulum (*ER*) and ribosomes. × 14 300

The *lipid-pigment-complexes* can be viewed as the ultrastructural correlate of the brown pigmentation observed in many cases. They occur very frequently in the inner zona fasciculata and zona reticularis. According to

CHRISTENSEN'S (1965) examinations of the Leydig cells of guinea pigs, these complexes consist of the following components: 1. the actual pigment, 2. a lipid vacuole, and 3. a lysosomal body. SZABO et al. (1967) were able to reveal the presence of acid phosphatase in these complexes thus proving the existence of lysosomal complexes. Descriptions such as "vacuolar or osmiophilic bodies" (HOLZMANN and LANGE, 1966) or "dense bodies" are used synonomously. Within the "dense bodies" of guinea pig adrenal cortex, peroxydase activity but no acid phosphatase could be observed. Therefore BLACK and BOGART (1973) characterized these bodies as peroxisomes. They appear in the fetal stage of the normal human adrenal cortex (McNUTT and JONES, 1970).

HOLZMANN and LANGE (1966) described enlarged *Golgi complexes* in cases of hyperplasia. MÄUSLE (1971) found conspicuous Golgi complexes in rats following ACTH stimulation.

In comparison to the normal adrenal cortex the *nuclei* in cases of hyperplasia are non-round and sometimes more heterochromatic and equipped with enlarged nucleoli. The space between the nuclear membranes is often dilated. Similar nuclear changes were also described in animal experiments after ACTH stimulation (ASHWORTH et al., 1959; MILLER, 1954; SANDRITTER and HUEBOTTER, 1954).

In cases of *nodular hyperplasia* collagenous fibrils appear in abundance between the cortical cells. The basement membranes also appear to be wider (MACKAY, 1969; TANNENBAUM, 1973). The clear cells of the noduli largely correspond to the cells in the zona fasciculata. The cell organelles however show obvious structural alterations (MACKAY, 1969).

In a particular case of bilateral nodular hyperplasia with increased secretion of cortisol, aldosterone and androgens, a more abundantly developed granular endoplasmic reticulum and a conspicuously developed smooth endoplasmic reticulum could be observed in addition to the above described findings. It was arranged in whorls or spirals (Fig. 7b) and appeared to be partially confluent with the outer mitochondrial membranes. The close relationship to the mitochondria is also emphasized by FLADERER et al. (1974) who described similar changes in a Leydig-cell tumor. We could not prove the existance of crystalline cytoplasmic inclusions similar to Reinke's crystals in Leydig cells as found by MAGALHAES (1972) in male adrenal cortices which seemed to be related to androgen secretion.

In addition, we could observe tuft-like and usually elongated membranes in the mitochondrial interior (Figs. 6b, 7a). They did not correspond to the electron-dense intramitochondrial granula, which have often been shown in compact cells in cases of hyperplasia (MACKAY, 1969) and which were also found in zona glomerulosa cells of sheep by LUTHMAN (1971). Similar paracrystalline formations were found by FLADERER et al. (1974) in the cells of an adrenal carcinoma and by GIACOMELLI et al. (1965) in the zona glomerulosa after sodium restriction. Such changes are viewed as an expression of increased hormone synthesis.

In this case we also found a nuclear inclusion consisting of several vacuoles (Fig. 6a). These are more often described as invaginations if surrounded by nuclear membranes—which, however, could not be observed here.

These ultrastructural deviations from the above described changes in adrenal hyperplasia could be related to a multihormonal secretion of steroid hormones. Thus, the ultrastructural examination of the adrenal cortex permits not only a differentiation between active and inactive cortical cells, but can also possibly yield evidence for the actual varying hormonal secretion in individual cases.

Ultrastructural alterations of adrenal cortical hyperplasia after therapy with adrenostatic drugs:

In cases of diffuse hyperplasia no particular alterations of the mitochondria could be shown after treatment with *Metyrapone*, an inhibitor of 11-β-hydroxylase (Mackay, 1969). By contrast, changes were observed in rats. The mitochondria showed a loss of cristae (Sekiyama and Yago, 1972). After treatment with *Aminoglutethimide* which inhibits the conversion of cholesterol to pregnenolone, numerous membrane-bound lipid vacuoles appeared. The mitochondria displayed extremely varied structures with circumscribed swellings and also diminutions and a more osmiophilic matrix. The smooth endoplasmic reticulum remained largely unaffected (Mackay, 1969).

After treatment of a nodular hyperplasia with o,p'-DDD the mitochondria showed a pronounced swelling with a lighter matrix and sparse internal structures (Mackay, 1969).

B. Adrenal Cortical Tumors

1. Adrenal Cortical Adenomas

a) Clear Cell Adenoma

A basement membrane is developed around the capillaries and adenoma cells. In contrast to the zona reticularis or to nodular hyperplasia, only sparse collagenous fibrils can be shown in the interstitium beside the capillaries (Mackay, 1969). The cell membranes are primarily elongated although twisting or microvillous projections can appear in circumscribed areas. The number of microvilli can be larger than in normal cortical cells (Mackay, 1969).

The clear cells are characterized ultrastructurally by numerous, densely placed and membrane-bound lipid vacuoles (Fig. 9). They can also be confluent with an interruption of the liposomal membranes. Cells rich in lipid globules contain only few and small mitochondria. These are anisomorphous with lamellar and tubular cristae. We also saw these granular vesicles at least partially deriving and seperating from the granular endoplasmic reticulum which developed in lipid-rich cells whereas the granular endoplasmic reticulum may also appear in circumscribed areas. The Golgi complexes are not prominent. Furthermore the cells contain small lipid-pigment complexes and the nuclei

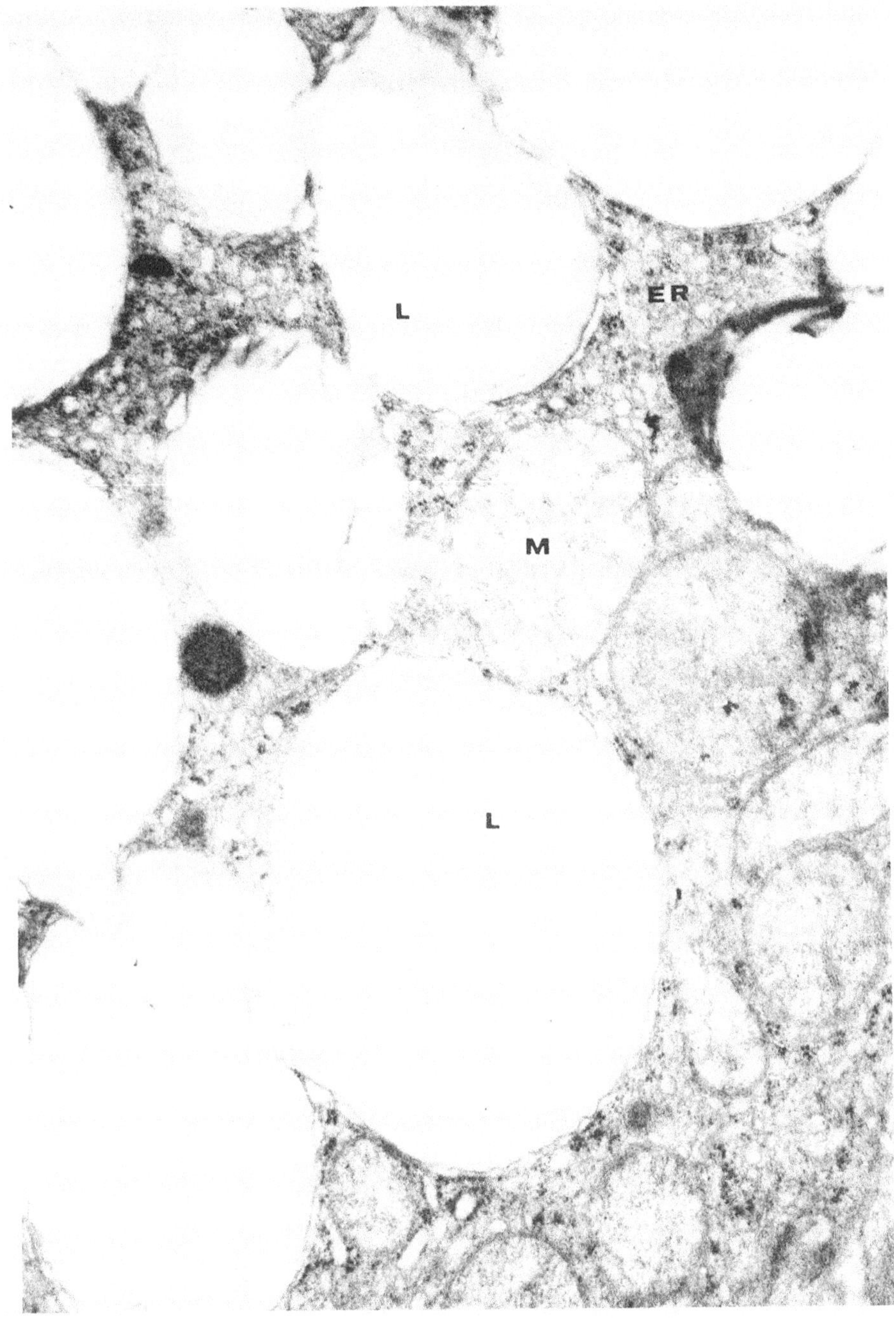

Fig. 9. Clear cell adenoma with large, membrane-bound and partially confluating lipid vacuoles (*L*), mitochondria (*M*) with pale matrix and rather few tubular cristae and a poorly developed agranular endoplasmic reticulum (*ER*). × 20950

can be irregularly configurated. The nucleoli of the clear adenoma cells are, however, not conspicuously enlarged.

In individual cases myelolipomatous formations may also be observed in circumscribed areas of clear cell adenomas. Ultrastructurally there is no connection between these foci and regressively altered adenoma cells. Moreover, it was not possible to definitely associate these formations to reticulohistiocytic cells.

b) Compact Cell Adenoma

In contrast to the interstitium where no alteration in the clear cell adenoma was observed, a conspicuous development of the steroid hormone producing organelle system could be noticed in the compact adenoma cells (BAHU et al., 1974; LUSE, 1967; MACKAY, 1969; MITSCHKE et al., 1973; NEVILLE and MACKAY, 1972; TANNENBAUM, 1973). The agranular endoplasmic reticulum in form of densely placed tubular and vesicular structures dominates the cytoplasm (Figs. 10, 11a). In comparison to hyperplasia the granular endoplasmic reticulum is also more conspicuously developed. In addition, numerous mitochondria can be observed which are anisomorphous, ranging from large to the development of giant mitochondria and primarily contain densely placed parallel cristae. Next to fragments of granular endoplasmic reticulum, numerous and partly aggregated ribosomes can also be observed. Characteristically, the compact adenoma cells contain only very few and small osmiophilic lipid vacuoles. According to MACKAY (1969), the lipids in less differentiated adenoma cells occur more frequently in free form, without membrane enclosure, as osmiophilic lipid droplets. The lipid-pigment complexes are conspicuously increased.

MACADAM (1970) proved the existence of cytoplasmic inclusions in a compact adenoma in a case of Cushing's syndrome. The inclusions, seen in cross–sections, had a cristalloid structure and were enclosed by a membrane. Their significance remained unclear since they did not correspond to the cristalline inclusion which MAGALHAES (1972) observed in individual peri-endothelial cells of male adrenal cortex.

The nuclei of compact cellular adenomas are in part very irregularly configurated with deep invaginations (BAHU et al., 1974; MACKAY, 1969; MITSCHKE et al., 1973) (Fig. 10) which, according to individual sections, can also appear as so-called nuclear inclusions. The space between the nuclear membranes is widened in circumscribed areas. In comparison to the clear cell adenoma and to hyperplasia the nucleoli are distinctly enlarged and very electron dense.

In the special case of a 30 g compact cell adenoma in a three-year-old girl with increased glucocorticoid- and androgen secretion, even more abundantly developed granular endoplasmic reticulum and large Golgi complexes could be observed thus deviating from the above described compact adenoma cells. By comparison, the smooth endoplasmic reticulum was rather reduced (Fig. 12). The numerous mitochondria were primarily ovoid or elongated with small

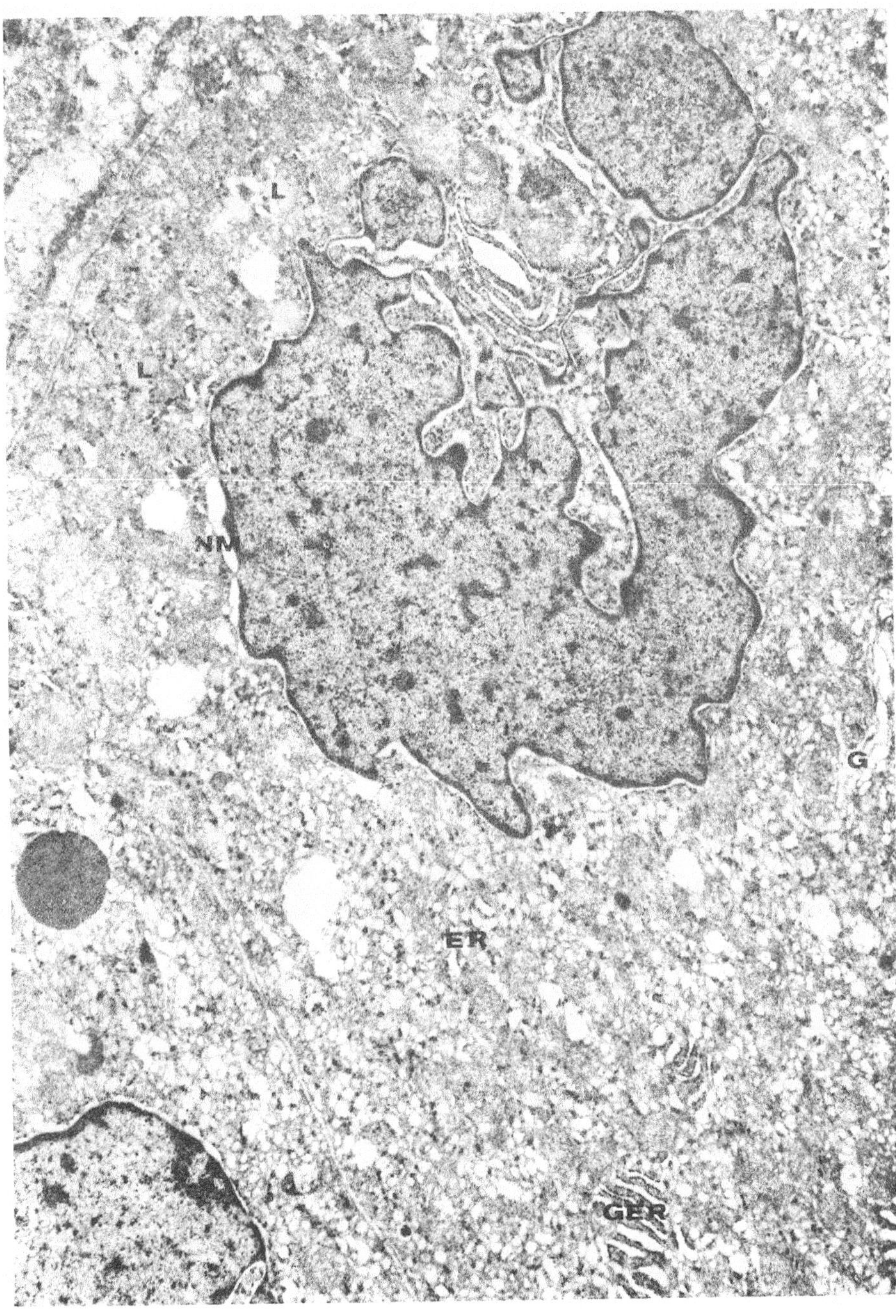

Fig. 10. Compact cell adenoma. The cells contain vera few lipid vacuoles (*L*). The agranular endoplasmic reticulum (*ER*) is increased, with stacks of granular endoplasmic reticulum (*GER*), a prominent Golgi complex (*G*) and numerous aggregated ribosomes. The nucleus shows a bizarre configuration with deep invaginations and a dilated space between the nuclear membranes (*NM*). ×8340

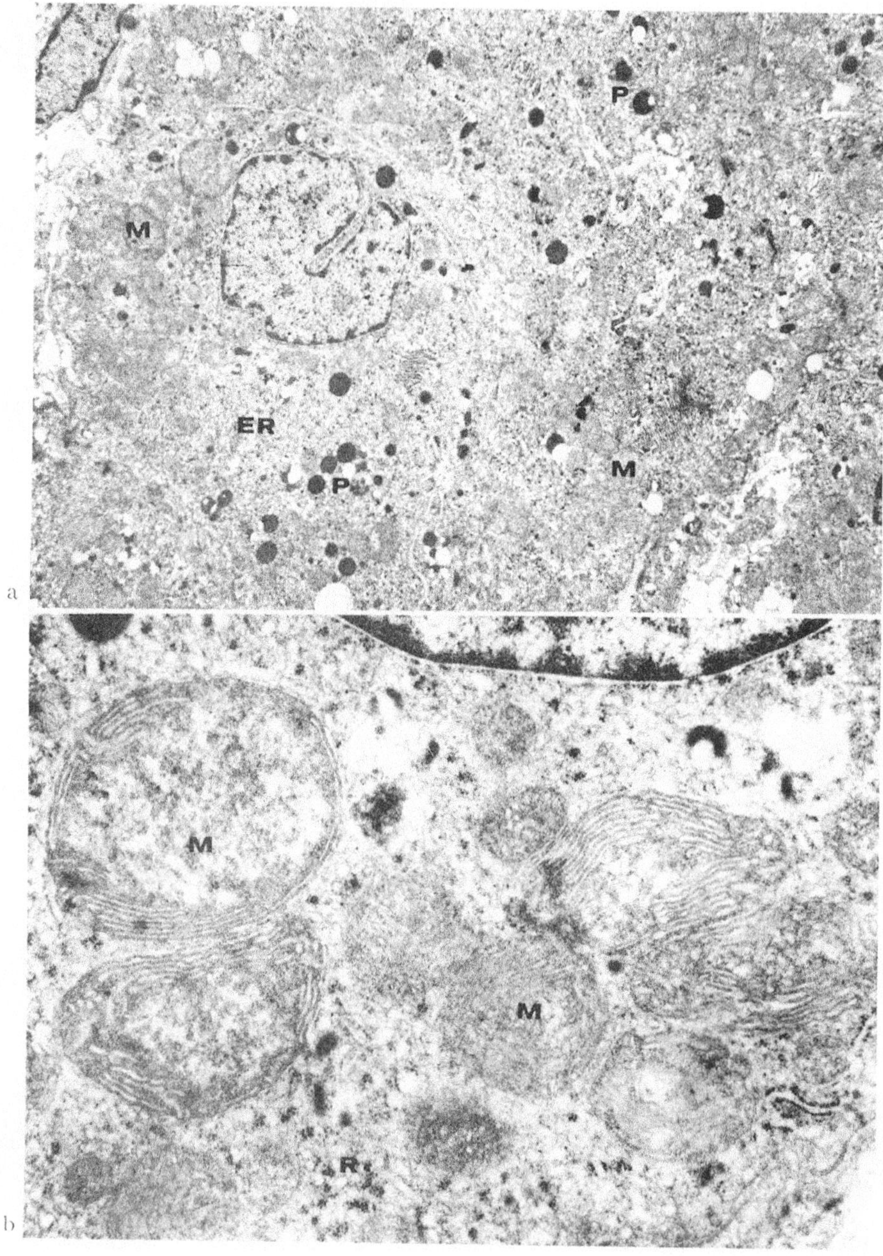

Fig. 11a and b. Compact cell adenoma. a Prominent agranular endoplasmic reticulum
(*ER*) besides numerous mitochondria (*M*) and multiple pigment complexes (*P*). ×4650.
b Demonstration of the variability of mitochondria with predominantly parallel internal
membranes (*M*) besides free and small fragments of membrane-bound ribosomes (*R*).
×13680

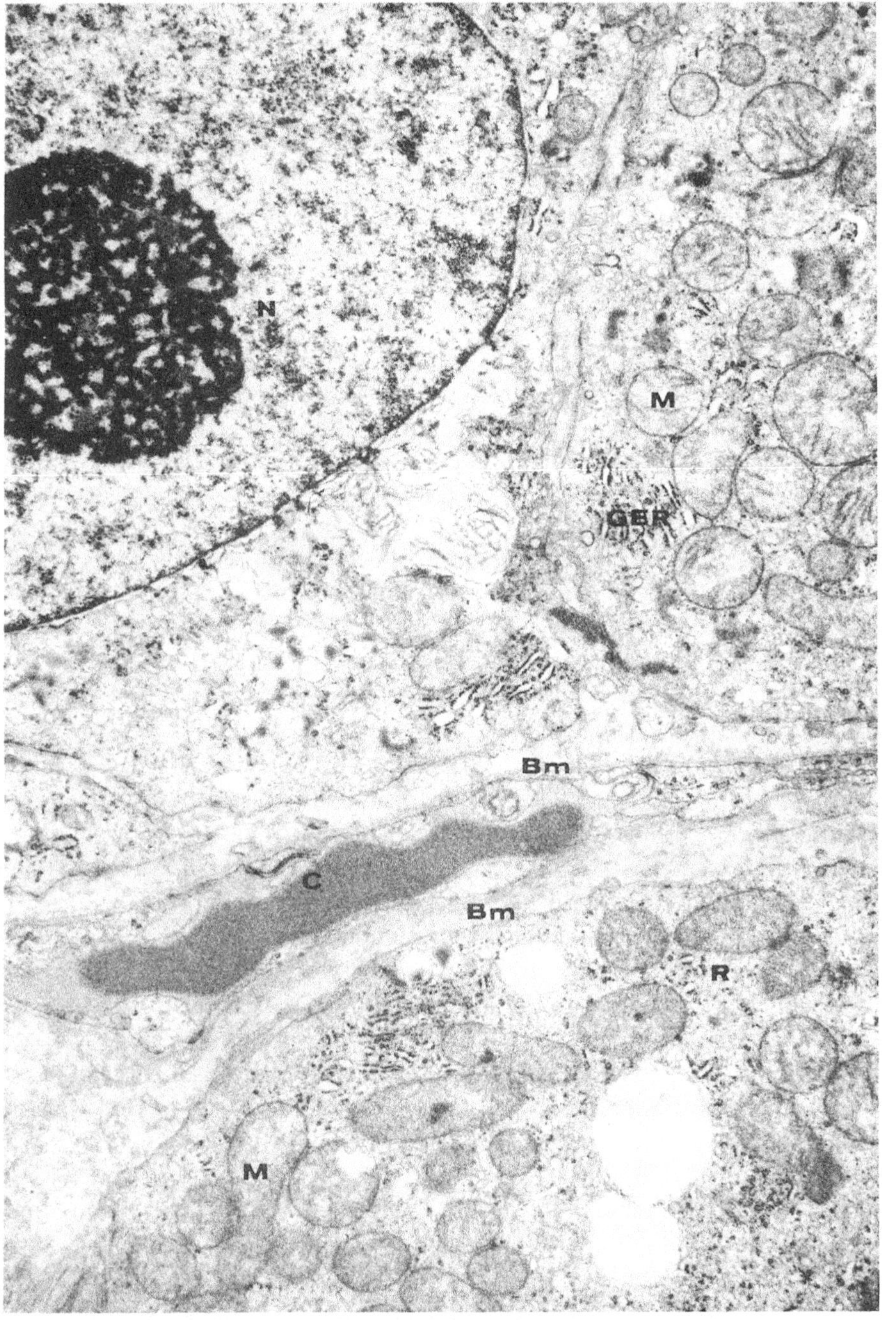

Fig. 12. Compact cell adenoma of a 3 year old girl with increased production of cortisol and androgens. The center is occupied by a capillary (C) with endothel cells and basement membranes (Bm). The tumor cells contain numerous, partially elongated mitochondria (M) with rather few, laminated cristae and occasionally intramitochondrial granules. The agranular endoplasmic reticulum seems diminished in contrast to a well-developed granular endoplasmic reticulum (GER) and many free ribosomes in addition to small pigment bodies. Nucleus (N) with a large nucleolus. × 8280

irregular cristae. Occasionally, they contained intramitochondrial granula. Lipid vacuoles were rare, and in addition, small bizarrely configurated pigment bodies could be observed. Cristalline cytoplasmic inclusions were not present. The ovoid, euchromatin-rich nuclei contained very large nucleoli. As evidence for the benign nature of this tumor one could observe a clear demarcation of the adenoma cells from the interstitium by basement membranes.

Further analogies to cells of the zona reticularis which—on the basis of ultrastructural examination of an androgen–secreting, masculinising adrenal cortical adenoma—were described by Fisher and Danowski (1973), could not be found in our case.

Fisher's and Danowski's (1973) findings of a swelling of the mitochondria with laminar cristae, the numerous lipofuscin bodies, the many free, aggregated ribosomes and the villiform surface enlargement of the cell membranes also occur in adenomas with Cushing's syndrome.

2. Carcinoma of the Adrenal Cortex

In contrast to the adenomas, the basement membranes around the tumor cells are not completely preserved (Mackay, 1969). The cell membranes show evidence of individual interdigitation. According to Tannenbaum (1973), the plasmalemma of the carcinoma cells have particularly complex invaginations.

In the literature one finds various accounts on the content of cell organelles in carcinoma cells. Neville and Mackay (1972) described variably formed steroid hormone producing organelle systems. Thiele (1974) was able to demonstrate an increase of smooth and granular endoplasmic reticulum, the mitochondria, and Golgi complexes. Our own examinations revealed primarily a reduction of the smooth endoplasmic reticulum and mitochondria (Mitschke et al., 1973) (Fig. 13). Mackay (1969), too, described a reduction of the agranular endoplasmic reticulum, whereby its development is parallel to the formation of other cytoplasmic organelles.

The equal distribution of cellular organelles is reversed in carcinoma cells. The mitochondria form clusters (Mackay, 1969; Tannenbaum, 1973), possibly because of rapid mitochondrial division without dispersion over the cytoplasm. They are anisomorphous and matrix-rich with sparse and irregular inner structures. Occasionally a giant mitochondrion can be observed (Thiele, 1974). In circumscribed areas condensation products of mitochondria can be observed which, in part, resemble structures produced in animal experiments (Magalhaes and Magalhaes, 1968) or, also, paracristalline inclusions (Fladerer et al., 1974; Mitschke et al., 1973) which are surrounded by circular cytomembranes. Similar structures were also described by Kimmel et al. (1974) in Snell adrenal carcinoma 494. The smooth endoplasmic reticulum encloses, in part, other cell organelles and, in circumscribed areas, is in direct continuity with the granular endoplasmic reticulum (Thiele, 1974). The latter occurs primarily in numerous short fragments and does not appear to be more

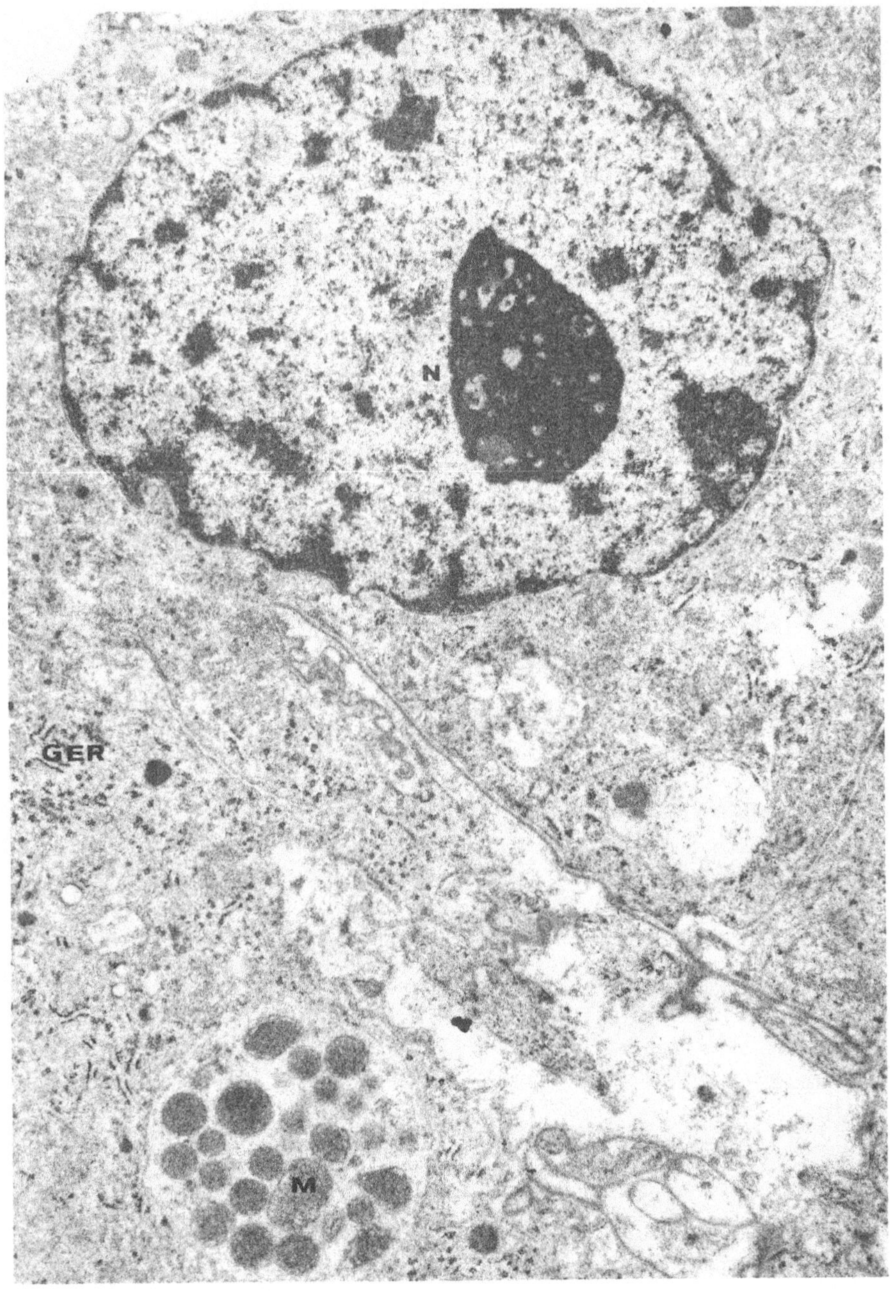

Fig. 13. Carcinoma of the adrenal cortex. The cytoplasmic process at the lower left corner contains clusters of mitochondria (*M*) with an electron-dense matrix. The cytoplasm shows only few organelles with scattered granular endoplasmic reticulum (*GER*) and polyribosomes. Nucleus (*N*) with an irregular, prominent nucleolus. × 15100

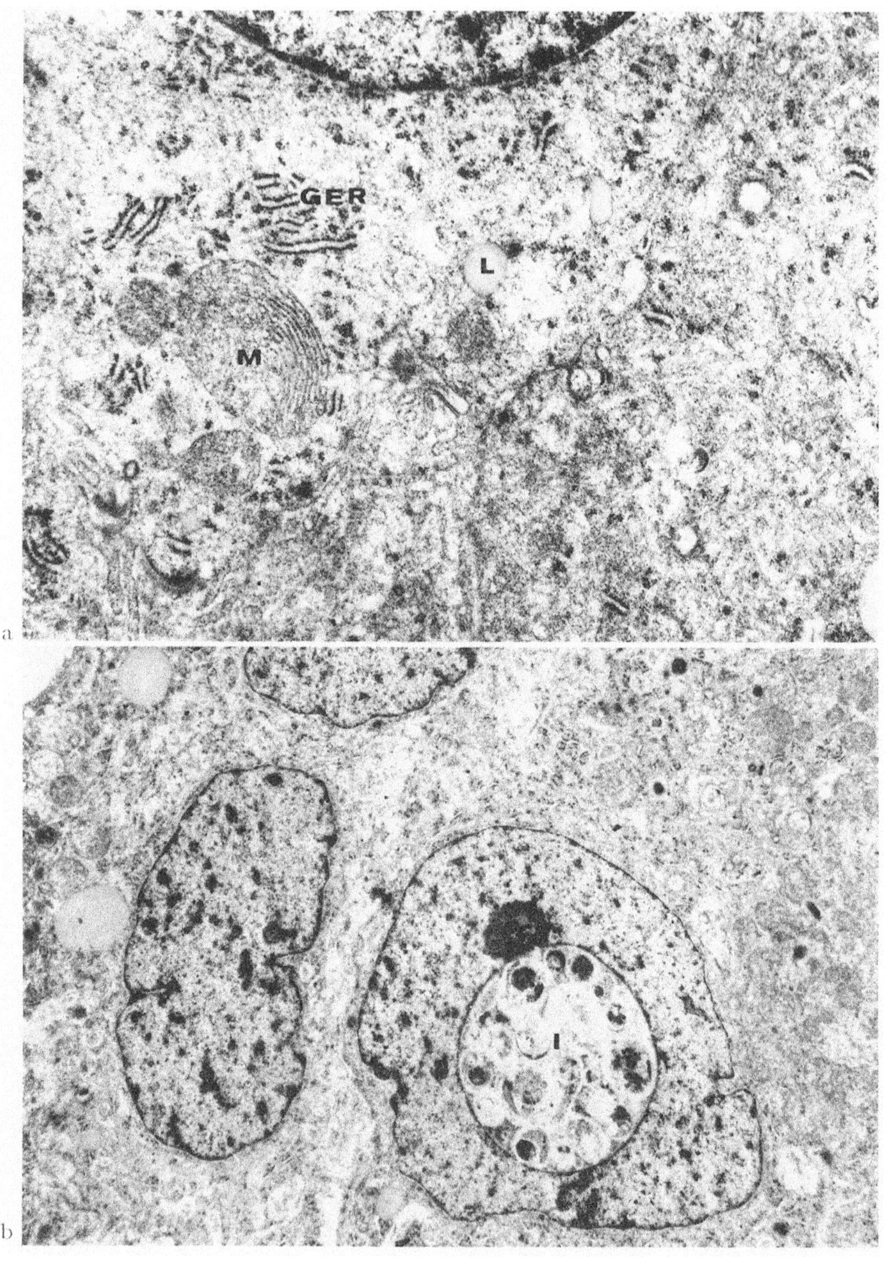

Fig. 14a and b. Carcinoma of the adrenal cortex. a The cytoplasm shows only a few atypical mitochondria (*M*), osmiophilic lipid vacuoles (*L*), scattered granular endoplasmic reticulum (*GER*) and polyribosomes. × 10125. b Nuclear invagination containing degraded cytoplasmic organelles. × 5400

conspicuously developed than in compact adenoma cells (Fig. 14a). By contrast, free and aggregated ribosomes can be observed in abundance and are distributed diffusely over the cytoplasm. THIELE (1974) described large Golgi complexes in carcinoma cells. Liposomes can be observed in equally small number and variable size as in compact adenoma cells. The distribution of pleomorphous lysosomal pigment complexes is also variable (MITSCHKE *et al.*, 1973; THIELE, 1974). The nuclei of carcinoma cells show a very bizarre configuration with deep invaginations and individual nuclear inclusions (Figs. 13, 14b) (MACKAY, 1969; MITSCHKE *et al.*, 1973; TANNENBAUM, 1973; THIELE, 1974). They contain very large, partially doubled and electron dense nucleoli which have lost their round form. Individual perichromatin granules may be observed in the area of the nuclear membrane.

An animal experimental model for the adrenal carcinoma exists in the adrenal carcinoma 494 which develops spontaneously and can be transplanted (SNELL and STEWART, 1959). It is ultrastructurally characterized by relatively sparse lipid vacuoles and mitochondria with a conspicuous granular and smooth endoplasmic reticulum as well as numerous polysomes (SHARMA and HASHIMOTO, 1972). The few mitochondria contain only sparse lamellar cristae (KIMMEL *et al.*, 1974).

3. Ultrastructural Signs for Differentiating Between Glucocorticoid and Mineralocorticoid Hormone Producing and Functionally Inactive Adenomas

Although with light microscopic examinations parallels appear to exist between clear and compact cortical cells and the corresponding tumor cells, quantitative and qualitative alterations of the cell organelles in adenoma as well as in carcinoma cells can be proven electronmicroscopically (MACKAY, 1969; MITSCHKE *et al.*, 1973; TANNENBAUM, 1973). These alterations are—in comparison to the normal adrenal cortex—more clearly evident in compact cell adenomas than in clear cell tumors.

They consist in a substantial increase of the smooth and granular endoplasmic reticulum, free ribosomes, and an increase and pleomorphism of mitochondria. These contain, at least in part, fewer tubulovesicular internal structures and rather lamellar cristae. The configuration of the nucleus is more variable and often bizarre, whereby in compact adenoma and carcinoma, cells with very large nucleoli can be observed.

By contrast, the *adenomas with Conn-Syndrome* are unanimously described as lipid-rich tumors. The cells contain numerous membrane-bound lipid vacuoles (CERVOS-NAVARRO *et al.*, 1965; KOVACS *et al.*, 1974; LUSE, 1967; MACKAY, 1969; NEVILLE and MACKAY, 1972; PROPST, 1965; REIDBORD and FISHER, 1969; TANNENBAUM, 1973; TSUCHIYAMA, 1967). It should be worth noting that the mitochondria are partially elongated and have lamellar cristae as in the normal cells of the zona glomerulosa (LONG and JONES, 1967b; LUSE, 1967; MACKAY, 1969). In aldosteronomas, however mitochondria with tubulovesicular cristae can be observed such as those in cortisol producing tumors, so that one may speak of hybrid cells with light microscopic characteristics of the zona fasciculata and a biochemical capacity to produce aldosterone (Reidbord and Fisher, 1969). The variability of the mitochondrial structures (Kovacs *et al.*, 1974; Mackay, 1969; Sommers and Terzakis, 1970) is also explained as a dependence of the internal membranes on stimulative and inhibitory influences (Kovacs *et al.*, 1974). In addition, numerous lysosomal bodies, an increase of the smooth and granular endoplasmic reticulum, focal lipid depletion and hypertrophy of the Golgi complexes were observed in aldosteronomas (Kovacs *et al.*, 1974).

Only a few ultrastructural examinations concerning *functionally inactive adenomas* or noduli exist (Reidbord and Fisher, 1969; Tannenbaum, 1973).

According to Reidbord and Fisher (1969), these adenoma cells correspond ultrastructurally to a great extent to normal cells of the zona fasciculata. In their opinion an electronmicroscopic examination of such lipid-rich adenomas can—taking into consideration the mitochondrial structures—differentiate between active adenomas with Conn-syndrome and functionally inactive adenomas. Tannenbaum (1973), however, demonstrated in individual inactive adenomas a reduction of the smooth and granular endoplasmic reticulum and an alteration of the mitochondria which did not show the typical internal structures of steroid hormone producing cells. They were located next to lipid vacuoles.

The occasionally observed brown-black pigmentation of adenomas is caused by a lipofuscin accumulation (Garrett and Ames, 1973; Robinson *et al.*, 1972). In view of the cell organelles observed in some of the so-called inactive nodules or adenomas, the concept of a functional inactivity appears questionable. Such adenoma cells are probably hypoactive. They may exhibit an autonomous behavior with regard to their growth but not with regard to their endocrine function.

Animal experiments on cortical noduli in the rat—however without correlating functional studies—gave evidence of an increase of mitochondria and smooth endoplasmic reticulum and enlargement of the Golgi complex in hyperplastic small cellular noduli which was even more conspicuous than in hypertrophic macrocellular ones. The lipid-rich type alone appears to exhibit an advanced phase of an inactive nodule (Sugihara *et al.*, 1973).

4. Ultrastructural Characteristics for Differentiation Between Adrenal Cortical Adenoma and Carcinoma

In the literature many references are made as to the difficulties of establishing a differential diagnosis between adenoma and carcinoma of the adrenal cortex (Kracht and Zimmermann, 1964; Mitschke *et al.*, 1973; Muller *et al.*, 1970; Rückert, 1970; Symington, 1969). In comparison to the adenomas, the carcinoma cells may in circumscribed areas exhibit a more primitive aspect with reduction of the steroid hormone–producing organelle system. The free ribosomes and the nucleoli in particular corresponding to the RNA increase are especially numerous and enlarged. This suggests an increased production of structural proteins and a heightened tendency of cell proliferation. In addition to light microscopic criteria such as vesicular nuclei, enlarged nucleoli, and necrosis, one can include the ultrastructural characteristics of focal clusters of primitive mitochondria and interruptions of the basement membranes (NEVILLE and MACKAY, 1972).

Absolutely reliable characteristics proving malignancy do not, however, exist with regard to the tumors in Cushing's syndrome. The absence of lipid, conspicuous ultrastructural abnormalities, decreased hormone biosynthesis and an increase in malignancy do not always correlate (MACKAY, 1969).

C. Ultrastructural Findings of the Atrophic Adrenal Cortex

Functionally autonomous adrenal tumors with hypercortisolism as well as an exogenous treatment with cortisol lead to an atrophy of the contralateral and the ipsilateral attached cortex. Since the secretion af aldosterone is not affected (BAYER et al., 1960; LUSE, 1967; MÜLLER et al., 1967; NORMAN et al., 1968; THOMAS and EL-SHABOURY, 1971), the term "dissociated secondary adrenal cortical insufficiency" was coined. Histologically and ultrastructurally the zona glomerulosa thus remains largely unchanged.

In the zona fasciculata which exhibits an obvious transformation of the normally fascicular cortical formations, large densely placed lipid vacuoles appear (LUSE, 1967; MACKAY, 1969; MITSCHKE and SAEGER, 1973) (Figs. 3 b, 15). Most of the large lipid globules appear empty, whereas the smaller ones still possess a weak osmiophilic content. The lipid vacuoles are confluent in part or closely packed in complexes. The suppressive effect of the increased, circulating steroid hormone levels effects a reduction of the endoplasmic reticulum and the mitochondria. The small, sparse mitochondria contain only stubby, tubular cristae. Agranular endoplasmic reticulum is almost entirely absent, whereas the granular endoplasmic reticulum can still be observed in fragments (LUSE, 1967; MACKAY, 1969; MITSCHKE and SAEGER, 1973). The nuclei are irregularly configurated with an increase of heterochromatin. We once observed a nuclear inclusion made up of concentric lamellae with varying electron density (MITSCHKE and SAEGER, 1973). PROPST (1970) described a similar finding in an aldosteronoma.

A zona reticularis cannot be defined within the small inner cortical layers. The cells here are characterized by numerous lipid-pigment complexes and elongated mitochondria. The lipid vacuoles are less numerous and the interstitial collagenous fibres are more abundant.

The atrophy of the steroid hormone producing organelle system can be explained on one hand by the decreased trophic effect of the reduced ACTH levels and on the other hand by a negative feed back mechanism in the adrenal

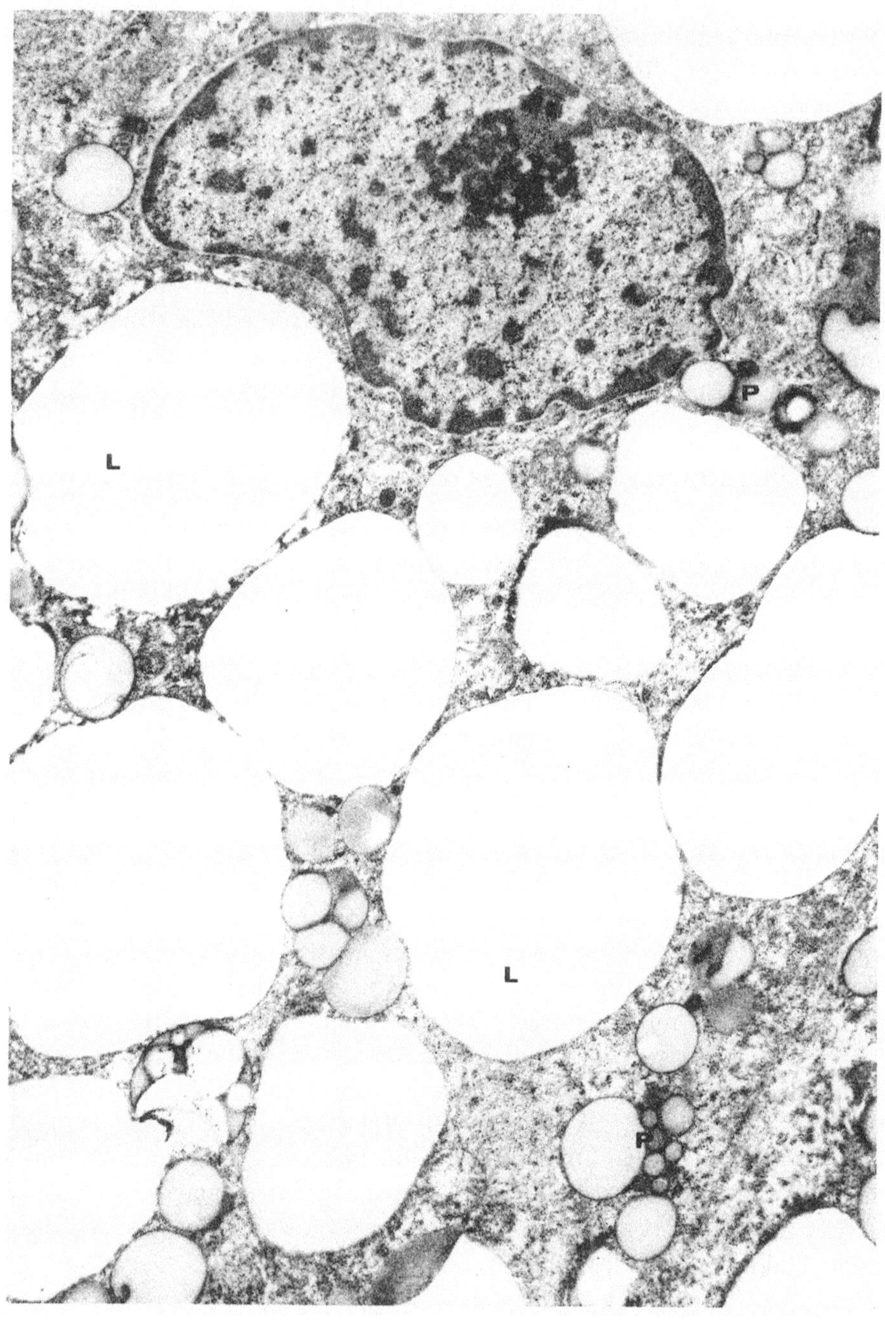

Fig. 15. Secondary atrophy of the adrenal cortex, attached to an adrenal tumor. The zona fasciculata cell demonstrates clusters of large, membrane-bound lipid vacuoles (*L*) besides lipid-pigment complexes (*P*) in addition to an obvious decrease of mitochondria and agranular endoplasmic reticulum. × 7890

cortex itself caused by the increased glucocorticoidhormone levels (Nuss-DORFER, 1970; NUSSDORFER and MAZZOCCHI, 1970, 1971a). In animal experiments these lead to a marked inhibition of protein synthesis in the cortical cells (KAHRI, 1973; UEBERBERG *et al.*, 1970).

Similar ultrastructural alterations comparable to the atrophic cortex in humans could also be shown in animal experiments after hypophysectomy (CANICK and PURVIS, 1972; FUJITA, 1972; IDELMAN, 1970), by exogenous corticoid administration (BOROWICZ, 1965; BRAUNSTEINER *et al.*, 1955; CANICK and PURVIS, 1972; NUSSDORFER, 1970; NUSSDORFER and MAZZOCCHI, 1970; RHODIN, 1971; WYLLIE *et al.*, 1973) or in rats bearing a corticosteron producing tumor (Snell 494 adrenal carcinoma) (NICKERSON, 1973).

In the inactive mitochondria which is partially fused into giant mito-chondria (CANICK and PURVIS, 1972), the matrix often appears empty with reduced cristae. Occasionally, bizarre mitochondrial configurations with para-cristalline-appearing lamellar systems can be noticed (Fig. 16).

As shown in tissue cultures, the altered mitochondria can be restored into the active form by ACTH administration (KAHRI, 1970). The endoplasmic reticulum is reduced (Figs. 16, 17a, 17b). The large lipid vacuoles represent the substrate of a greatly diminished conversion of cholesterol into pregnenolone in the absence of ACTH stimulation. This increase and enlargement of the lipid vacuoles right up to fatty degeneration of cortical cells was also described following hypophysectomy (FUJITA, 1972; IDELMAN, 1970). RHODIN (1971) found cristalline configurated lipid inclusions next to lysosomal bodies. KOVACS *et al.* (1971) also described similar structures following the administration of aniline which led to alterations of cortical cells analogous to those following aminoglutethimide.

The contradictory findings concerning an increase (RHODIN, 1971) or decrease (NUSSDORFER, 1970) of lipid vacuoles following exogenous adminis-tration of corticoid hormones are possibly caused by a varying dose of hormone and varying duration of the experiment. In our studies with rats using 10 mg corticosterone/kg body weight, a focally accentuated increase of lipid vacuoles could be observed after daily intraperitoneal application, whereby the mem-branes were partially disintegrated and formed myelinic figures. The mito-chondria were not substantially reduced in number although they did show a reduction of their tubulovesicular internal membranes (Fig. 17b). An in-crease of glycogen (RHODIN, 1971) and a reduction of the Golgi complexes (FUJITA, 1972) have also been described in inactive cortical cells. After hypo-physectomy, the lipid-pigment complexes are more numerous (LUSE, 1967). An obvious reduction of the granular endoplasmic reticulum or the ribosomes was not observed in our experiments. The cell nuclei are smaller and irregularly configurated. In animal experiments following hypophysectomy, nuclear pyknosis in degenerating cortical cells was observed (IDELMAN, 1970). A decrease in the number of cells in the inner cortical layers by apoptosis (WYLLIE *et al.*, 1973) was also induced following ACTH suppression.

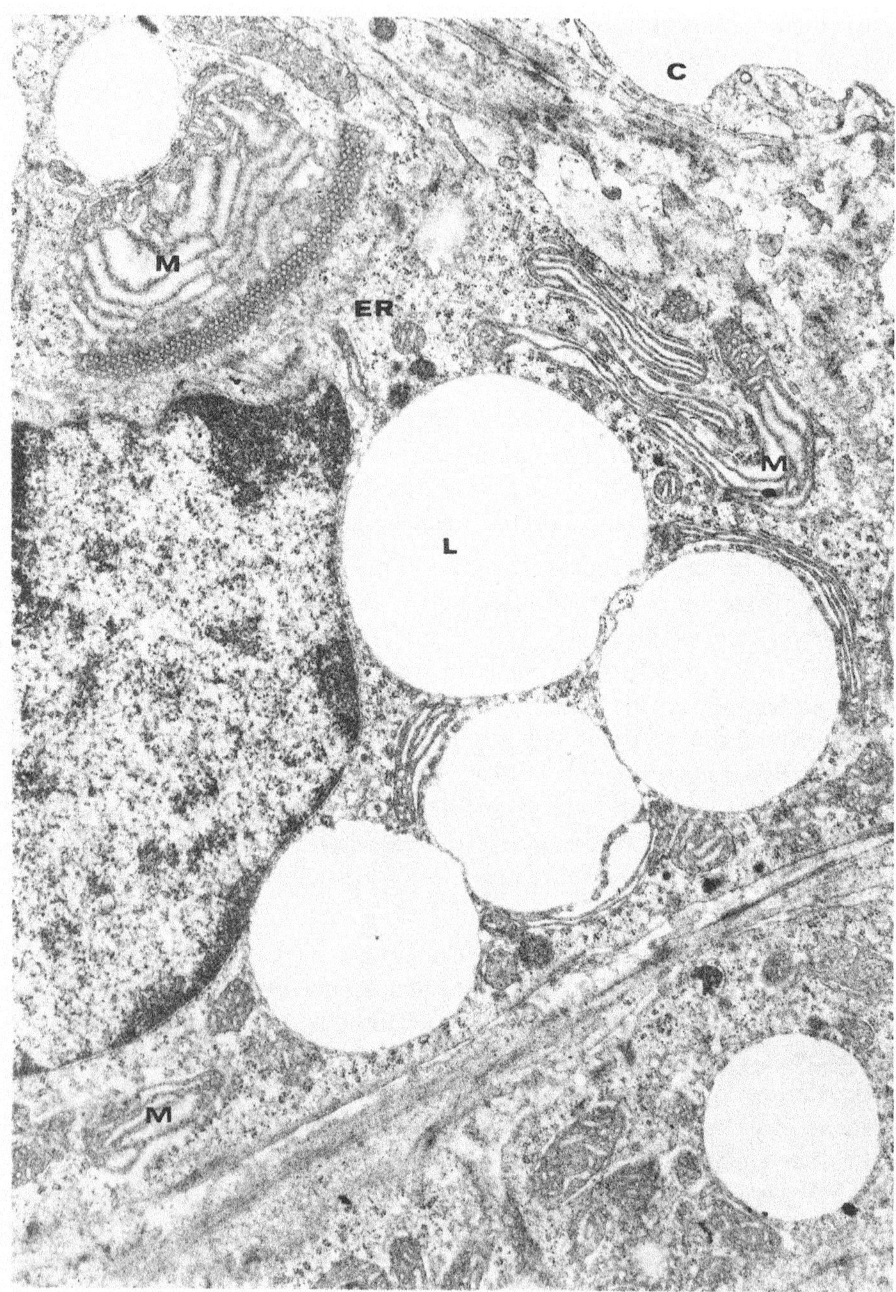

Fig. 16. Zona fasciculata of rat adrenal cortex after hypophysectomy. The cytoplasm contains large, membrane-bound lipid vacuoles (*L*) and irregular configurated mitochondria (*M*) with a peculiar arrangement of the internal structures. An obvious reduction of the agranular endoplasmic reticulum (*ER*) can be noticed. Capillary (*C*) with basement membranes. × 14400

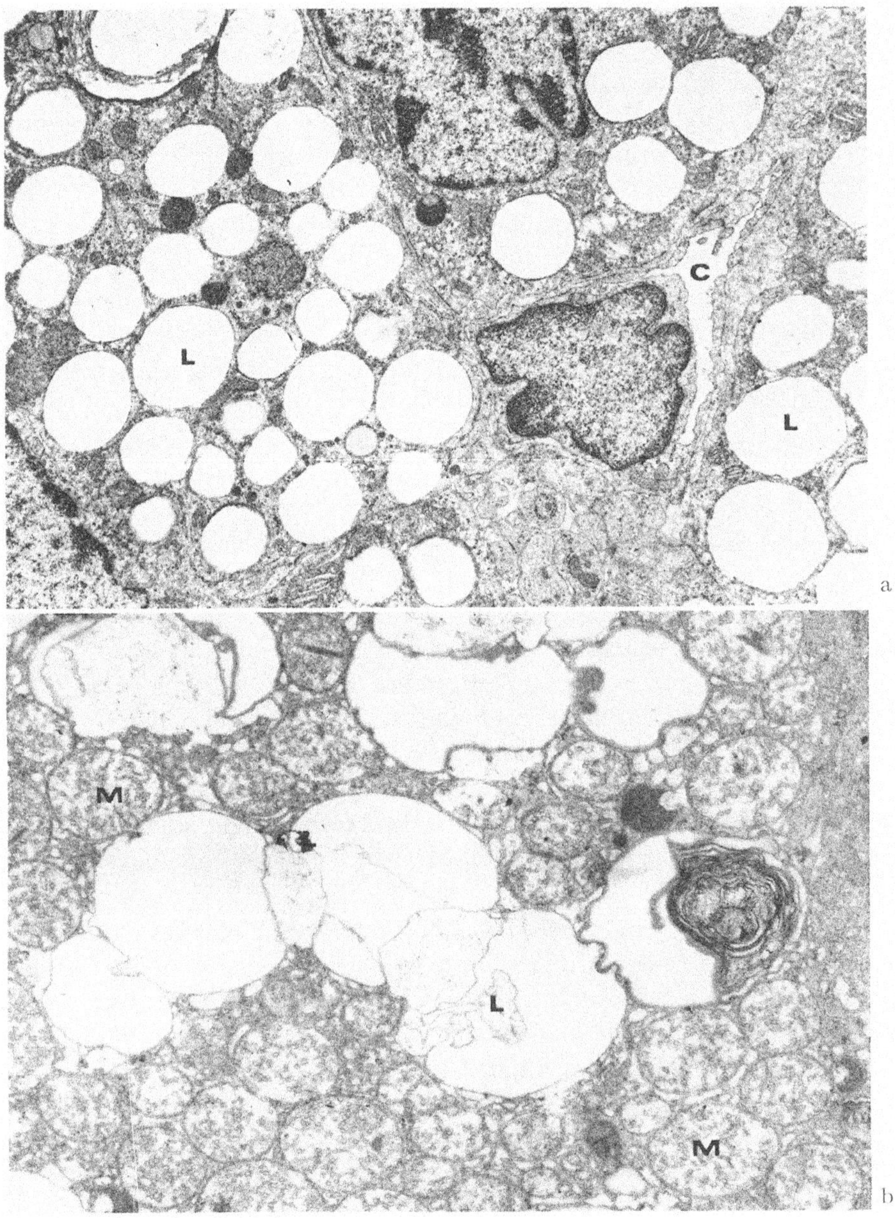

Fig. 17a and b. Zona fasciculata of the rat adrenal cortex after (a) hypophysectomy. The cytoplasm demonstrates numerous membrane-bound lipid vacuoles (L) and a remarkable reduction of the ultrastructural features engaged in the steroid biosynthesis. Capillary (C) with endothelial cells. × 7630. b Zona fasciculation of the rat adrenal cortex after treatment with corticosterone. This part of cell illustrates a confluence of membrane-bound lipid vacuoles (L) with a myelinated body. The mitochondria (M) appear to be relative numerous. They demonstrate however a reduction of their tubulo-vesicular internal structures. The agranular endoplasmic reticulum is diminished. × 12540

D. Correlations Between Ultrastructure and Function of the Adrenal Cortex

The lipids in the form of cholesterol ester reach the cortical cells by capillaries through endothelial pores. The lipid enters the cytoplasm by pinocytosis from the interstitium—the coated vesicles being a morphological gauge of the pinocytose processes (Mackay, 1969).

Cholesterol is stored in the lipid vacuoles; it is the only steroid in storage form in the adrenal cortex (Holzbauer et al., 1973; Makin and Trafford, 1972). The number and size of the lipid globules thus can be viewed as a morphological criterium for the conversion rate of cholesterol to pregnenolone. In addition to synthesis, the utilization and resorption will affect the content of the intracellular lipid. Therefore only very few and small lipid vacuoles are contained in the compact cells, particularly in compact cell adenomas and carcinomas, whereby even the small compact cell adenoma can exhibit a high rate of steroid hormone biosynthesis in relation to the weight of the tumor. In the atrophic cortex the metabolisation is very slight and thus explains the abundance of lipid stores.

Correlative clinical and ultrastructural examinations have shown that lipid-rich clear cell adenomas are capable of an increase in cortisol synthesis following ACTH administration (Mitschke et al., 1973). According to this behavior such adenomas possess only limited functional autonomy. In compact cell adenomas no increase of cortisol excretion following the administration of ACTH could be observed. The ultrastructural correlate for this varying behavior is likely to be based on the abundance of lipid stores of the clear adenoma cells and, possibly, also on the varying density of ACTH receptors within the cell membranes.

The reduction of lipids following ACTH stimulation manifests an increased cortisol synthesis which can be recognized morphologically by a reduction of lipid stores. Animal experiments revealed a substantial increase of lipid vacuoles after aminoglutetimide which inhibits the conversion of cholesterol into prenenolone (Magalhaes and Magalhaes, 1972).

The following conversion of cholesterol into pregnenolone passing hydroxy- and dihydroxy-cholesterol takes place in the mitochondria (Makin and Trafford, 1972). In this connection the role of ACTH in regulating cortisol synthesis is to be mentioned. In hyperplasia and in animal experiments following ACTH administration very numerous and enlarged mitochondria with densely placed internal membranes were observed. The simultaneous increase of RNA in the mitochondria is associated with increased enzyme synthesis (Nussdorfer and Mazzocchi, 1971 b).

The further steps take place in the so-called microsomal fraction which includes the granular and agranular endoplasmic reticulum and the free ribosomes. In addition to isomerisation with conversion of pregnenolone into progesterone the successive hydroxylation ensues in 17α- and 21-position. The following hydroxylation in 11β-position, by contrast, occurs in the mitochondria (MAKIN and TRAFFORD, 1972; VOLK, 1971a). These microsomal enzyme systems are probably normally located in the agranular endoplasmic reticulum.

The particularly close and morphologically demonstrable relations between the mitochondria and the agranular endoplasmic reticulum were emphasized by VOLK (1971 b), among others, in the form of mitochondrial tubular membranes. ACTH appears to effect an intra- as well as extramitochondrial protein synthesis in the adrenal cortex of the rat. The rapid hormonal reaction of the adrenal glands to ACTH stimulation is probably due to an increased permeability of the mitochondria for pregnenolone (NUSSDORFER et al., 1971).

In correlation to an increase of the mitochondria, whereby not only their number but also the extent and configuration of the internal membranes plays a significant role in steroidgenesis (MACKAY, 1969), a conspicuous development of the agranular endoplasmic reticulum can be observed with increased cortisol synthesis.

At least in animal experiments an enlargement of the nuclei and nucleoli was induced by stimulating the adrenal cortex with ACTH (KJAERHEIM, 1968; MÄUSLE, 1971; SANDRITTER and HÜBOTTER, 1954). MACKAY (1969) did not notice an immediate connection between the nuclear structure and secretory activity in his ultrastructural examinations of human adrenal glands. Autoradiographically NUSSDORFER and MAZZOCCHI (1971 b) demonstrated a distinct increase in nuclear RNA synthesis.

The substantially enlarged nucleoli found in adenomas—particularly in compact cells and even more in carcinomas—may correlate to an increased cellular activity, for example, in cell growth and mitoses. These alterations of the nuclei and nucleoli thus offer a parameter for the proliferatory tendency and ultimately for development of malignancy. The differences in nuclear structure between compact cell adenomas and carcinomas are, however, not clear cut with sometimes only minor variations at the ultrastructural level.

Summary

In *Cushing's syndrome* the alterations of the adrenal cortex may consist in diffuse or nodular hyperplasia in an adenoma or carcinoma with secondary atrophy of the attached and contralateral adrenal cortex.

The increased synthesis of glucocorticoid hormones correlates to characteristic ultrastructural findings of the cell organelles. These deviations from the normal ultrastructure are more quantitatively expressed in the forms of adrenal hyperplasia, whereas in adenomas and carcinomas significant qualitative changes can be demonstrated.

In the *hyperplastic adrenal cortex* the number of compact cells in the inner zona fasciculata and reticularis with their higher secretory activity is usually increased. The cytoplasm contains abundant smooth endoplasmic reticulum and mitochondria with varying and more closely arranged internal membranes.

In addition these cells possess increased lipid-pigment complexes. The clear cells in the outer zona fasciculata are characterized by closely arranged membrane-bound lipid vacuoles and rather few hormone-producing cell organelles.

The *adenomas of the adrenal cortex* can be differentiated into predominantly clear and compact cell adenomas.

The *clear cell adenomas* contain numerous large membrane-bound lipid vacuoles. The mitochondria and the agranular endoplasmic reticulum are only slightly developed.

A conspicuous increase of the hormone-producing organelle system can be demonstrated, however, in the *compact cell adenomas*. The smooth endoplasmic reticulum is tightly packed. The pleomorphic mitochondria often contain lamellar cristae. Only very few and small osmiophilic lipid vacuoles can be found in compact cells, whereas the pigment bodies are very numerous. An obvious increase in size of the nuclei and especially of the nucleoli is evident. There is also a higher content of the granular endoplasmic reticulum and ribosomes, indicating an increased synthesis of structural proteins.

The nuclear and nucleolar alterations are even more evident in the *adrenal carcinoma*. In addition the cell organelles show a considerably variable distribution with marked pleomorphism of the mitochondria. In contrast to the adenomas, the basement membranes surrounding the sinusoidal-like capillaries are interrupted in carcinoms.

The cells of the *atrophic adrenal cortex*—with exception of the zona glomerulosa—in correlation to the suppressed steroid hormone synthesis contain barely demonstrable agranular endoplasmic reticulum and very few mitochondria, but do contain numerous large lipid vacuoles with storage of the precursor lipids.

With electron microscopic studies of the adrenal cortex the hormonal activity of individual cells can be assessed, with the agranular endoplasmic reticulum and the number and structure of the mitochondria serving as the most important parameters. These findings in human adrenal glands correlate to experimental studies in different animal species. The ultrastructural features for differentiating adenomas with Cushing's syndrome from adenomas with Conn's syndrome are discussed. In mixed syndromes with increased androgen or aldosterone secretion in addition to hypercortisolism, the ultrastructural findings of whorled-like membranes of the smooth endoplasmic reticulum, the increase of the granular endoplasmic reticulum with alterations of the mitochondria and crystalline-like intramitochondrial inclusions can possibly be looked upon as the morphological correlate for a multihormonal steroid production.

References

Ashworth, C. T., Race, G. J., Mollenhauer, H. H.: Study of functional activity of adrenocortical cells with electron microscopy. Amer. J. Path. **35**, 425–438 (1959).
Bahu, R. M., Battifora, H., Shambough, G.: Functional black adenoma of the adrenal gland. Light and electron microscopical study. Arch. Path. **98**, 139–142 (1974).

Bayer, J. M., Holtmaier, H. J., Breuer, H.: Cushing-Syndrom; langdauernde disso-
ziierte Rindeninsuffizienz nach operativer Entfernung eines Nebennierenrindenadenoms. Chirurg 31, 529–534 (1960).

Besser, G. M., Edwards, C. R. W.: Cushing's syndrome. In: Clinics in endocrinology
and metabolism, vol. I/2. London-Philadelphia-Toronto: W. B. Saunders 1972.

Bierich, J. R.: Diskussionsbemerkung in: Verh. dtsch. Ges. Path. 55, 146 (1971).

Black, V. H., Bogart, B. I.: Peroxisomes in inner adrenocortical cells of fetal and
adult guinea pigs. J. Cell Biol. 57, 345–358 (1973).

Borowicz, J. W.: Some ultrastructural changes in adrenocortical cells of rats after
hypophysectomy. Beitr. path. Anat. 132, 441–468 (1965).

Braunsteiner, H., Fellinger, K., Pakesch, F.: Elektronenmikroskopische Beobachtungen der Mitochondrien in der Zona fasciculata der Nebennierenrinde. Wien.
Z. inn. Med. 36, 281–288 (1956).

Brenner, R. M.: Fine structure of adrenocortical cells in adult rhesus monkeys. Amer.
J. Anat. 119, 429–454 (1966).

Canick, J. A., Purvis, J. L.: The maintenance of mitochondrial size in the rat adrenal
cortex zona fasciculata by ACTH. Exp. molec. Path. 16, 79–93 (1972).

Carr, I.: Microvilli of the cells of the human adrenal cortex. Nature (Lond.) 182, 607
(1958).

Carr, I.: The ultrastructure of the human adrenal cortex before and after stimulation
with ACTH. J. Path. Bact. 81, 101–106 (1961).

Cervós-Navarro, J., Tonutti, E., Garcia-Alvarez, F., Bayer, J. M., Fritz, K. W.:
Elektronenmikroskopische Befunde an zwei Conn'schen Adenomen der Nebennierenrinde. Endokrinologie 49, 35–52 (1965).

Christensen, A. K.: The fine structure of testicular cells in guinea pigs. J. Cell Biol.
26, 911–935 (1965).

Christensen, A. K., Fawcett, D. W.: The fine structure of testicular interstitial cells
in mice. Amer. J. Anat. 118, 551–572 (1966).

Fisher, E. R., Danowski, T. S.: Ultrastructural study of virilizing adrenocortical
adenoma. Amer. J. clin. Path. 59, 480–489 (1973).

Fladerer, H., Auböck, L., Binder, M., Vilits, P.: Zwischenzellgeschwulst des
Hodens. Zbl. allg. Path. path. Anat. 118, 510–518 (1974).

Fujita, H.: On the fine structure of alteration of the adrenal cortex in hypophysectomized
rats. Z. Zellforsch. 125, 480–496 (1972).

Garret, R., Ames, R. P.: Black-pigmented adenoma of the adrenal gland. Report of
three cases including electron microscopic study. Arch. Path. 95, 349–353 (1973).

Giacomelli, F., Wiener, J., Spiro, D.: Cytological alterations related to stimulation
of the zona glomerulosa of the adrenal cells. J. Cell Biol. 26, 499–522 (1965).

Hartemann, P., Leclere, J., Mollet, E., Talancé, N. de, Grignon, G., Duminy, F.,
Cheval, M. C.: Syndrome de Cushing par hyperplasie surrénale bilatérale et adénome
sécrétant unique. Discussion nosologique. Ann. Endocr. (Paris) 32, 788–800 (1971).

Hashida, Y., Kenny, F. M., Yunis, E. J.: Ultrastructure of the adrenal cortex in
Cushing's disease in children. Human Path. 1, 595–614 (1970).

Holzbauer, M., Bull, G., Youdim, M. B. H., Wooding, F. B. P., Godden, U.: Subcellular distribution of steroids in the adrenal gland. Nature (Lond.) New Biol. 242,
117–119 (1973).

Holzmann, K., Lange, R.: Zytologische Beobachtungen an der hyperplastischen Nebennierenrinde des Menschen. Z. Zellforsch. 69, 80–92 (1966).

Horvath, E., Kovacs, K.: Effect of temporary ischemia on the fine structure of the rat
adrenal cortex. Path. europ. 8, 43–60 (1973).

Idelman, S.: Ultrastructure of the mammalian adrenal cortex. Int. Rev. Cytol. 27,
181–281 (1970).

Kadioglu, D., Harrison, R. G.: The functional relationships of mitochondria in the
rat adrenal cortex. J. Anat. (Lond.) 110, 283–296 (1971).

Kadioglu, D., Harrison, R. G.: The pleomorphism of mitochondira in the rat adrenal
cortex. J. Endocr. 52, 203–204 (1972).

Kahri, A. I.: Selective inhibition by chloramphenicol of ACTH-induced reorganization
of inner mitochondrial membranes in fetal adrenocortical cells in tissue cultures.
Amer. J. Anat. 127, 103–130 (1970).

Kahri, A. I.: Inhibition of ACTH-induced differentiation of cortical cells and their mitochondria by corticosterone in tissue culture of fetal rat adrenals. Anat. Rec. **176**, 253–272 (1973).

Kawaoi, A.: Ultrastructural zonation of the human adrenal cortex. Acta path. jap. **19**, 115–149 (1969).

Kimmel, G. L., Péron, F. G., Haksar, A., Bedigan, E., Robidoux, W. F., Lin, M. T.: Ultrastructure, steroidogenic potential and energy metabolism of the Snell adrenocortical carcinoma 494. A comparison with normal adrenocortical tissue. J. Cell Biol. **62**, 152–163 (1974).

Kjaerheim, A.: Studies of adrenocortical ultrastructure. 3. Effects of dexamethasone and medroxyprogesterone on interrenal cells of the domestic fowl. Z. Zellforsch. **91**, 456–474 (1968).

Kovacs, K., Blaschek, J. A., Yeghiayan, E., Hatakeyama, S., Gardell, C.: Adrenocortical lipid hyperplasia induced in rats by aniline. Amer. J. Path. **62**, 17–34 (1971).

Kovacs, K., Horvath, E., Delarue, N. C., Laidlaw, J. C.: Ultrastructural features of an aldosterone-secreting adrenocortical adenoma. Hormone Res. **5**, 47–56 (1974).

Kracht, J., Tamm, J.: Bilaterale kleinknotige Adenomatose der Nebennierenrinde bei Cushing-Syndrom. Virchows Arch. path. Anat. **333**, 1–9 (1960).

Kracht, J., Zimmermann, D.: Die Nebennierenrinde bei endogenem Hypercortisolismus. Symp. dtsch. Ges. Endokr. **11**, 185–189 (1964).

Labhart, A., Hedinger, C., Kistler, G., Müller, J., Prader, A., Siebenmann, R., Töndury, G., Zachmann, A.: Die Nebennierenrinde. In: Labhart, A. (Ed.), Klinik der inneren Sekretion. Berlin-Heidelberg-New York: Springer 1971.

Liebegott, G.: Die Pathologie der Nebennieren. Verh. dtsch. Ges. Path. **36**, 21–68 (1952).

Long, J. A., Jones, A. L.: The fine structure of the zona glomerulosa and the zona fasciculata of the adrenal cortex of the opossum. Amer. J. Anat. **120**, 463–487 (1967a).

Long, J. A., Jones, A. L.: Observations on the fine structure of the adrenal cortex of man. Lab. Invest. **17**, 355–370 (1967b).

Luse, S.: Fine structure of adrenal cortex. In: The adrenal cortex (ed. Eisenstein, A. B.). Boston: Little, Brown & Co. 1967.

Luthman, M.: Intramitochondrial bodies in sheep adrenal zona glomerulosa cells. Z. Zellforsch. **121**, 244–248 (1971).

Macadam, R. F.: Fine structure of a functional adrenal cortical adenoma. Cancer (Philad.) **26**, 1300–1310 (1970).

Mackay, A.: Atlas of human adrenal cortex ultrastructure. In: Th. Symington (ed.), Functional pathology of the human adrenal gland. Edinburgh-London: Livingstone 1969.

Mäusle, E.: Geschlechtsunterschiede in der Ultrastruktur der Nebennierenrinde der Ratte. Z. Zellforsch. **116**, 136–150 (1971).

Magalhaes, M. C.: A new crystal-containing cell in human adrenal cortex. J. Cell Biol. **55**, 126–133 (1972).

Magalhaes, M. C., Magalhaes, M. M.: Ultrastructural alterations produced in rat adrenal by aminoglutethimide. A stereologic and cytochemical study. Endocrinology **90**, 444–452 (1972).

Makin, H. L. J., Trafford, D. J. H.: The chemistry of the steroids. In: Clinics in endocrinology and metabolism, vol. I/2. London-Philadelphia-Toronto: Saunders 1972.

Marek, J., Thoenes, W., Motlik, K.: Lipoide Transformation der Mitochondrien in Nebennierenrindenzellen nach Aminoglutäthimid. Virchows Arch. Abt. B **6**, 116–131 (1970).

McNutt, N. S., Jones, A. L.: Observations on the ultrastructure of cytodifferentiation in the human fetal adrenal cortex. Lab. Invest. **22**, 513–527 (1970).

Miller, R. A.: Quantitative changes in the nucleolus and nucleus as indices of adrenal cortical secretory activity. Amer. J. Anat. **95**, 497–522 (1954).

Milner, A. J.: ACTH and the differentiation of rat adrenal cortical cells grown in primary tissue culture. Endocrinology **88**, 66–71 (1971).

Mitschke, H., Saeger, W.: Zur Ultrastruktur der atrophischen Nebennierenrinde bei dissoziierter, sekundärer Nebennierenrindeninsuffizienz. Virchows Arch. Abt. A **361**, 217–228 (1973).

MITSCHKE, H., SAEGER, W., BREUSTEDT, H.-J.: Zur Ultrastruktur der Nebennieren-rindentumoren beim Cushing-Syndrom. Virchows Arch. Abt. A **360**, 253–264 (1973).

MITSCHKE, H., SAEGER, W., DONATH, K.: Zur Ultrastruktur der Nebennierenrinde beim Cushing-Syndrom. Virchows Arch. Abt. A **353**, 234–247 (1971).

MÜLLER, J., FROESCH, E. R., MEYER, U. A., LABHART, A.: Persistierende Störung der ACTH-Sekretion nach Operation eines Nebennierenrindenadenoms bei drei Fällen von Cushing-Syndrom. Schweiz. med. Wschr. **97**, 861–865 (1967).

MULLER, M., STEINER, H., RUEDI, B.: Diagnostic et traitement du carcinome cortico-surrénalien. Schweiz. med. Wschr. **100**, 1478–1485 (1970).

NAKAMURA, K.: An electron microscopic observation on RE-cells of the rat adrenal cortex with respect to the nature of lipid globules. Tohoku J. exp. Med. **109**, 205–221 (1973).

NEVILLE, A. M., MACKAY, A. M.: The structure of the human adrenal cortex in health and disease. In: Clinics in Endocrinology and metabolism, vol. I/2. London-Philadelphia-Toronto: Saunders 1972.

NEVILLE, A. M., SYMINGTON, T.: The pathology of the adrenal gland in Cushing's syndrome. J. Path. Bact. **93**, 19–35 (1967).

NICKERSON, P. A.: Adrenocortical cells in rats bearing a corticosterone secreting tumor. Virchows Arch. Abt. B **13**, 297–305 (1973).

NORMAN, N., REKSTEN, K. R., VOGT, J. H.: Steroid determinations in six cases of hyperplasia and three cases of tumour of the adrenal cortex. Acta med. scand. **183**, 41–48 (1968).

NUSSDORFER, G. G.: Effects of corticosteroid-hormones on the smooth endoplasmic reticulum of rat adrenocortical cells. Z. Zellforsch. **106**, 143–154 (1970).

NUSSDORFER, G. G., MAZZOCCHI, G.: Correlated morphometric and autoradiographic studies of the effects of corticosterone on adrenocortical cells of intact and hypo-physectomized ACTH-treated rats. Z. Zellforsch. **111**, 90–105 (1970).

NUSSDORFER, G. G., MAZZOCCHI, G.: Effects of corticosterone on nuclear and mito-chondrial DNA-dependent protein synthesis of adrenocortical cells of hypophys-ectomized ACTH-treated rats. Steroidologia **2**, 244–256 (1971a).

NUSSDORFER, G. G., MAZZOCCHI, G.: Effect of ACTH on mitochondrial RNA synthesis of rat adrenocortical cells. Z. Zellforsch. **118**, 35–48 (1971b).

NUSSDORFER, G. G., MAZZOCCHI, G.: A stereologic study of the effects of ACTH and cyclic 3',5'-AMP on adrenocortical cells of intact and hypophysectomized rats. Lab. Invest. **26**, 45–52 (1972).

NUSSDORFER, G. G., MAZZOCCHI, G.: Effects of 3',5'-cyclic nucleotides on adrenocortical cells of hypophysectomized rats. A stereologic and autoradiographic study. Lab. Invest. **28**, 332–342 (1973).

NUSSDORFER, G. G., MAZZOCCHI, G., REBONATO, L.: Long-term trophic effect of ACTH on rat adrenocortical cells. An ultrastructural, morphometric and autoradiographic study. Z. Zellforsch. **115**, 30–45 (1971).

NUSSDORFER, G. G., REBUFFAT, P., MAZZOCCHI, G., BELLONI, A. S., MENEGHELLI, V.: Investigations on adrenocortical mitochondria turnover. I. Effect of chronic treatment with ACTH on the size and number of rat zona fasciculata mitochondria. Cell Tiss. Res. **150**, 79–94 (1974).

PROPST, A.: Elektronenmikroskopie der Nebennierenrinde bei primärem Aldosteronismus. Beitr. path. Anat. **131**, 1–21 (1965).

PROPST, A.: Über konzentrisch geschichtete Kerneinschlüsse in einem menschlichen Nebennierenrindenadenom. Virchows Arch. Abt. B **4**, 263–266 (1970).

REIDBORD, H., FISHER, E. R.: Electron microscopic study of adrenal cortical hyper-plasia in Cushing's syndrome. Arch. Path. **86**, 419–426 (1968).

REIDBORD, H., FISHER, E. R.: Aldosteronoma and nonfunctioning adrenal cortical adenoma. Comparative ultrastructural study. Arch. Path. **88**, 155–161 (1969).

RHODIN, J. A. G.: The ultrastructure of the adrenal cortex of the rat under normal and experimental conditions. J. Ultrastruct. Res. **34**, 23–71 (1971).

ROBINSON, M. J., PARDO, V., RYWLIN, A. M.: Pigmented nodules (black adenomas) of the adrenal. An autopsy study of incidence, morphology, and function. Human Path. **3**, 317–325 (1972).

Ross, M. H., Pappas, G. D., Lanman, J. T., Lind, J.: Electron microscope observations on the endoplasmic reticulum in the human fetal adrenal. J. biophys. biochem. Cytol. **4**, 659–661 (1958).

Rückert, U.: Zur Frage der Carcinomentstehung auf dem Boden eines kompensatorisch-hyperplastischen NNR-Regenerates. Chirurg **41**, 417–419 (1970).

Sabatini, D. D., Robertis, E. D. P. de, Bleichmar, M. B.: Submicroscopic study of the pituitary action of the adrenocortex of the rat. Endocrinology **70**, 390–406 (1962).

Saeger, W., Mitschke, H.: Zur Pathologie des Cushing-Syndroms. Dtsch. med. Wschr. **98**, 1272–1274 (1973a).

Saeger, W., Mitschke, H.: Licht- und elektronenoptische Untersuchungen an der Zona glomerulosa der Rattennebenniere nach Carbenoxolon. Virchows Arch. Abt. A **358**, 45–59 (1973b).

Saito, A., Fleischer, S.: Intramitochondrial tubules in adrenal glands of rat. J. Ultrastruct. Res. **35**, 642–649 (1971).

Sandritter, W., Hübotter, F.: Über die Bedeutung des Nucleolus in der Nebennierenrinde. Frankfurt. Z. Path. **65**, 219–229 (1954).

Sekiyama, S., Yago, N.: A study on the correlation between function and ultrastructure in the rat adrenal cortex. Acta path. jap. **22**, 77–98 (1972).

Sharma, R. K., Hashimoto, K.: Ultrastructural studies and metabolic regulation of isolated adrenocortical carcinoma cells of rat. Cancer Res. **32**, 666–674 (1972).

Snell, K. C., Stewart, H. L.: Variations in histological pattern and functional effects of a transplantable adrenal cortical carcinoma in intact, hypophysectomized and newborn rats. J. nat. Cancer Inst. **22**, 1119–1132 (1959).

Sommers, S. C., Terzakis, J. A.: Ultrastructural study of aldosterone-secreting cells of the adrenal cortex. Amer. J. clin. Path. **54**, 303–310 (1970).

Sugihara, H., Kawai, K., Tsuchiyama, H.: Pathology of intracortical nodules in rat adrenal glands, especially on their fine-structure. Acta path. jap. **23**, 253–260 (1973).

Symington, T.: Functional pathology of the human adrenal gland. Edinburgh-London: Livingstone 1969.

Szabo, D., Stark, E., Varga, B.: The localisation of acid phosphatase activity changes in lysosomes in the adrenal zona fasciculata of intact and hypophysectomized rats following ACTH administration. Histochemie **10**, 321–328 (1967).

Tannenbaum, M.: Ultrastructural pathology of the adrenal cortex. Pathology Annual **8**, 109–156 (1973).

Thiele, J.: Feinstrukturelle Untersuchungen an einem endokrin aktiven Carcinom der Nebennierenrinde. Virchows Arch. Abt. B **17**, 51–62 (1974).

Thomas, J. P., El-Shaboury, A. H.: Aldosterone secretion in steroidtreated patients with adrenal suppression. Lancet **1970I**, 623–625.

Tonutti, E.: Experimentelle Untersuchungen zur Pathophysiologie der Nebennierenrinde. Verh. dtsch. Ges. Path. **36**, 123–158 (1952).

Tsuchiyama, H.: Morphological studies of human adrenal cortex under pathologic conditions. Acta path. jap. **17**, 155–170 (1967).

Ueberberg, H., Stöcker, E., Städtler, F.: Zur zellulären Nucleinsäure- und Protein-Synthese der Nebennierenrinde von Ratten nach Dexamethason-Applikation. Virchows Arch. Abt. B **6**, 97–106 (1970).

Volk, T. L.: Alterations of the adrenal cortex of rats treated with progesterone. Virchows Arch. Abt. B **9**, 206–217 (1971a).

Volk, T. L.: Mitochondrial-tubular membrane interconnections in the rat adrenal cortex. Lab. Invest. **25**, 349–355 (1971b).

Wyllie, A. H., Kerr, J. F. R., Macaskill, I. A. M., Currie, A. R.: Adrenocortical cell deletion: the role of ACTH. J. Path. **111**, 85–94 (1973).

Pathology Department, Ludwig-Aschoff-Haus, University of Freiburg,
Freiburg i. Br., West Germany

DNA in Human Tumors: A Cytophotometric Study

N. Böhm* and W. Sandritter

With 6 Figures

Contents

* Supported by Deutsche Forschungsgemeinschaft (DFG) Grant No. Bo 395/1/2.

A. Introduction

A quarter century ago, Vendrely and Vendrely (1949) and Mandel *et al.* (1950) determined on the basis of biochemical measurements that the DNA content in the nucleus of human and various mammalian cells is practically identical, and that it amounts to circa 6×10^{-12} g. This is all the more surprising considering that the chromosome count among various placental mammals—which was determined only much later (Atkin *et al.*, 1965)—is highly variable.

Boivin *et al.* (1948) observed that within the same species the cell nuclei in various organs contain the same amount of DNA. They proposed that the genetic endowment of every cell is the same, and that each gene corresponds to a particular quantity of DNA (Boivin's Hypothesis).

The prophetic intuition of these gifted scientists has since—at least in part—been confirmed. The genetic code has been deciphered. Today we understand the triplet combinations of purine and pyrimidine bases which specify the placement of particular amino acids of the molecular level of the gene. Thus the sequence of bases in the DNA macromolecule specifies the amino acid sequences of cellular proteins—enzymes, hormones, etc.

Thus, we can generally say that the genetic activity and function of a cell is determined by the DNA present in the nucleus. This results in a constant mass relationship between the nucleus and its corresponding cytoplasm (nuclear/cytoplasmic ratio) which is maintained in normal cells under physiological conditions.

The chromosome count ($2n = 17$–18 in the field mouse, $2n = 40$ in the white mouse, $2n = 46$ in man, $2n = 64$ in the horse, and $2n = 78$ in the dog, Atkin *et al.*, 1965) apparently plays a subordinate role. The total quantity of genetic material, i.e., DNA, is functionally more important and biologically more significant (Atkin and Richards, 1956). In fact, many investigators can demonstrate a remarkably uniform proportionality between chromosome count and DNA content within the same animal, whereas tumor cells show deviations, the mean DNA content for tumor chromosomes being increased up to 22% (Atkin *et al.*, 1966). This phenomenon may result from the appearance of abnormally large and striking chromosomes (marker chromosomes, Atkin and Baker, 1966). Hypodiploid and pseudodiploid chromosome counts can also lead to hyperdiploid DNA values (Atkin and Richards, 1956). The tight proportionality between chromosome count and DNA content is no longer borne out for tumor cells. Thus it seems more meaningful to determine the DNA content directly as the biologically and functionally more important parameter in tumors, rather than through the intermediary of chromosome counts. DNA content in tumor nuclei is usually increased, but the question as to whether this is a cause or effect of malignant transformation remains open. The further consequences of elevated DNA are largely unknown.

Since it is assumed that not all cells in tumor tissue contribute to growth, several authors have measured chromosome counts (Atkin, 1971; Atkin,

1973; ATKIN *et al.*, 1974) and DNA content in metaphase plates to determine the proliferating stem cell population (STICH and STEELE, 1962). This approach appears problematical, however, since it is known that metaphase plates can revert back to interphase nuclei without dividing (c-mitoses). Thus metaphase plates are not representative of the actual dividing cell population. This appears to hold especially for cells with a chromosome count which deviates from the stem cell population, since the DNA values measured in metaphase show a significantly higher variance than those measured in anaphase (BADER, 1959; STICH and STEELE, 1962). One must also take into account the fact that a tumor can increase in size quite considerably by polyploidy in the absence of cell divisions. This phenomenon is also observed in normal tissues, such as hepatic parenchyma (SWARTZ, 1956) and myocardium (SANDRITTER and SCOMAZZONI, 1964). It must certainly play an important role in the high-ploidy tumors with multiple duplication levels. We are therefore convinced that cytophotometric measurements of nuclear DNA contain more information than chromosome counts, and that this information permits us to reach conclusions regarding the functional activity and degree of differentiation of the tumor cells, as well as predictions of the proliferation capacity and prognosis of a given tumor. Finally, DNA measurements can assist in tumor diagnosis and in the selection of treatment modalities. For this purpose, one requires the greatest possible number of DNA values taken from the greatest possible number of nuclei in a tumor. It is not enough to determine only the most frequent DNA value, as representing the DNA stem line of the tumor, since the non-stem line and nonproliferating cells also belong to the tumor.

Consistent with this point of view, we have surveyed the literature on cytophotometric measurements of DNA content in human tumors, assembled them in tables, and compared them with our own investigations. We make no claims for the completeness of our selection of publications. We have tried to review those papers accessible to us.

B. Materials and Methods

The comparison of results from different laboratories is always problematical when different preparation, staining, and measurement techniques have been employed. In the early years of cytophotometry, the technical facilities now available to us had not been developed. Thus the early results of STOWELL (1945, 1946) and SANDRITTER (1952) do not qualify as genuine cytophotometric measurements in the present day sense, since the absorption and extinction of many cells in a section were measured together through a photometer opening and a mean extinction per cell nucleus was obtained through division by the nucleus count. Obviously no DNA histograms were possible with these methods, which were fraught with other technical errors. Thus these results are not appropriate for our tables. We shall now discuss briefly the various other cytophotometric staining and measurement methods for determining nuclear DNA content.

1. Cytophotometric Staining and Measurement Methods Employed in the Literature

Preparation techniques include imprint and smear preparations from fresh, unfixed tumors, as well as thick paraffin sections usually from formalin fixed tissue. The most widely used staining method for the quantitative, histochemical representation of DNA is the Feulgen reaction with basic pararosaniline, in which a variety of conditions of acid hydrolysis have been chosen.

Sandritter et al. (1963) and Greisen (1971) employed DNA staining with gallocyanine-chromalaun following RNAse treatment. The staining follows that of Einarson (1951). Sandritter and Kleinhans (1964) reported comparison measurements with UV absorption, gallocyanine-chromalaun, and Feulgen staining in bronchial carcinoma. Absorption cytophotometry, at varying levels of technical precision, is by far the most popular measurement apparatus. Measurements are made by

1. the plug method,
2. the 2-wave length method after Ornstein (1952) and Patau (1952),
3. the scanning method with integrating microdensitometer after Deely (1955),
4. the Zeiss UMSP I and
5. the Vickers apparatus.

Details are listed in Table 1.

2. Personal Staining Method with Acriflavine-Feulgen

In earlier papers (Böhm and Sprenger, 1968; Böhm, 1972) we demonstrated that cytophotometric measurements of the fluorescence intensity in cell nuclei after Feulgen staining with acriflavine-SO_2 (Feulgen-DNA fluorescence cytophotometry) exhibit a limited proportionality to stain concentration, which is sufficient for the quantitative determination of Feulgen DNA up to extinction values of 0.2–0.25. Integrating absorbance and fluorescence cytophotometric measurements led to identical results (Böhm and Sprenger, 1968; Böhm et al., 1970).

Source of tumors: Material used in these studies was in part from surgical specimens, in part from autopsy material no more than 24 hours post mortem. Carefully cleaned and defatted slides were smeared with a fresh cut surface of unfixed tumor tissue and immediately wet-fixed.

Fixation: The fixation fluid consists of 85:10:5 volume percent methanol: commercial formalin:glacial acetic acid. This mixture has proved itself especially suitable for the fixation of cell smears (Böhm et al., 1968). The fixation period is 1 hour. Afterwards the slides are rinsed 10 minutes in aqua dest., and either immersed in the acid hydrolysis bath or else briefly dried in 96% ethanol and stored up to 14 days dust-free at room temperature in the dark. During this time, other cases are collected, so that all may be hydrolyzed together following a 10 minute hydration in aqua dest.

Hydrolysis: Acid hydrolysis proceeds in 4N HCl at 28°C in a thermostatically controlled water bath (± 0.2°C). Duration of hydrolysis is limited to 60 minutes, whereas we previously hydrolyzed for 100 minutes (Böhm, 1968; Böhm and Sprenger, 1968) to achieve maximal staining intensity.

Staining with Acriflavine-SO$_2$: The Schiff reagent is prepared with 0.01% acriflavine (Serva, Heidelberg, West Germany). A leukobase cannot be produced with the Schiff-type acridine dyes so that decolorization with activated charcoal is omitted. Acriflavine-Schiff reagent is stored in a tightly sealed flask in the refrigerator at 2–4°C and warmed to room temperature before use.

The smears remain for 1 hour in the staining bath at room temperature. Then they are rinsed six times, 5 minutes apiece, in SO$_2$ water, dehydrated in 70%, 96%, absolute alcohol, and xylol (at least 5 min), and finally mounted in non-fluorescing Cargille Oil (Cargille Laboratories, Cedar Grove, N.Y., USA) with a refraction index of $n_D^{20°} = 1.54$. Cover slips were sealed with nail polish.

The finished slides were stored in closed slide jackets in the dark until being measured. Slides remain fresh under these conditions almost indefinitely.

3. Personal Fluorescence Cytophotometric Measurement Methods and Conditions

The fluorescence cytophotometric measurements were carried out on a Leitz MPV I (Leitz Co., Wetzlar, West Germany) under epi-illumination conditions (excitation filter BG 12, 5 mm and GB 38, 4 mm; 50% beam splitter; barrier filter 590 nm) with a phase contrast objective (Pv Fl 70X, n.a. 1.15). The following improvements have been made since our previous, detailed description of the measuring device (Böhm and Sprenger, 1968):

a) A shutter built in the light path allows us to limit the exposure time with short wave length excitation light to a constant 250 msec. Thus, the rapid fluorescence fading of acridine dyes has only a minimal and uniform influence upon the measuring values. Double exposures of the same nucleus or measurements of the immediately neighboring nuclei are avoided.

b) Instead of the light-spot galvanometer, we employ a digital display (ADW 2-, DA 2, Wandel & Goltermann, Reutlingen, West Germany) with a 200X magnification, 200 msec delay interval, and a display area of 5000.

The registered values are read out on a printer (Sprenger and Böhm, 1971).

4. Diploid Reference Value

Cytophotometric measurements, regardless of technique, require a reference value with a known DNA content, which is then used to calculate the true DNA content on measured nuclei in relative or absolute units. Since histochemical reactions exhibit an unavoidable variation from one experiment to the next even under optimally standardized preparation and staining conditions, it follows that nuclei suitable for reference values (e.g., sperm, lymphocytes, granulocytes, diploid liver cells) should if possible be on the same slide, but at least treated in the same hydrolysis and staining bath as the tumor cells being evaluated.

Even so there are problems. Sperm exhibit varying hydrolysis properties from other somatic cells under certain conditions and should only be used as a standard with caution (Böhm et al., 1968). The same holds for lymphocytes and granulocytes, which have the advantage, however, that they appear naturally in practically every tumor preparation, and are easy to identify by phase contrast. Here we are dealing with mature, euploid, postmitotic cells, i.e., with a homogeneous, nonproliferating, diploid cell population, from which we can expect a mean DNA content corresponding to the diploid chromosome complement (2c-value).

Investigations by Atkin and Richards (1956), Hale (1963), Garcia (1964), and Mayall (1969) have shown, however, that the measured Feulgen value in granulocytes and lymphocytes can lie 5–15% under the expected diploid value. The exact reason for this is currently unknown (Garcia, 1969; Sullivan and Garcia, 1970; James, 1973). Nonetheless, lymphocytes and granulocytes are most often used for calculation of the diploid 2c value (Table 1). Atkin's group increases the measured value for lymphocytes and fibroblasts by 10% in order to achieve the 2c value for normal epithelial cells (Atkin and Richards, 1956). Levi et al. (1969) consider the Feulgen DNA value for lymphocytes unsuitable for the calculation of the diploid DNA standard. In a previous paper (Böhm et al., 1968), we made an intensive study of proportionality errors in Feulgen hydrolysis. Although lymphocytes and granulocytes exhibit significantly lower measured values (minus 5–17%) than the diploid liver cells after alcohol fixation along the entire course of the hydrolysis curve, this error is reduced to circa 4% when methanol:formalin: glacial acetic acid fixation is employed. A similar effect was observed by Mayall (1967) with this fixative and the gallocyanine-chromalaun stain. Thus we employ methanol:formalin:glacial acetic acid volume percent 85:10:5 as our fixative and use the mean DNA content of lymphocytes and granulocytes which appear among the tumor cells without further correction as our 2c reference value. We are aware, however, that this value is more likely too low than too high.

C. Results

1. Definition of DNA Ploidy and DNA Stem Line

It should be emphasized that the concepts 2c, 3c, 4c, etc. express a Feulgen DNA value (*DNA ploidy*) which is two, three, or four times as large as the base value 1c. 1c corresponds to half the mean Feulgen value for lymphocytes and granulocytes.

A normal human somatic cell in interphase contains $2 \times 23 = 46$ uncoiled and invisible chromosomes in its nucleus. The DNA content of such a normal euploid set of chromosomes is referred to as euploid or diploid (2c) amount of DNA. Prior to mitosis the nucleus has to double its DNA content. During mitosis the DNA strands are coiled and microscopically visible as chromosomes. The metaphase plate of a normal human somatic cell thus comprises 46 *double*-chromosomes which contain altogether a tetraploid (4c) amount of DNA. The karyotype of such a cell, however, is named euploid or diploid or 2n (*chromosome ploidy*). This must be clearly kept in mind in order to avoid confusion.

In 1963 SEIDEL and SANDRITTER coined the term "DNA stem line" of a tumor. They defined it as the DNA content of the most prominent peak in the DNA distribution pattern of the tumor cell population (SANDRITTER, 1964). The term had been chosen as analogous to "chromosome stem line" introduced by MAKINO and KANO (1952) and LEVAN and HAUSCHKA (1952) to describe the specific number of metaphase chromosomes dominating in a given tumor. Since the total amount of DNA is distributed among the chromosomes it was assumed that a change (usually an increase) in the number of chromosomes, called *chromosomal aneuploidy*—as it is often found in malignant tumors—should also result in an increased amount of DNA (*DNA aneuploidy*).

The tight proportionality between number of chromosomes and DNA content holds only, if the size and the DNA content of each individual chromosome remains the same. In malignant tumors, however, an augmented amount of DNA per chromosome was found (ATKIN *et al.*, 1966) besides a more or less increased number of chromosomes so that the close relation between number of chromosomes and amount of DNA is no longer valid for tumors.

BADER (1959), STICH *et al.* (1960) and MANOCHA (1969) used the term "DNA stem line" for the proliferating tumor cell population (growth fraction) assuming that the metaphases they measured were a reliable means for that purpose. There are, however, objections against this concept which we have discussed in an earlier subsection.

In the present paper we apply the expression "DNA stem line" only when the tumor reveals a distinct *bimodal* DNA histogram with a basic DNA value (= stem line) and a concommitant duplication peak. The duplication peak or secondary mode is usually formed by proliferating cells in G_2-phase, but may also comprise a tetraploid (4c) tumor cell population, especially if there are some few cells found in the octoploid (8c) range as well.

In undifferentiated tumors with broad unimodal DNA distribution patterns almost all of the cells should be proliferating with a high number of atypical mitoses so that a specific proliferating stem line can no longer be recognized. The mean DNA value of such a broad unimodal DNA histogram in our opinion should not be called a "DNA stem line".

2. Display of Results

We have tried to assemble the data on human tumors in the briefest and most synoptic possible format. We make no claims for completeness due to the wealth of published material. For brevity, DNA histograms have been reduced to a code in which peaks are represented with ploidy numbers and off-peak values with points (see Legend to Table 3).

Each "DNA distribution code" corresponds to a DNA histogram which, in our studies, encompasses 40–100 nuclei for benign tumors and 250–600 nuclei for malignant tumors. Means and standard deviations were calculated for clearly separated peaks on the histogram. These peaks can be given in detail, however, only for some histograms, which are fully displayed in Figs. 1–6. A portion of the results has been displayed in an earlier communication (Böhm et al., 1971).

Next we divided the tumors into benign and malignant, then subdivided the malignant tumors according to organ systems. We further grouped our own data according to the histological degree of differentiation of the tumors. The age and sex of the tumor patient is noted, as well as the specimen source (surgical or autopsy). The total number of cases (tumor patients) and biopsy specimens, subdivided according to organ systems, are given in Table 2.

The mean value for each frequency distribution was obtained, and ploidy values were designated in half-ploidy intervals according to the principle that 25% of the 2c value equals a half-ploidy interval. Mean values between 87.5% and 112.5% of the 2c value were designated 2c; mean values between 112.5% and 137.5% of the 2c value were designated 2.5c; mean values between 137.5% and 162.5% of the 2c value were designated 3c; etc.

3. Benign Tumors

It is often not possible to achieve an exact, conceptual boundary between an autonomous, benign tumor and a by and large hormonally induced hyperplasia without additional information such as hormonal status. We have therefore decided not to distinguish benign tumors and hyperplasias and have classified them rather as a common group to be contrasted with malignant transformations.

There is relatively little literature on benign tumors (Table 3). Benign tumors are usually included only as incidental, individual cases in larger studies of malignant tumors. We ourselves have studied a total of 8 benign tumors from various locations (Table 5). The DNA histograms uniformly show a unimodal distribution with a peak in the 2c range (Fig. 1a; T46 in Table 5). The variations is small so that only relatively few nuclei must be measured to achieve reliable, reproducible mean values. Incidental nuclei found in the 4c region correspond either to diploid cells in G2 phase or to hypertrophied, tetraploid cells in G1 phase. S-phase cells with a Feulgen DNA value between 2c and 4c are seldom encountered. They exist, however, in a proliferating uterine leiomyoma (T1 in Table 5) and in a papillary polyp in the rectal mucosa (Fig. 1b and T50 in Table 5). Histologically these tumors also show individual mitoses as an expression of a certain proliferation activity.

Exceptions to the 2c rule are observed by Izuo et al. (1971a) in several cases of fibrous-cystic breast disease, where aneuploid, widely scattered DNA

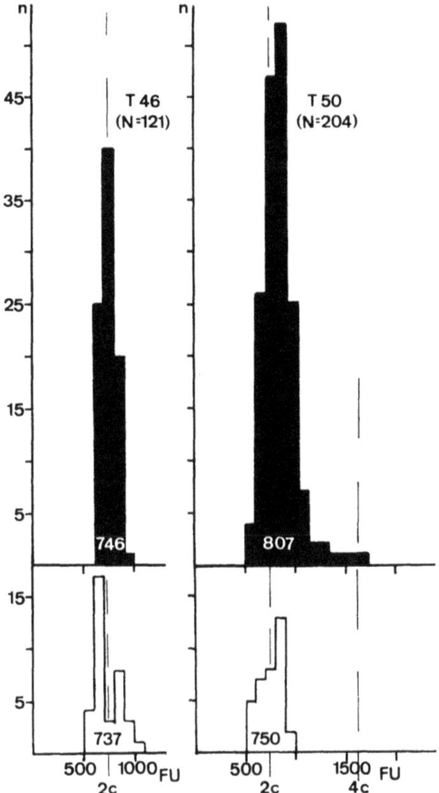

Fig. 1. Left side: Narrow 2c histogram obtained from a *cystic hyperplasia of the breast (mastopathia)* with an average nuclear DNA content of 746 FU which is in close agreement with the 737 *FU* measured from the diploid leukocytes. Right side: Unimodal DNA histogram of a *papillary polyp of the rectum*. Proliferative activity is shown by the few nuclei with a DNA content up to 4c which is enough to cause a slight increase in the average nuclear DNA content (807 *FU*) above the diploid leukocytes (750 *FU*). *N* Number of nuclei measured; *FU* relative nuclear DNA content in terms of fluorescence units

distributions and 3c peaks are seen (Table 3). All these' women developed mammary carcinoma in subsequent clinical followup, suggesting that one was already possibly dealing with a mammary carcinoma *in situ* in these intraductal papillomas and apocrine metaplasias.

An exceptional finding, confirmed by UV absorption measurements and chromosome counts, was noted by HAEMMERLI (1970) in nodular changes in the thyroid (Table 4). Whereas normal and macrofollicular thyroid nodules always exhibited a relative DNA content in the 2c range, the microfollicular and oncocytic nodules showed aneuploid and often highly elevated DNA values in a high percentage of cases. The authors concluded that these nodules should be regarded as potentially malignant. The DNA content in follicular and solid carcinomas, however, appeared at the 2c value in a majority of cases.

4. Colon Carcinoma

It seems rather difficult to compare our own measurements of colon carcinoma (Table 7) with those in the literature. The preparational and technical specifications are very different. Stich *et al.* (1960) measured only metaphase plates on 10 cases. The measurements thus average out twice as large as those for interphase nuclei made by other authors. Although mitotic figures were measured, a substantial variation was observed. Insofar as one can disregard variation due to technique alone (e.g. chromosome measurements on histological sections!), this finding leads us to conclude that the proliferating cell population is not very homogenous.

Comparable measurements from the same laboratory on telophase figures in colon carcinoma (Table 6, Stich and Steele, 1962) and from numerous other malignant tumors show, however, a markedly smaller variation in telophase measurements. We conclude from this that not all metaphase nuclei terminate in division, rather a portion revert back to interphase nuclei, especially those whose chromosome count deviates strongly from that of the "tumor stem line". They contribute to tumor growth through these c-mitoses and incidentally give rise to a wider variation and an elevated DNA content in the interphase population, which is expressed in the corresponding measurements.

In most cases we are dealing with well-differentiated adenocarcinomas as seen daily by the practicing pathologist. Anaplastic colon carcinomas are only seldom seen and apparently haven't been measured yet. It is remarkable, then, that the majority of these differentiated adenocarcinomas exhibit their first frequency peak at 2.5c and a smaller, duplication peak at 5c. This finding is even more striking in our own 12 carcinoma cases (Table 7) than in the literature cases (Table 6). For the most part, then, colon carcinomas have a hyperdiploid 2.5c DNA stem line with a corresponding duplication peak at 5c. Individual tumors also show higher DNA values at 3c, 3.5c, and 4c, in which here also a duplication peak is seen (bimodal DNA distribution, Fig. 2).

Only the results of Zank and Krug (1970), which in contrast to all the other studies are taken from two autopsy cases, deviate somewhat from the general trend. A bimodal, partially trimodal DNA distribution is indeed clearly observed in this investigation, but the measurements for the DNA stem line is seen distinctly lower (1.5c) in one case and substantially higher (5c) in another case by comparison to our own measurements and those of all other authors. Since both lymph node metastases resulted in DNA histograms very different from those of the primary tumor, the possibility of a measuring error must be considered.

5. Endometrial Carcinoma

DNA measurements on a large number of endometrial carcinomas have thus far been reported mainly from Atkin's laboratory (Table 8). Unfortunately in Atkin's (1959) comprehensive study, DNA histograms are not shown for a majority of cases, only the "basic DNA value". We cannot determine the magnitude of variation and the character of bimodal or trimodal DNA peaks from the publication. The presence of the DNA peaks, however,

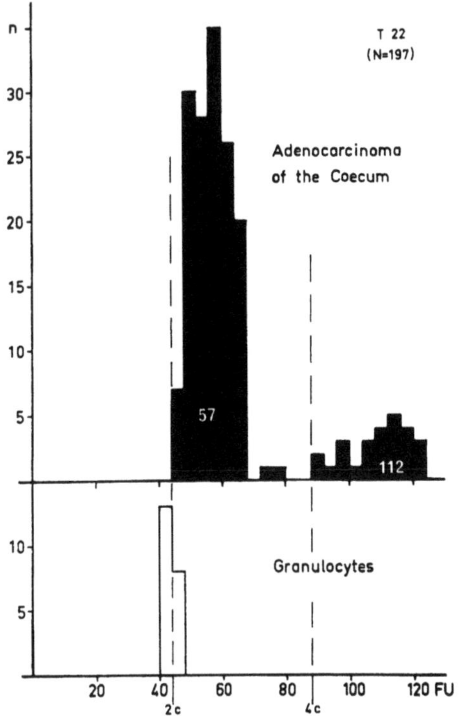

Fig. 2. Bimodal DNA distribution in a histogram of a *well differentiated adenocarcinoma of the coecum*. The second peak reveals a mean nuclear DNA content of 112 *FU* which is an exact duplication of the stem line peak with 57 *FU*

is discussed in the text. It seems probable to us, however, that Atkin's data and our own (Table 9) are largely in agreement, considering that the large majority of tumors in our series exhibit a Feulgen DNA value at 2.5c and a duplication peak at 5c, while Atkin usually finds a diploid basic DNA value in his series. The discrepancies may be technical. We compare our measurements directly to the mean value for lymphocytes and granulocytes whereas Atkin applies a 10% correction to his reference value. Atkin also observes 2 cases with a hypodiploid DNA content. He states there are two major tumor groups: a hyperdiploid and a tetraploid group, where the tetraploid group is substantially smaller. His complete series of highly differentiated adenocarcinomas (7 cases) was either diploid or hypodiploid.

Highly differentiated adenocarcinomas show a very uniform picture in our series with a DNA stemline at 2.5c and a duplication peak at 5c (Table 9). The occasional intermediate values represent proliferating cells. One tumor showed a 3c DNA value with a 6c duplication peak. The bimodal and trimodal DNA distribution demonstrates the presence of polyploid tumor cells. We have often observed such aneuploid-polyploid DNA histograms in differentiated carcinomas and regard them as an expression of orderly and hence regulated proliferation and growth, since polyploid cells are observed to a certain extent in normal organs and in benign tumors (euploid-polyploid DNA histograms).

Two of our cases (T125/126, T161) both from autopsies, were poorly or undifferentiated histologically. The DNA values were higher (5c, 6c) with a wide variation and no corresponding duplication peak. The same holds for endometrial carcinosarcoma (T41).

Insofar as the marginal areas and central portions of the same tumor were studied (4 cases), identical DNA distributions were observed (T 73/74, T 77/78, T 82/81, T 94/95 in Table 9). Identical DNA histograms were also found in a omentum and lymph node metastasis of a papillary adenocarcinoma (T125/126). The primary tumor in this case was excized two years prior to death. The patient was treated with x-irradiation and cytostatic drugs. She expired from cachexia secondary to disseminated metastases.

Recently GRANBERG *et al.* (1974) reported chromosome counts on 4 cases of endometrial carcinoma. Two DNA histograms were shown from these adenocarcinomas, in which a bimodal or even trimodal DNA distribution could be distinguished (Table 8).

6. Bronchial Carcinoma

The DNA distribution in bronchial carcinomas shows a substantially higher variability than the other carcinomas discussed so far, both in our studies (Table 11) and in those from the literature (Table 10). Clean, bimodal histograms are rare. Only STICH and STEELE (1962) could demonstrate up to 4 duplication levels as an expression of tumor cell polyploidy in their measurements on mitotic figures. In fact their basic value showed a hypodiploid DNA content (1.5c), whereas the highest metaphase values reached 24c. SANDRITTER and KLEINHANS (1964) also observed a small cell bronchial carcinoma with a 1.5c DNA content at the principal peak, and revealed scattered values up to a DNA content of 8c.

In marked contrast to the carcinomas of the bowel and endometrium, 3c stem lines with a 6c duplication peak were frequently seen in bronchial carcinomas. GREISEN noted this peculiarity in 1971. No less than 15 of his 31 tumor cases had a triploid or near-triploid DNA value. The remaining 16 tumors were diploid or near-diploid. Tetraploid DNA stem lines were not seen. Unfortunately, GREISEN doesn't give complete histograms, only the DNA ploidy level for the tumor stem line. A high proportion of 3c DNA histograms (8 out of 29 tumor cases) has also been reported by ADAMS and DAHLGREN (1968) (Table 10).

We also observed a 3c stem line with a duplication peak at 6c and occasional values up to 12c in two differentiated squamous cell carcinomas (T 28, T 72 in Table 11). Bimodal DNA distributions with 2,5 c and 5c peaks were demonstrated in another differentiated squamous cell carcinoma both in the primary tumor and in a liver metastasis. However, two further metastases from the same tumor in lymph node and pleura showed a unimodal 4c peak with scatter up to 8c (T 106–109). Tumor tissue in these metastases was histologically undifferentiated. Relatively low DNA values at 2,5c and 3c were also measured

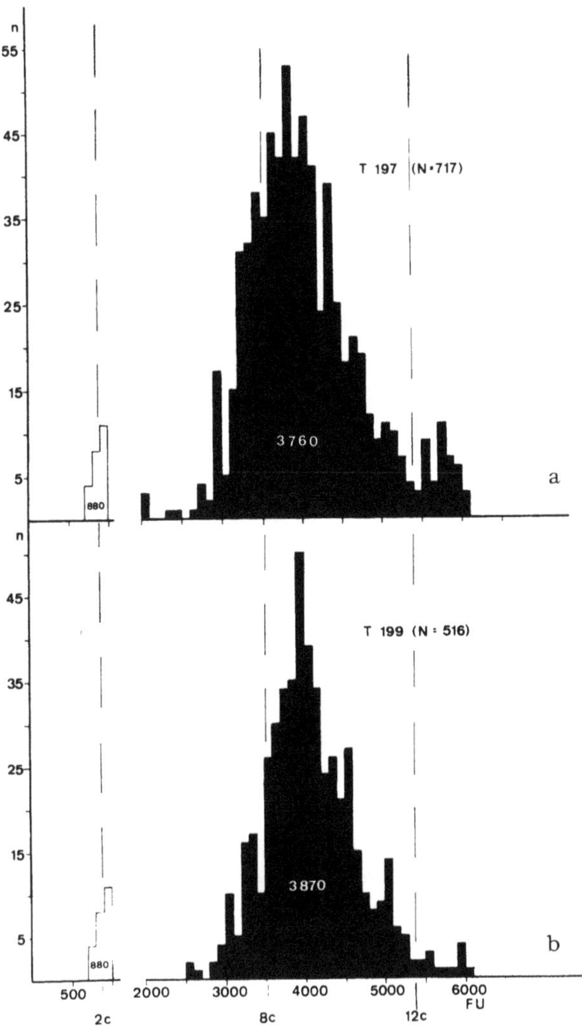

Fig. 3. Broad unimodal DNA histogram in an *anaplastic bronchial carcinoma*. The material was obtained from an autopsy case. The DNA distribution of the *primary lesion (a)* and the *liver metastasis (b)* are congruent. The mean nuclear DNA content is very high (9c)

on small cell bronchial carcinomas (T 153/156, T 170/171). One tumor showed a 2c peak with minimal scatter up to 4c, both in the primary tumor and liver metastasis (T 165/166). The undifferentiated adenocarcinomas and the anaplastic carcinomas, which like the small cell carcinomas in our series were taken only from autopsy material, showed a unimodal DNA distribution with broad peaks and high DNA contents which varied from tumor to tumor (Table 11). Primary tumors and metastases from various locations almost always exhibited comparable distribution patterns (Fig. 3).

The measurements of GREISEN (1971) on the semimalignant carcinoids and multiple cylindromas of the bronchial mucosa must be regarded as benign tumors both on the basis of their histology and their 2c DNA content.

Hährer's and Kaffenberger's (1962) UV-photometric measurements on bronchial carcinoma yield total amounts of nucleic acids (DNA and RNA together) and, therefore, cannot be compared with our results.

7. Mammary Carcinoma

Relatively extensive DNA measurements have been made on mammary carcinomas. The results are highly variable (Table 12). Bimodal and unimodal DNA histograms are seen in nearly equal proportion. Classification by particular histological carcinoma forms or degrees of differentiation is not possible since the specifications for the histology of these carcinomas are too imprecise. It is taken for granted, however, that the majority of "adenocarcinomas" or "mammary carcinomas" represent solid, undifferentiated tumors since these comprise circa 80% of all carcinomas. 3c stem lines are relatively uncommon among mammary carcinomas (single cases noted by Leuchtenberger et al., 1954; Meek, 1961; and Emson and Kirk, 1966). This agrees with the studies of Atkin (1972) on 67 mammary carcinomas. We cannot include the results of this paper in our tables since no DNA histograms were given, only the positions of each frequency maximum. Atkin determined from his rather extensive collection that the "DNA modes" for his carcinoma cases separate into two, discrete groups—a near-diploid and a triploid-tetraploid group. In terms of 8-year survival rates, the near-diploid group shows a significantly better prognosis than the triploid-tetraploid group. Similar findings were seen with ovarian carcinomas (Atkin, 1971).

The 14 mammary carcinomas which we studied (Table 13) were all taken from mastectomy operations except for 2 autopsy cases (T 114/115, T 158–160). Mammary carcinomas with a 2c DNA content had been observed by the Leuchtenberger's (1954) and Sachs (1971) but were not seen in our series. Part of the cases showed clear, bimodal DNA distributions with a 2,5c or 3,5c stem line and a 5c or 7c duplication peak. T 68, a medullary mammary carcinoma, showed a 4,5c stem line with a 9c duplication peak and DNA scatter up to 18c. The remaining carcinomas, including the two autopsy cases, exhibited broad, unimodal DNA histograms with substantial scatter, in which on occasion very high nuclear DNA values were reached (e.g. in an anaplastic carcinoma, T 215). 3c peaks were seen, however, only in two unimodal DNA distribution curves obtained from a pleural and a vertebral metastasis (T 159/160). The corresponding primary tumor, a scirrhous carcinoma, exhibited a very broad 4c peak (T 158). In all remaining cases the DNA histograms for the metastases agreed by and large with those of the primary tumor, as seen also by Meek (1971).

8. Gastric Carcinoma

Our group of eleven gastric carcinomas is larger than the total number of cases reported in the literature (Tables 14 and 15). The DNA measurements are extraordinarily variable. An undifferentiated adenocarcinoma with a 2c stem line and a 4c duplication peak was observed both by us (T 7/6 in Table 15) and by LEUCHTENBERGER *et al.* (1954). The scatter in these tumors was substantially greater than in the euploid (2c) benign tumors (Tables 4, 5). However, higher DNA values at 3c, 3,5c, 4c, 4,5c, and even 7c, in the major cell population often predominated. Although the histologically differentiated carcinomas exhibited a bimodal DNA distribution (T 8/9), the majority of poorly or undifferentiated carcinomas yielded a unimodal DNA histogram with broad scatter. Corresponding DNA histograms in the primary tumor and lymph node metastases were observed both in our 3 cases and in those of ZANK and KRUG (1970). The shift of the main peak from 4c to 2c in the first case of ZANK and KRUG is probably a measurement error; apparently lymphocytes were measured rather than tumor cells.

A shift of low DNA values in the primary tumor to higher values in the metastasis was reported by LEUCHTENBERGER *et al.* (1954) (2c to 3c). We observed an autopsy case in which the difference in DNA content between primary tumor and metastasis was even more marked (T 213/212) and simultaneously showed a change in the histological picture (Fig. 5). The primary tumor, a differentiated, mucous gastric adenocarcinoma, showed a bimodal distribution with 4c stem line and 7c duplication peak, whereas the liver metastases of this tumor revealed an undifferentiated polymorphocellular carcinoma and exhibited a very broadly scattered unimodal DNA histogram with a peak at 7c (Fig. 4). Here we see quite clearly another undifferentiated cell population present than in the primary tumor. A double carcinoma was ruled out by autopsy.

9. Hypernephroid Renal Carcinoma

DNA measurements on hypernephroid carcinomas are known only for 2 cases to date. LEUCHTENBERGER *et al.* (1954) determined a unimodal DNA distribution with 4c peak, whereas SANDRITTER *et al.* (1966) obtained a narrow, 3c peak.

Our DNA measurements on 6 surgically excized hypernephroid carcinomas (Table 16) yielded bimodal DNA distributions for the differentiated tumors and unimodal histograms with highly scattered DNA values for the poorly differentiated and anaplastic carcinomas. Of particular interest is a differentiated clear cell carcinoma with a 2c stem line and appropriate duplication peak. Corresponding histograms were seen in the center and edge of this 8 cm diameter tumor. The histograms of these malignant tumors are undistinguishable from a proliferating population of normal cells or a benign tumor.

10. Bladder and Ureteral Carcinoma

We have only measured one undifferentiated transitional cell carcinoma of the bladder from an autopsy case. It shows a broadly scattered unimodal

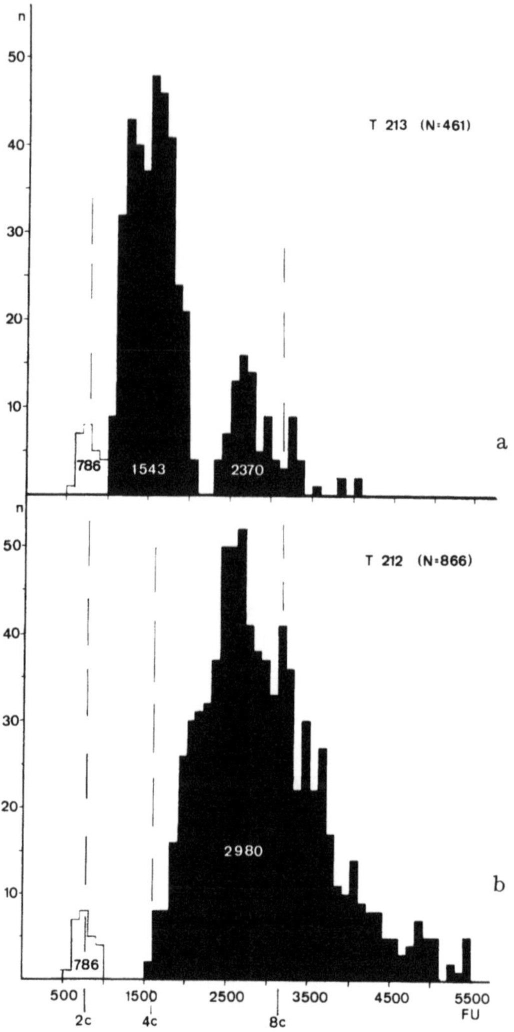

Fig. 4. DNA histograms obtained from a *gastric carcinoma*. The *well differentiated primary lesion (a)* reveals a bimodal DNA distribution, while the *anaplastic liver metastasis (b)* resulted in a broad unimodal DNA histogram with a much higher nuclear DNA content, the peak of which, however, is congruent with the secondary mode of the primary lesion

DNA distribution with a 4c peak (T 101 in Table 18). The majority of bladder carcinomas reported in the literature exhibit a 2c stem line and are hardly distinguishable from normal bladder epithelium, which according to Levi *et al.* (1969) can show tetraploid and octoploid DNA values in addition to the predominant diploid line. All authors agree that well differentiated tumors predominantly exhibit a 2c peak, whereas the nuclear polymorphy and DNA content of the dominant cell population increase with decreasing degree of differentiation. Levi *et al.* (1969) even suggest that bladder tumors originate as diploid cell populations and progress to hypotetraploid and finally to fully aneuploid carcinomas.

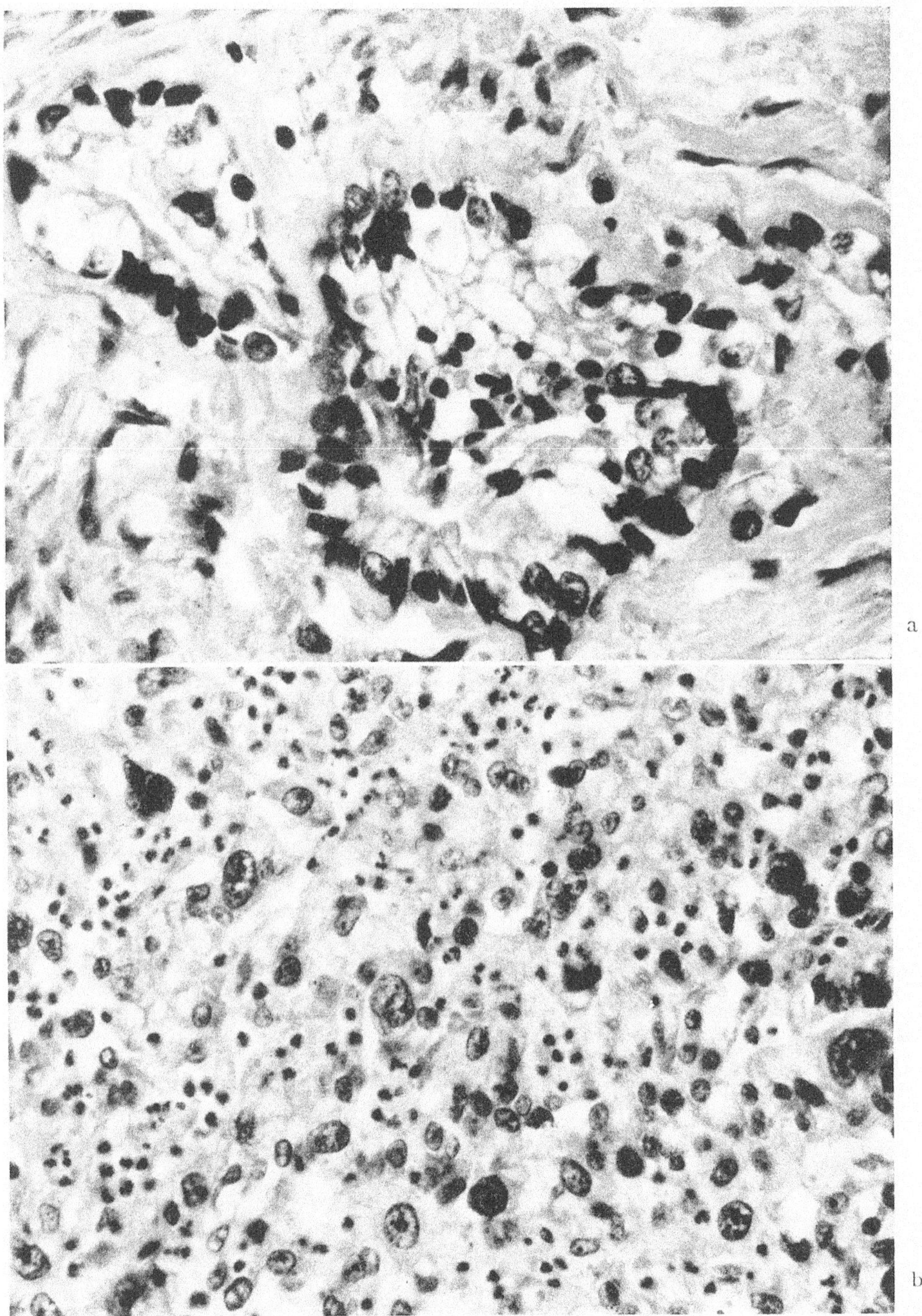

Fig. 5a and b. Histological appearance of the *gastric carcinoma* T 213/212 the histograms of which are shown in Fig. 4. a Differentiated mucous secreting adenocarcinoma in the primary lesion near the cardia. H and E, magn. × 320. b Anaplastic tumor tissue in the liver metastasis. H and E, magn. × 320

Tavares *et al.* (1966) studied 62 bladder carcinomas. They gave no histograms, however, only the c-values of the tumors, and found 35 tumors which they designated as diploid or tetraploid (group 2–4c) and 27 which they designated as triploid-hexaploid (group 3–6c). The first group had a substantially better prognosis than the second.

Four ureteral carcinomas exhibited a diploid (2c) DNA content despite various degrees of histological differentiation (Levi *et al.*, 1969).

11. Prostate Carcinoma

Except for a comprehensive paper by Jacobson (1968), who investigated 135 prostate carcinomas in a monograph unfortunately not available to us, there are only a few, sporadic reports on DNA histograms of prostate carcinoma.

Zank and Krug (1970) showed a 4c stem line with a clear 8c duplication peak in the primary tumor and a similar DNA distribution in the metastasis, except the proportion of 8c cells was larger in the metastasis.

Sprenger *et al.* (1974d) reported DNA measurements on imprint preparations and punch biopsies of the prostate. When inflammation (prostatitis) was present, they found a unimodal 2c population with scatter to 4c in prostatic adenomyomatosis. Widely scattered DNA values between 2c and 4c with a 3c peak and a distinct 6c duplication peak were measured in an anaplastic prostatic carcinoma. Individual measurements reached to 12c. After estrogen therapy a diploid (2c) tumor cell population with a small 4c duplication peak predominated, giving a histogram similar to an adenomyomatosis with prostatitis. Individual measurements still reached to 8c (Sprenger *et al.*, 1974).

We ourselves measured only a single prostatic adenocarcinoma from an autopsy case. It showed a unimodal distribution with a 2,5c peak and values reaching to 5c (T 157 in Table 18).

Tavares *et al.* (1966) studied 35 prostate carcinomas (once again without giving the histograms) and determined that the tumors separate into two groups—a 2–4c group with a better prognosis and a 3–6c group with a poorer prognosis. This prognostic difference is based upon the observation that 22 of 24 patients with a euploid-polyploid tumor in the 2–4c group responded well to estrogen therapy whereas 8 of 9 patients from the aneuploid 3–6c group responded poorly.

12. Ovarian Carcinoma

Our series includes only two papillary adenocarcinomas of the ovary (T 26, T 244 in Table 18), both from surgical excisions. Both show rather broadly scattered DNA values which begin at 2.5c and reach up to 16c in one tumor. The dominant cell population in T 26 has a DNA content of 4.5c, in T 244 of 2.5c. We are dealing with unimodal distribution curves without a genuine DNA stem line.

A broad scatter of DNA values is also observed by BADER (1959, 1960) (Table 19). In his series the dominant cell population usually exhibited a 2c DNA content. Of particular interest are the interphase, metaphase, and telophase measurements made on the same tumor. Although interphase and metaphase nuclei each exhibited very broadly scattered DNA distributions with values up to 13c, measurements on anaphase nuclei in 5 tumors all gave only 2c values. BADER concluded that the genuine proliferating stem cell population whose mitoses were actually completed exhibit a 2c DNA content.

In 1971, ATKIN published another study on 61 ovarian carcinomas. He gave only the chromosome count or modal DNA value for each tumor, no histograms. The carcinomas separate into two discrete groups. A low ploidy (near-diploid) group which had less often extended beyond the ovary exhibited a significantly better prognosis than the high-ploidy (near triploid-tetraploid) group. The low-ploidy group was for the most part only minimally better differentiated than the high ploidy tumors.

13. Thyroid Carcinoma

HAEMMERLI (1970) reported on 17 carcinomas in her study of DNA measurements on nodular changes in the thyroid, including 14 with a 2c value, two with a 2.5c value, and one with a 3c value (Table 4). The histological type and degree of differentiation of these carcinomas was not stated.

An anaplastic thyroid carcinoma reported by SANDRITTER *et al.* (1966) showed a unimodal DNA distribution with a 3.5c peak. We also observed unimodal DNA histograms in each of our 3 autopsy cases of anaplastic thyroid carcinoma (Table 18), including a 3c, a 4c, and a 4.5c tumor. In each case the DNA values were widely scattered, reaching to 10c and 12c. Metastases, measured in two cases, showed essential agreement with the DNA distribution of the corresponding primaries (T 122–124, T 239–242).

Little is available on chromosomal findings in early thyroid tumors in the human. Frank cancers of the thyroid have been invariably found to be aneuploid. No two tumors had identical chromosomal changes (SANDBERG and SAKURAI, 1974).

14. Cervical Carcinoma and Precancers

Without even mentioning chromosome analysis, the literature on DNA content in premalignant and malignant changes in the uterine cervix are almost too numerous to review. Several reasons must underly this unusual interest by scientists: (1) the organ is easily accessible; (2) clearly bounded stages of precancerous disease are discernible, so that the development of a carcinoma from its precursors can readily be observed and controlled; (3) nuclear changes in exfoliated cervical cells play a decisive role in the diagnosis and management of cervical carcinoma.

Thus DNA measurements on cervical epithelium are of special interest both to cancer researchers and to practicing clinical gynecologists.

Since there are already so many published articles (Table 20) in this area, including those from our own group, we did not carry out any further DNA measurements on cervical changes in the present series. Nonètheless we shall attempt to show a sequence of changes in this organ which lead from normal tissue, regulated by the genome, to a malignant, autonomous neoplasm which finally destroys the patient.

Although it is difficult to achieve an overview from the large amount of measurements obtained by many authors with differing methods of preparation and measurement and varying precision, some tendencies seem to emerge. Among dysplastic changes we usually find a 2c or 4c DNA stem line in which further duplication peaks at 8c, 16c, and even 32c are observed. The DNA values are usually widely scattered, so that one requires relatively many cells to discern distinct peaks. In a comprehensive paper by SACHS *et al.* (1972), we find no peaks at all in most of the tumor histograms (i.e., most intervals contain fewer than 10 cells!) We couldn't use these histograms in our table. The same holds for the paper by LAUMONIER *et al.* (1963).

The euploid polyploidy in dysplastic cervical epithelium observed both by ourselves (BÖHM *et al.*, 1971), BRANDAO (1969), and WAGNER *et al.* (1972), is a remarkable finding, which is distinctly different from the results with carcinoma *in situ* and invasive carcinoma. Euploid polyploidy, i.e. bimodal, trimodal, and polymodal DNA distributions with a 2c base and multiple duplication peaks at 4c, 8c, 16c, and 32c, is also seen in the functional acceleration of a normal organ, e.g. in heart hypertrophy (ADLER and SANDRITTER, 1971; PFITZER, 1971), phenobarbital-induced hepatomegaly (BÖHM and MOSER, 1975), or in hormonal cell stimulation, e.g. in the Arias-Stella reaction of endometrium (WAGNER and RICHART, 1968), the granulosa-lutein cells of the corpus luteum (STANGEL *et al.*, 1970), and in lactating breast (IZUO *et al.*, 1971). This finding in cervical epithelium would thus mean that dysplastic cell and nuclear changes, in contrast to carcinoma *in situ*, represent benign changes possibly due to the influence of estrogen. The same concept was discussed by LAUMONIER *et al.* (1963) and WILBANKS *et al.* (1967) on the basis of cytophotometric measurements.

DNA histograms in carcinoma *in situ* and invasive carcinoma are not distinguishable, according to SANDRITTER and FISCHER (1962), and LAUMONIER *et al.* (1963). We are dealing for the most part with a unimodal DNA distribution with a 2.5c or 3c peak and broad scatter to higher DNA values, however without genuine duplication peaks.

In carcinoma *in situ*, surgically managed either by hysterectomy or an excisional cone biopsy of the cervix, a painstaking histological workup comprising numerous sections at various levels reveals normal epithelial cells, inflammatory areas, dysplastic regions, and frank carcinoma *in situ* which itself is divisible into progressive stages of change, such a "simple replacement", "coarse proliferation in glands, "early stromal invasion", and "microcarcinoma". SANDRITTER and FISCHER (1962) found identical DNA histograms with a 2.5c peak in all four stages of carcinoma *in situ* within a single case. In a second case, the DNA values for "simple replacement" and "coarse proliferation in glands" (6c and 5c peaks) were double the DNA values for early stromal invasion and microcarcinoma (2.5c with duplication peaks). This finding of "ploidy reduction" in the progression from precancerous to invasive carcinoma seems especially interesting to us. SACHS *et al.* (1972) made similar observations. SANDBERG and SAKURAI (1974), independently, mentioned a reduction of the chromosome number, when they compared carcinoma *in situ* and invasive cancer of the cervix. "Ploidy reduction" is perhaps mediated by a selection mechanism in which a cell of lower, near-diploid DNA content is selected from a larger pool of higher aneuploid cells of the carcinoma *in situ* (STEELE *et al.*, 1969), and serves as the stem cell from which a tumor clone arises. This tumor cell population gives rise to a unimodal DNA distribution up to 6c, later a bimodal distribution, and finally, especially after radiation therapy, to a broadly scattered DNA histogram with high DNA values (see also Table 27). Management with cytostatic drugs, by contrast, appears to have no influence on the DNA histogram (HOLZNER and GOLOP, 1968).

ATKIN (1964) observed a 2c stem line with a 4c duplication peak in half his carcinoma cases. Biopsy DNA histograms agreed with cytological smear DNA histograms in all cases.

Since it is possible to map Papanicolaou-stained cervical smears photographically and to follow up with consecutive Feulgen staining (WIED *et al.*, 1966), it is possible to amplify a cytological decision of pseudodyskaryosis or dyskaryosis on a single cell with a nuclear content measurement on the same cell (BÖHM *et al.*, 1971; WAGNER *et al.*, 1972; SPRENGER *et al.*, 1974b). The results of SANDRITTER *et al.* (1960, 1964) with gallocyanine chromalaun staining of vaginal cytological material are not comparable since pretreatment with RNAse was not carried out. Fluorescence cytophotometry on vaginal cytologic material carries a special significance, since it has proven to be a practical, automatic prescreening procedure for gynecological cytology (SPRENGER *et al.*, 1971a, 1971b; SPRENGER *et al.*, 1972; SPRENGER *et al.*, 1974a, 1974c).

15. Skin Carcinoma and Cutaneous Precancers

The results of DNA measurements on basal cell carcinoma of the skin are contradictory. MANOCHA (1969) observed 2c anaphase and 4c metaphase DNA content exclusively on his measurements of mitotic figures. In most tumors the measurement variation was hardly larger than the comparison population of lymphocytes. Only 5 of 15 basal cell carcinomas gave a bimodal DNA distribution with 4c and 8c peaks in the metaphase plates. All others were unimodal. A substantial portion of values between 4c and 8c were found only in 3 of the bimodal DNA histograms. A basal-squamous carcinoma gave an aneuploid 6c value for metaphase DNA.

On the other hand, EHLERS (1968) observed only unimodal, relatively broadly scattered DNA values, with aneuploid frequency maxima consistently greater than 2c in 14 basal cell carcinomas of various histological types.

In a later paper, MANOCHA *et al.* (1969) compared DNA histograms from metaphase plates of skin carcinoma *in situ* (this classification is unclear to us) to those of squamous epithelial carcinoma, including a "self-healing carcinoma" (keratoacanthoma). While the predominant cell population almost always showed diploid metaphase plates (4c DNA content) with occasionally very high DNA measurements, squamous epithelial carcinoma regularly exhibited broadly scattered DNA histograms with maxima in the 5c to 10c regions (measured on metaphases) (Table 21). Bimodal and even trimodal DNA histograms with maxima inconsistent with a geometric series, i.e. inconsistent with simple polyploidy, were seen as the expression of a mosaic mixture of tumor from multiple tumor cell stem lines. From this "genetically heterogeneous collection of cells with no dominant cell type", a "more vigorous" stem line is selected which subjects the predominant cell mass to invasion by proliferation. "The formation of a stem line seems to be almost a prerequisite to establish a tumor or to make it invasive" (MANOCHA *et al.*, 1969). The epidermoid carcinomas measured by EHLERS and HERBSTREIT (1973) exhibited hyperdiploid (2.5c) and triploid (3c) DNA maxima almost exclusively, with scatter reaching to very high DNA values.

In contrast to the epidermoid carcinomas, facultative and obligate precancers of the skin (EHLERS and STEPHAN, 1972a, 1972b) resulted in a higher DNA content throughout, including some unimodal, some bimodal histograms, with peaks localized at 4c, 5c, 6c, and even 7c, and 8c. The scatter in all measurements was considerable, so that cell populations highly heterogeneous with respect to the DNA complement must be presumed. Similar findings were observed by SACHS (1970) (Table 21).

The high DNA content in precancers of the skin and the lower hypodiploid to triploid DNA content in invasive squamous epithelial carcinoma underscores the hypothesis of ploidy reduction discussed in the previous subsection, which may appear in the progression of precancer to invasive carcinoma.

DNA measurements on a mycosis fungoides of the skin were recently published (VAN VLOTEN *et al.*, 1974). Most skin changes showed a bimodal DNA distribution with 2c and 4c peaks, the euploid or euploid-polyploid DNA patterns, which are unusual for malignant tumors. Since polyploid nuclei are so rare in the skin, however, the authors feel that 5% or more nondiploid cells should serve as a criterion for malignancy. Since the early stages of mycosis fungoides are difficult to determine histologically, this could prove to be an ancillary diagnostic tool.

16. Carcinomas in Different Locations

The DNA distribution in differentiated adenocarcinoma of the pancreas seems to resemble that of the gastrointestinal tract quite strongly. The few cases currently available exhibit a near-diploid (2c, 2.5c) peak, frequently with a duplication peak at 5c. LEUCHTENBERGER *et al.* (1954) determined a 1.5c DNA value with a 4c duplication peak in a pancreatic adenocarcinoma (Table 22).

Our own studies include only 2 pancreatic carcinomas (Table 18), a differentiated glandular tumor with a 2.5c peak and a 5c duplication peak and an undifferentiated signet ring carcinoma exhibiting a unimodal, broadly scattered DNA distribution maximal in the 6–8c region. The metastases for each carcinoma agree with the corresponding primaries (T103–105, T192–194).

This also holds for two squamous epithelial carcinomas of the esophagus and their satellites. The DNA contents for these poorly and undifferentiated carcinomas, respectively, were relatively high at 3.5c and 4c, including scatter to 10c (T117–119, T200–202). As for the pancreatic carcinomas, the esophagus carcinomas were both from autopsy cases.

A rare, highly differentiated adenocarcinoma of the ileum with lymph node metastases, exhibited a DNA histogram consistent with benign proliferation (T24 in Table 18). A distinct 2c stem line with 4c duplication peak was seen (Fig. 6). Only the occasional values exceeding 4c on the histogram expose the underlying malignancy of this tumor.

The literature contains only scattered reports on testicular tumors (Table 22). All are either seminomas or pseudoseminomas (synonym for seminoma+malignant teratoma?). Unimodal DNA distributions with 3c, 4.5c, and 2.5c maxima and scatter up to 7c are described. We found a 2.5c principal peak, 5c duplication peak, and measurements reaching to 10c in the seminoma we studied (Table 18).

ATKIN (1973) reported a large series of chromosome counts and DNA measurements on 103 seminomas and malignant testicular teratomas in which hyperdiploid and triploid chromosome counts predominated. Three origins are possible for the 3n chromosome counts: 1. repeated nondisjunction, 2. endoreduplication with chromosome loss, 3. tumor origin from a triploid epithelial germ line.

17. Malignant Lesions of Blood and Hematopoetic System

DNA measurements on malignant tumors of the hematopoietic system have been heretofore carried out only on blood and bone marrow smears from leukemia patients (Table 23). Findings reported in the literature make it clear that DNA content in leukemic cells differs little or not at all from that in normal human leukocytes. Cases of chronic myelogenous and lymphatic leukemia measured by HALE (1959) are diploid except for a purposely measured population of primitive cells (blastic crisis?) which exhibited 4c DNA values with considerable variation.

All other authors, without exception, report acute leukemias with 2c or 2.5c, i.e. near-diploid. Bimodal DNA histograms were reported only by OBRECHT *et al.* (1970), including a case with 4.5c, another case with 5c DNA stem lines (Table 23). It is interesting that leukemic cells with an elevated

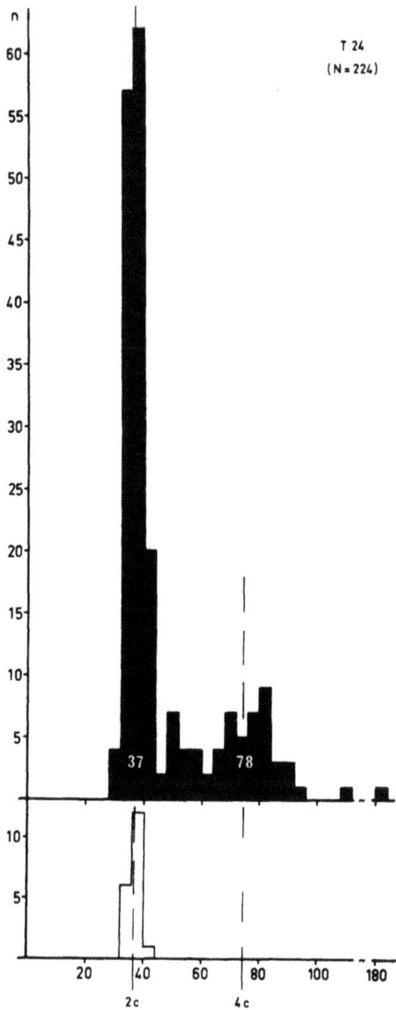

Fig. 6. Bimodal DNA distribution of a *well differentiated adenocarcinoma of the ileum*. The 2c stem line peak (37 *FU*) is narrow, and the duplication peak (78 *FU*) is only slightly more prominent than one would expect from a normal proliferating tissue. The pattern is virtually indistinguishable from that of a benign tumor. Only two nuclei were found with a DNA content far beyond the 4c value

DNA content responded better to cytostatic therapy and thus exhibited a better prognosis than leukocytes with a 2c DNA content (LAMPERT, 1967; OBRECHT *et al.*, 1970).

Our own studies concern tumor changes in the hematopoietic system (Table 24), not leukemia cells in blood smears. The number of cases is limited and should be expanded. We determined a 3c stem line with 6c and 12c duplication peaks in a lymphogranulomatosis (Hodgkin's disease) of mixed type. Intermediate values were almost never observed.

A chronic lymphadenosis showed a 3c cell population in a periaortic lymph node and two 2.5c populations in an axillary and an iliac lymph node, all with narrow variation.

Post mortem material from two cases of plasmacytoma was investigated in three locations apiece. In one patient we found a 3c stem line with 6c duplication peak, in the other a 2.5c DNA histogram with scatter up to 5c. In both cases the tissue samples from various locations agreed with respect to the DNA histogram (T110–112 and T145–147 in Table 24). Since this is usually observed in solid tumor metastases, we cannot conclude from this that plasmacytoma is inherently a systemic 'disease. The finding, however, underscores the monoclonal nature of this disease.

18. Sarcomas

Malignant mesenchymal tumors have heretofore only been studied as isolated cases (Table 25). The DNA histograms are highly variable. Unimodal and bimodal DNA distributions are seen. In differentiated osteosarcoma stem lines at 3.5c and 5c have been described, with duplication peaks at 7c and 10c, respectively.

We ourselves measured a total of 7 sarcoma cases from various locations and various degrees of differentiation (Table 26). A desmoid tumor of the fascia lata of the thigh in a 12 year old girl showed an aneuploid 2.5c DNA content with a 5c duplication peak. The monomorphic cellular picture in a differentiated liposarcoma of the leg was reflected in the narrow, 2.5c DNA peak. A monomorphic spindle cell sarcoma and a rhabdomyosarcoma resulted in 2.5c stem lines with 5c duplication peaks.

Broadly scattered unimodal DNA histograms were seen in 2 undifferentiated sarcomas (leiomyosarcoma of the myometrium and endometrial sarcoma).

A 17 cm diameter uniformly undifferentiated nephroblastoma (Wilms tumor) from a 6 year old boy showed a unimodal DNA distribution with rather broad scatter, in agreement at 5 locations.

D. Discussion

1. Benign Tumors

The DNA histograms from benign tumors and tumor-like hyperplasias, whether measured initially by us or taken from the majority of relevant literature, exhibit a narrowly scattered, 2c distribution. This is seen both in epithelial and mesenchymal tumors. The narrowly distributed, 2c DNA content, which agrees with diploid leukocytes in these benign tumors, coincides with the monomorphic histological and cytological appearances of these growths. As soon as one sees some proliferative activity histologically, either as mitotic figures or as inflammatory activation, the DNA histogram shows occasional values reaching to 4c. These are expressions of a nuclear DNA synthesis (S-phase cells), which prepares the cell for division. If a sufficient number of cells are chosen at random in a histogram of sufficient precision, then we can even determine the proportions of G1, S, and G2 phase cells.

A bimodal DNA distribution with a clearly discernible 4c peak would thus indicate a prolonged G2 phase, possibly the expression of an early, euploid polyploidization, which we see for example in dysplasia of cervical epithelium (q.v.).

Euploid polyploidizations with repeatedly duplicated DNA levels up to 32c (geometric series) are also seen in benign phaeochromocytoma, as Lewis (1971) could show in 12 cases (Table 4). Histologically these hormonally active tumors, which usually arise in the adrenal medulla, exhibit an extraordinary cellular and nuclear polymorphy, so that one anticipates a malignancy at first glance. Since we are dealing with an autonomous growth, there is no chance that we are seeing simply a hormonally controlled hyperfunctional hypertrophy with nuclear polyploidization, which we recognize for example in the granulosa-lutein cells of the corpus luteum (Stangel et al., 1970), in the Arias-Stella cells of the endometrium (Wagner and Richard, 1968), and in the beta cells of the islets of Langerhans seen in fetopathia diabetica (Böhm, unpublished results). It is nonetheless interesting and remarkable that euploid polyploidizations arise typically in endocrine organs, and almost invariably are associated with elevated function, i.e. increased hormone production. This is also true for the autonomous phaeochromocytoma (Lewis, 1971), in which paroxysmal release of epinephrine and norepinephrine leads to the pathological hypertensive crises in these patients.

The few cases seen by Izuo et al. (1971a) of mastopathy with aneuploid 1.5c and 3c DNA content all eventually developed a mammary carcinoma, so that we were dealing already with a carcinoma *in situ* at the time of measurement, or else an aneuploid DNA content in a histologically benign tumor has a poor prognosis in the long run. In the final analysis, both interpretations amount to the same thing.

In marked contrast to the generally reliable rule of a euploid or euploid-polyploid DNA content in benign tumors and tumorous hyperplasias, the findings of Haemmerli (1970) on nodular changes in the thyroid stand alone. We are dealing again with an endocrine gland which exhibits remarkable properties. Haemmerli determined that normal adult thyroid tissue, fetal thyroid tissue, and normo- and macrofollicular nodular changes in the thyroid in all 210 cases she studied exhibited a 2c DNA content, whereas microfollicular and oncocytic thyroid nodules had an elevated DNA content at 2.5c, 3c, even 3.5c, in over three-fourths of cases (Table 4). The cytophotometric measurements could be substantiated by cytogenetic studies of chromosome counts.

From the viewpoint of general pathology, in dealing with microfollicular and especially with oncocytic nodules in the thyroid, we are talking about adenomas, i.e., TSH independent, autonomous thyroid tumors, for which the pathologist using histology alone, often experiences considerable difficulties in determining the character of the growth in the absence of an invasive factor. Haemmerli interprets the elevated DNA content as evidence for a early locally limited, noninvasive carcinoma or at least a precancerous stage,

and the experience of the pathologist teaches us that the degeneration rate
to genuine invasion and metastatic thyroid carcinoma is quite low. A remarkable and currently unexplained discrepancy in this evaluation is the fact that
14 of 17 invasive thyroid carcinomas measured by HAEMMERLI have a 2c DNA
content. Is this another realization of the "ploidy reduction principle" in the
transformation of a precancer into an invasive carcinoma?

2. Malignant Tumors

Tumors which have the histological and biological criteria of malignancy
usually exhibit an aneuploid DNA content (deviating from the diploid 2c)
in a majority of nuclei. This rule is not without exceptions. In 4 of 97 tumors
we investigated, i.e., in 4% of cases, we determined a 2c DNA stem line. All
other tumors had an aneuploid or polyploid DNA content. Hypodiploid stem
lines were not seen. On closer examination the four "outliers" were 2 highly
differentiated carcinomas—a hypernephroid carcinoma (T96/97 in Table 16)
and an adenocarcinoma of the ileum (T24 in Table 18)—and 2 undifferentiated
carcinomas—a small cell bronchial carcinoma (T165/66 in Table 11) and a
solid gastric carcinoma (T7/6 in Table 15). All carcinomas distinguished
themselves histologically as having a monotonous cellular and nuclear picture.
The malignancy of the intestinal tumors was established by the presence of
regional lymph node metastases, and that of the hypernephroma by the size
of the tumor (8 cm diameter). Both patients are alive after 4 years with no
recurrence. The small cell bronchial carcinoma resulted from an autopsy case,
and the 65 year old patient with the gastric carcinoma expired a few months
later with uncontrolled tumor dissemination.

The DNA histograms in these carcinomas are similar to those of benign
tumors. The scatter in these tumors was somewhat greater than that in
diploid benign tumors, however. Except for the unimodal small cell bronchial
carcinomas, all DNA histograms showed a 4c duplication peak. In the intestinal and gastric carcinomas, some DNA values were seen reaching to 6c
and 8c. These aneuploid measurements over 4c constitute important evidence
of malignancy.

The literature contains more frequent reports of malignancies with a 2c
DNA content. In certain organs such as the bladder (Table 17) and the ovary
(Table 19), and also to a certain extent in differentiated squamous epithelial
carcinomas of the cervix (ATKIN, 1964; in Table 20), they seem to appear
more often. Intermediates between benign and distinctly malignant, tumors
are well known for papillary neoplasias of the bladder and ovary, which can
be expressed in terms of cytologic criteria for "grading" of tumor malignancy.

Recently LEDERER et al. (1972) reported that there is a correlation between
the grade of a papillary tumor and its nuclear DNA content. Thus cytophotometric DNA determinations may offer a method for solving differential
diagnostic problems in the gray area between benign and malignant growth.

We hesitate to recommend this method because of the insufficient discriminatory power and the relatively high margin of error in cytophotometric preparations and measurement methods. Too many bladder cell carcinomas with 2c DNA content have been described (Tavares et al., 1966; Levi et al., 1969; Fossa, 1975).

The relationships for papillary-serous adenocarcinoma of the ovary, especially as described by Bader (1959), are entirely analogous. The great majority of tumor cells exhibit a 2c DNA content, even in grade III carcinomas. High DNA measurements reaching beyond 4c were seen in practically every tumor, however. Thus we feel that aneuploid DNA values lying above 4c constitute a surer sign of distinction between benignness and malignancy than the "DNA stem line". This is especially important in the evaluation of flowthrough fluorescence cytophotometric DNA data (Sprenger et al., 1974c).

We have already gone over Haemmerli's (1970) 2c thyroid carcinomas. A great number of cases with a dominant 2c population have been determined in malignancies of the hematopoietic system (leukemia and plasmacytoma, Table 23), in which only a minimal variation of values is seen, consistent with the monotonous morphological appearance in leukemia and plasmacytoma cells. The tumorous changes in our series on the hematopoietic system all showed a low, aneuploid, 2.5c or 3c DNA content (Table 24).

van Vloten et al. (1974) recently reported on the euploid-polyploid DNA values in mycosis fungoides in the skin. These authors feel that more than 5% nondiploid reticulum cells serve as a criterion for malignancy in this particular tumor location in the skin.

We wish to summarize these findings with the concept that a dominant 2c tumor population in no way rules out malignancy. Thus the postulate that malignant transformation is always accompanied by a quantitative change in genetic material should be dispelled. When atypical mitotic figures lead to an unequal distribution of chromosomes and thence to the appearance of cell nuclei with an aneuploid DNA content, one should ask why these mitotic errors occur. The cells must be altered or damaged in some fashion. The point of attack of spindle poisons and mitotic inhibitors is understood. Gene and chromosomal mutations have been discussed as mechanisms in the initial carcinogenesis. Thus it is clear that a qualitative change in the chromatin must precede the quantitative change in the sense of a multiple step progression in carcinogenesis. The quantitative changes in DNA content of tumor cells are not the cause but rather a result or associated finding in malignant transformation (specific and coincidental changes as discussed by Atkin and Baker, 1966). An elevated DNA content doesn't represent a necessary prior condition for malignant tumor growth. It is simply a phenomenon often observed in tumor cells which plays an important role in the histological evaluation of tumor tissue as an index of nuclear hyperchromasia. Carcinomas and sarcomas with a diploid (2c) DNA content are seen nonetheless, and with regularity in certain organs.

3. Histological Differentiation and Bimodal DNA Histograms

As we have stated several times, in our own series the DNA distribution of tumor tissue is faithfully expressed in the monomorphy or polymorphy of the histological picture. The measurement of nuclear DNA content simply confirms a finding which the eye of the histologist has long regarded as a valid criterion of malignancy.

Furthermore the histological degree of differentiation in tumors has been determined by pathologists for many years, where it is often the case that poorly or undifferentiated malignancies exhibit a polymorphic cellular and nuclear picture. We have further noted, especially in our own material, that *differentiated carcinomas*, regardless of location but especially colon and endometrial adenocarcinomas, usually *exhibit bimodal DNA distributions* (Table 7 and 9). The dominant cell population usually has a 2.5c DNA content. The corresponding duplication peak appears at 5c, and even a third frequency peak at 9–10c is noted in several highly differentiated carcinomas (T44, T57, T65 in Table 7). Only in these bimodal or trimodal DNA histograms can we speak about a "DNA stem line" in the strict sense, since we see here both the "basic DNA content" and the proliferating cell population of the tumor. The appearance of aneuploid-polyploid frequency maxima ("secondary modes") is evidence for a normal DNA duplication in the S phase and for predominantly regularly terminating mitoses in these differentiated tumors. The duplication peaks arise from cells in the G2 phase or from endomitotic nuclei in the G1 phase (polyploid tumor cells). Thus the proliferation kinetics of these tumors resembles by and large the kinetics of a normal, proliferating tissue. In these differentiated tumors both the histological picture and the DNA distribution point to a process of cell growth which is, at least in part, ordered and controlled.

4. Undifferentiated Carcinomas with Unimodal DNA Histograms

Usually the nuclear DNA content in undifferentiated malignant tumors is more highly elevated than in differentiated tumors. There are exceptions, expecially in small cell bronchial carcinomas. *DNA histograms are usually unimodal* with a single, very broadly scattered frequency maximum, often spanning several ploidy levels. *A "DNA stem line" cannot be distinguished* in these undifferentiated, anaplastic carcinomas. Most of these tumor cells are obviously capable of proliferation. Atypical mitoses are numerous. They lead to an enormous heterogeneity in the tumor cell population which is seen histologically in the form of a significant cellular and nuclear polymorphy. Althouth many tumor cells perish, the tumor grows rapidly. In contrast to the differentiated tumors, a controlled organization is not recognizable either histologically or at the level of proliferation kinetics. Unrestrained, self-destructive growth is seen.

We have noted these unimodal, broadly scattered DNA histograms principally in our autopsy cases, and we feel that these fully autonomous and wildly growing tumors often represent the *end stages of neoplastic disease,* which are unresponsive to further therapy.

5. Precancers

Precancerous changes have been studied on the uterine cervix and on the skin. Because of the great significance which attaches to nuclear changes in the cytologic evaluation of exfoliated cells from the cervix, there is a great interest in DNA measurements on vaginal cytologic material. There are numerous published articles (Table 20). While unambiguous separation of dysplasia of the cervical epithelium from carcinoma *in situ* is not possible cytologically, these two precancerous changes can readily be distinguished on histological section. The DNA histograms likewise show characteristic differences. Whereas the dysplasias with their euploid-polyploid DNA distributions spanning sometimes to extremely high values (up to 32c) more closely resemble precancers of the skin, the DNA histograms for carcinoma *in situ* are in most cases undistinguishable from those for invasive carcinoma. In other words, the precancerous "so-called carcinoma *in situ*" corresponds more to a late stage invasive carcinoma as regards its DNA complement. The first important step in the direction of malignancy is thus the transformation of the euploid-polyploid DNA distribution of dysplasia into a heterogeneous, aneuploid cell population of carcinoma *in situ*. The second, biologically decisive step is the invasion of the stroma. In the cervix, where we can observe the stages of tumor development directly, the alteration in DNA content precedes the invasive stage of the carcinoma. Thus DNA elevation is the prelude to carcinoma invasion. Invasive squamous epithelial carcinomas in the cervix, however, are usually diploid or hyperdiploid in their dominant cell population (Table 20). Thus a reduction in DNA content ("ploidy reduction") may accompany the initiation of invasive growth with selection of a near-diploid stem line. Sandritter and Fischer (1962) were able to show this in a case of carcinoma *in situ* with early stromal invasion using DNA measurements in different regions with progressive stages of invasion. In another case, however, they found a preservation of the DNA peak in the transition from carcinoma *in situ* to invasive carcinoma. Thus ploidy reduction is not seen in all cases. There are also near-tetraploid (3.5c, 4c, 4.5c) cervical carcinomas which have obviously arisen through selection of a higher ploidy cell clone.

Ehlers and Stephan (1972a, 1972b) could not demonstrate any differences in the DNA histogram between facultative and obligate precancers of the skin. Here they observed some bimodal, some unimodal DNA histograms with broad scatter and high or very high DNA values (Table 21), whereas unimodal hyperdiploid and triploid DNA maxima were observed almost exclusively in epidermoid carcinomas (Ehlers and Herbstreit, 1973, in Table 21). It is an open question whether the principle of ploidy reduction plays a role in the appearance of invasive skin carcinomas from their earlier stages.

6. Mosaic Composition of Tumors

STICH and STEELE (1962) and STICH (1963) determined the DNA content for interphase, metaphase, and telophase nuclei within the same tumor. The values for interphase nuclei and to an extent also for metaphase nuclei were widely scattered and often exhibited no stem line, whereas the telophase plates always showed little scatter in the DNA values. The authors concluded that "most of the sarcomas and carcinomas exhibited various degrees of mosaic composition, which may be limited to nondividing cells but may be present also in the dividing cell population." In this broad context, all tumors with a bimodal or even with a broadly scattered unimodal DNA distribution exhibit a "mosaic composition", which is simply the expression of a variable DNA complement in a heterogeneous tumor cell population.

We wished to understand the concept of mosaic composition more closely and asked ourselves whether similar or varying DNA distribution patterns were present at different locations. We took tissue samples from the same tumor at various places, usually in the center or periphery, and studied them histologically and cytophotometrically. The tumor histology as well as the DNA histograms were almost always in agreement (Fig. 3, Table 9, 16, 24). Only on occasion did we detect minor variations in the DNA histogram from place to place (T88/89 in Table 7; T85/86 in Table 15).

In a predominantly sarcomatous, 16 cm diameter, large nephroblastoma from a 6 year old boy we measured practically identical DNA distributions at 5 different points in the tumor (Table 26). Genuine, "coarsely granular mosaics" with distinct cell populations (clones) in different sections of the same tumor seem to appear only rarely.

These "cross-sectional studies" of a tumor, which can only show the condition of the tumor disease at a single point in time, are supplemented by simultaneous DNA measurements on primary tumors and metastases. Usually the DNA histograms in metastases agree with those in the primary tumor, both in the literature (MEEK, 1961, in Table 12) and in our own studies (Tables 13, 15, 18). Several cases showed deviations, especially in metastatic bronchial carcinoma (Table 11), where in certain autopsy cases the patient had a primary tumor and some metastases in agreement, whereas other metastases showed a different DNA distribution and sometimes even a different histological appearance (e.g., 106–109 in Table 11).

An egregious example of this heterogeneity is seen in the gastric carcinoma T213/212 in Table 15 and Fig. 4. While the primary tumor presents itself as a poorly differentiated, mucoid, glandular carcinoma with a bimodal DNA histogram and 4c maximum, the liver metastases of this tumor is undifferentiated and polymorphocellular with a broadly scattered unimodal DNA histogram and 7c peak. Based on our own material, we have the impression that, with regard to the DNA histogram, lymph node metastases are more closely connected with the primary tumor than hematogenous metastases. The number of cases is too meager for a definite pronouncement. Perhaps only a few, especially resistant cells can survive from the numerous tumor cells shed into the blood, where the selective pressure is heavier than in the lymphatics, whose cytotoxic properties against tumor cells are obviously more limited. Zank and Krug (1970) have found diverging DNA distributions more frequently in primary tumors with metastases.

When one considers DNA measurements on metastases as part of the picture, there is unquestionably a mosaic composition in certain tumor diseases conditioned by multiple coexisting cell clones. Stich and Steele (1962) and Stich (1963) have pointed this out.

7. Changes of DNA Ploidy in the Progression of Neoplastic Disease

DNA photometric data from "longitudinal studies", i.e., repeat DNA measurements in the temporal course of a neoplastic disease have not been carried out both for technical reasons and the impracticality of repeated biopsies. We can only attempt to answer the question of DNA ploidy changes, i.e., whether a fully developed tumor can spontaneously alter its DNA complement.

Stich (1963) devoted a paper to this question and concluded that "preneoplastic lesions and malignant neoplasms consist of various cell types with chromosome complements and DNA values which deviated from those in cells of normal tissues. This change from a genetically homogeneous cell populations into a heterogeneous one can take place in the early stage of carcinogenesis. The data also indicate that only few of these genetically abnormal cells acquire malignant properties."

We should like to substantiate and enlarge upon this determination in that we feel thatf ully developed, malignant neoplasms, too, can undergo certain, regular changes in the DNA complement, especially when they reach the end stages of the tumor disease. We have collected these concepts of DNA kinetics in Table 27 and illustrated them with the example of premalignant and malignant transformations in the cervix. An aneuploid cell population with a broadly scattered DNA histogram without a characteristic stem line develops either directly via the appearance of atypical mitoses or through the indirect route of a euploid polyploidization (dysplasia). This anenploid condition in the cervix corresponds to carcinoma *in situ*. I.e., we are dealing here with a carcinoma precursor (the DNA aneuploidy notwithstanding), not with a full blown carcinoma. The disease can remain quiescent in this stage for years without progressing. When a stem line first develops through selection from this heterogeneous cell population, the basal membrane is broken through and an autonomous, invasive carcinoma with a bimodal DNA histogram develops. This DNA stem line can be hypodiploid, hyperdiploid, or even euploid. When the number of atypical mitoses increases, for example as a result of therapeutic measures, especially irradiation, a unimodal, aneuploid, genetically fully heterogeneous tumor cell population can once again arise, where practically all cells are capable of division. This is the terminal stage of tumor disease, which we have seen predominantly in autopsy cases.

This generalized progression theory of cancer can be demonstrated especially well on the example of the cervix. We feel that this has general validity and can be extended to carcinomas in other locations. Skin cancers, which often develop from an existing precancer, show an analogous frequency of DNA changes. Corresponding studies on precancers in the internal organs, such as carcinoma *in situ* of the breast or early cancer of the stomach, are not available. We can easily observe the end stages, however. Carcinomatous tissue surgically excized soon after its initial discovery almost always exhibits a bimodal DNA histogram and a distinct DNA stem line which belongs to the tumor cell population. In the terminal stages of tumor disease, however, such as we see in autopsies, there is only a broadly scattered DNA histogram without a well-delimited stem line. These tumors are usually undifferentiated, and we cannot decide whether this final situation is not actually a result of therapy which the patients had undergone for months and years before they died of their tumor diseases.

8. Chromosomal Karyotype and Nuclear DNA Content

The karyotypes obtained from various benign and malignant human tumors are in close agreement with the results obtained by DNA cytophotometry. The cytogenetic picture of benign neoplasms reveals almost always a normal diploid $(2\,n)$ chromosome count (SANDBERG and SAKURAI, 1974) which matches well with the cytophotometrically obtained 2c DNA histograms of benign tumors and hyperplasias.

The increased DNA values, observed in the majority of malignant tumors, run just so parallel with the morphological changes of the metaphase karyograms in which numerical aberrations as well as morphological deviations of chromosomes may occur. Several additional, abnormally large "marker" chromosomes are not unusual in cancer cells and almost invariably indicate the presence of a malignant neoplastic process. The appearance of additional normal chromosomes and "marker" chromosomes in the karyogram of tumor cells must be considered the direct sequel of the increased amount of nuclear DNA, and *vice versa*. Nothing is known so far about the genetic activity of "marker" chromosomes and their role in the abnormal biochemistry of the cancer cell. Nothing is known about the significance of additional amounts of DNA in the tumor cells. There is, however, no specific 'tumor' chromosome, and the large array of chromosomal changes in human cancer and the seemingly endless variety of karyotypic pictures are probably secondary phenomena to the cancerous state and not its primary cause (SANDBERG and SAKURAI, 1974).

In experimental chemical carcinogenesis the general opinion is that most, if not all, of the tumors start out as diploid. Karyotypic changes become evident with either biological progression of the tumor, transformation to a more malignant phase, or in the metastases of the tumor. Heterochromatically altered regions in chromosomes, generated during carcinogen-induced malignant transformation, may be responsible for nondisjunction of chromosomes, leading to nonrandom rearrangement of chromosomal complement with an abnormal DNA content and neoplastic characteristics of proliferation (Sugiyama, 1971).

In breast nodules benign lesions always revealed a diploid chromosome count, while lobular carcinoma *in situ* contained mostly diploid karyotypes with a few aneuploid ones. The presence of multiple abnormalities in the karyotype of breast cancers tends to be associated with a poorer prognosis of the tumor because of its higher malignancy. The preponderant number of adenomas of the colon was found to have a diploid karyotype when the histology was benign and no clinical evidence for malignant transformation was detected (Sandberg and Sakurai, 1974).

At least 50% of the cases with acute human leukemias do not have any recognizible cytogenetic changes in the tumor cells. An equally large number of diploid DNA distribution patterns was found in cytophotometric investigations. Thus, acute leukemia is the best example of a neoplastic disease which may not be associated with deviations of the DNA content and karyotype from diploidy. There is, however, evidence of an altered DNA arrangement (higher DNA packing ratio) in chromosomes of malignant lymphoma (Lampert, 1971).

9. Therapy and Prognosis

Therapy and prognosis seem to have an intimate relationship to ploidy resp. aneuploidy. Tavares et al. (1966) determined this for 35 prostate carcinomas. Whereas 22 of 24 patients with DNA content in the 2–4c group responded well to estrogen therapy, 8 of 9 carcinomas in the aneuploid 3–6c group proved to be resistant. The five year survival rates in these groups were significantly different. A similar finding is seen for bladder tumors.

Nitze (1969) observed an increased nuclear DNA content and a considerable broader scatter of measurement values in a keratinized epidermoid carcinoma of the larynx after x-irradiation of the tumor.

After cytostatic treatment of a cutaneous angioblastic reticulosarcoma, a reduction of the DNA content occurred with a 2c DNA value in the residual tumor cell moiety (Ehlers et al., 1971). A similar effect leading to a decrease of the mean DNA content of the tumor cells was reported by Urasinski et al. (1971) after treatment of acute leukemias by a combination therapy of 6-mercaptopurine and prednisolone. Müller (1971) saw a temporary decrease of the Feulgen DNA values in leukemias when glucocorticoids alone had been given. A slight augmentation of the nuclear DNA content after cytostatic treatment with 'Bleomycin' of various malignant skin tumors has been reported recently (Ehlers, 1975) which was accompanied by histologic signs of dedifferentiation in some of the tumors.

Independent of therapeutic modality (irradiation or operation) ATKIN and RICHARDS (1962) showed a better prognosis in squamous epithelial carcinoma of the cervix in carcinomas with a high ploidy (4c) DNA content. NG and ATKIN (1973) confirmed and extended this observation. Large cell cervical carcinomas show a 5 year survival rate of 51.8%, small cell cancers only 10%. In carcinomas of the endometrium, breast, and ovary, the results are reversed. Here carcinomas with a lower, near diploid DNA content had a better prognosis than the high ploidy ones (ATKIN et al., 1959; ATKIN, 1972; ATKIN et al., 1973).

OBRECHT et al. (1970) after combined chemical therapy of acute leukemias in adults found a poorer response to treatment in cases with a diploid DNA content when compared with tetraploid and hypertetraploid ones.

Our own studies are not informative with respect to prognosis, except that we classify carcinomas with a broad, unimodal, high ploidy DNA histogram, the usual stage found at autopsy, as tumors with a bad prognosis.

E. Summary

Feulgen cytophotometric measurements were obtained from tissue smears of various human tumors. The fluorescence cytophotometric technique (BÖHM and SPRENGER, 1968; BÖHM, 1972) was employed using the strongly fluorescent acriflavine as a substitute for the weekly fluorescent pararosaniline in the Schiff reagent.

250 tissue smears were prepared from unfixed human tumors partly obtained from surgical material, partly from autopsy cases no longer than 12 hours after death. From each tissue specimen which had been used for a smear a microscopic slide was made for histological diagnosis. 165 smears from 105 different tumor cases could be evaluated cytophotometrically. The residual ones had to be eliminated because of insufficient material, loss of cells during hydrolysis and necrobiosis of tumor cells.

The frequency distribution of the nuclear Feulgen DNA values of each individual tumor smear was plotted as a DNA histogram from which the DNA ploidy of the tumor could be determined by comparison with the measurement values of lymphocytes and granulocytes (internal 2c reference value). Finally, the DNA histograms were reduced into a "DNA distribution code" in order to save printing space. The details are given in the Legend of Fig. 3.

The pertinent literature was carefully reviewed. The literature results were collected into tables as well and compared with our own measurement data.

From this information we have drawn the following conclusions:

1. Benign human tumors have identical diploid DNA stem lines. Occasionally a few nuclei may be found up to 4c, thus indicating some proliferative activity.

2. The vast majority of the malignant tumors exhibits nuclear DNA values more or less beyond the diploid DNA amount. Only 4% of the total number

of malignant tumors investigated in our own study were found to have a diploid DNA stem line. It is, therefore, evident that aneuploidy and increased nuclear DNA contents are rather dependable signs of malignancy.

3. Among the malignant tumors, the well differentiated ones, in particular the differentiated adenocarcinomas of the colon and the endometrium and the differentiated hypernephroid carcinomas, revealed DNA stem lines in the hyperdiploid and triploid range with concommitant duplication peaks with a 5c and 6c DNA content. In such tumors the histological appearance as well as the DNA distribution pattern disclose some degree of orderly and regulated growth with normal cell divisions resulting in a bulk of G1-cells which are pooled into the stem line peak, and some G2-cells forming the duplication peak. Some tumors were found to give rise to three modes, the mean DNA contents of which were forming a geometrical series indicating polyploidization of the aneuploid tumor stem line.

4. The undifferentiated anaplastic tumors, on the other hand, do not form a distinct tumor stem line. They exist with widely scattered DNA values forming one broad peak which is usually located in the tetraploid and hyper-tetraploid DNA range. Histologically these tumors lack differentiated structures. Atypical mitoses are commonly found indicating an irregular distribution of chromatin during cell division which must obscure distinct DNA stem lines.

5. Undifferentiated tumor histology and widely scattered DNA histograms were more often found in autopsy cases than in surgical material. We may, therefore, conclude that undifferentiated tumors with no discernible stem line formation in their histograms represent the end stage of tumor disease.

6. There is some evidence also that in an individual malignant tumor the histological appearance as well as the DNA distribution pattern remain constant, at least for some time, because some specimen excised from different sites of the main tumor and from metastases resulted in congruent DNA histograms. However, some cases were found in which the DNA histograms obtained from different sites of the primary tumor or from primary tumor and metastases did not follow the same pattern. In such cases the distinct tumor histology did reveal some shift, too, usually towards a lower degree of differentiation in the outer parts of the tumor or in the secondaries.

7. Precancerous conditions of the uterine cervix and the skin often exhibit euploid polyploidizations with some very high DNA values of individual nuclei up to 32c which may progress into broad unimodal aneuploid tumor cell populations of carcinoma *in situ*. If the carcinoma starts to grow invasively, a low ploidy tumor stem line may be selected (ploidy reduction) which is maintained as long as the tumor is differentiated histologically. In the late stage, dedifferentiated invasive carcinoma again predominates as unimodal aneuploid DNA histograms.

Table 1. Source of material, preparation and staining techniques, methods of cytophotometric measurement, instruments and reference values employed by various authors

1 Reference. 2 Material obtained by surg(ery), aut(opsy), biop(sy). 3 Preparation. 4 Staining (F = Feulgen; GCA = gallocyaninchromalaun; UV = UV-absorbance). 5 Method of measurement (scan. = scanning, t.w. = two wave lengths, flu. = fluorescence). 6 Instrument. 7 Phase of cell cycle (int. = interphase, meta = metaphase, ana = anaphase, telo = telophase). 8 Reference value (ly = lymphocyte, leuk = leukocyte, gran = granulocyte).

1	2	3	4	5	6	7	8
ATKIN and RICHARDS, 1956	surg.	smear	F	scan.	Deeley	int.	leuk ($+10\%$)
ATKIN et al., 1959	surg.	smear	F	scan.	Deeley	int.	leuk ($+10\%$)
ATKIN, 1964	biop. +	vag. sm.	F	scan.	Deeley	int.	ly ($+10\%$)
BADER, 1959, 1960	surg. ?	sect.	F	plug. + t.w.	Leitz	int.	ly
BÖHM et al., 1971a	—	vag. sm.	F	flu.	Leitz	int.	gran. + norm. epith.
BÖHM et al., 1971b	surg.	smear	F	flu.	Leitz	int. + meta	ly + gran
BRANDAO, 1969	surg.	sect.	F	scan.	Deeley	int.	fibrobl. + norm. epith.
CASPERSSON, 1964	—	vag. sm.	F, UV	scan.	Caspersson	int.	leuk ($+10\%$)
COLE and McKALEN, 1960	surg.	impr.	F	plug	Leuchtenberger	int.	norm. epith.
EHLERS, 1968	biop.	sect.	F	scan.	Deeley	int.	ly, sperm
EHLERS and SOLL, 1971	surg.	smear	F	scan.	Deeley	int.	ly
EHLERS and STEPHAN, 1972a, b	biop.	sect.	F	scan.	Deeley	int.	ly
EMSON and KIRK, 1966	surg.	sect.	F	t.w.	?	int.	ly
FÖDISCH et al., 1974	biop. surg.	smear	F	scan.	Deeley	int.	?
FOSSA, 1975	surg.	impr.	F	scan.	SMPO5 (Zeiss)	int.	ly
GRANBERG et al., 1974	surg.	smear	F	flu.	Leitz	int.	leuk
GREISEN, 1971	aut.	sect.	GCA	plug	Leitz	int.	norm. epith.
GRUNDMANN et al., 1961	cone biop.	sect.	F	plug	self contr.	int.	ly
HALE and WILSON, 1959	blood	smear	F	scan.	Deeley	int.	norm. leukocytes
HAEMMERLI, 1970	surg.	impr.	F	scan. + UV	Deeley + UMSP	int.	leuk + ly
HAOUR and CONTI, 1958	—	vag. sm.	F	plug	Lison	int.	epith. from the mouth
HOLZNER and GOLOB, 1968	biop.	smear	F	t.w.	Leitz	int.	ly
HRUSHOVETZ and LAUCHLAN, 1970	biop.	sect.	F	t.w.	Reichert	int.	ly
INUI and OOTA, 1965	surg.	sect.	F	scan.	Olympus	int.	norm. epith.
IZUO et al., 1971a, b	surg.	sect.	F	plug	Leitz	int.	ly
KOTHER and SANDRITTER, 1964	surg.	sect.	F	plug	self constr.	int. + meta	ly
LAMPERT, 1967	bone marr.	smear	F	scan.	Deelsy	int.	ly
LEDERER et al., 1972	surg.	impr.	F	scan.	Deeley	int.	ly

Table 1 (Cotinued)

1	2	3	4	5	6	7	8
Leuchtenberger et al., 1954	surg. + aut.	sect.	F	plug.	Caspersson	int.	norm. epith.
Levi et al., 1969	surg.	susp. sm.	F	scan.	Deeley	int.	ly
Lewis, 1971	surg.	sect.	F	scan.	Vickers M 85	int.	ly
Manocha, 1969	biop.	sect.	F	t.w.	?	ana + meta	ly
Manocha et al., 1969	biop.	sect.	F	t.w.	Swift	int. + meta	ly
Meek, 1961	surg.	smear	F	scan.	Deeley	int. + meta	leuk
Müller, 1969	blood + b.m.	smear	F	scan.	Zeiss USMP	int.	ly
Mundy, 1973	blood + b.m.	smear	F	scan.	Deeley	int.	gran
Nitze, 1969	surg.	smear	F	scan.	Deeley	int.	ly
Nodskov-Pedersen, 1971	biop.	squash	UV	plug	Pollister	int.	norm. epith.
Obrecht et al., 1970	blood	smear	F	scan.	UMSP	int.	ly
Ojima et al., 1960	surg.	sect.	F	plug	?	int.	embryonic liver
Petrakis, 1953	blood + b.m.	smear	F	plug	Pollister	int.	ly, spermatids
Pfitzer, 1970	sputum	smear	F	scan.	UMSP I	int.	ly
Pfitzer and Pape, 1971	surg.	smear	F	scan.	UMSP II	int.	ly
Rabotti, 1959	surg. + aut.	sect.	F	plug	?	int.	ly
Reid and Singh, 1960	surg. + aut.	smear	F	plug	Lison	int.	sperm
Sachs, 1970	biop.	sect.	F	plug	Leitz	int.	liver I
Sachs, 1971, 1972	surg.	sect.	F	plug	Leitz	int.	ly, norm. epith.
Sandritter and Fischer, 1962	surg.	sect.	F	plug	self constr.	int. + meta	norm. epith. + sperm
Sandritter et al., 1966	surg.	smear	F	scan.	Deeley	int.	ly
Seidel and Sandritter, 1963	surg. + aut.	sect.	F	plug	self constr.	int.	ly + norm. epith.
Sprenger et al., 1974b	biop.	impr.	F	flu.	Leitz	int.	leu
Stich et al., 1960	surg.	sect.	F	t.w.	Swift and Rasch	meta	ly, norm. epith.
Stich and Steele, 1962	surg.	sect.	F	t.w.	Swift and Rasch	int. meta, telo	ly + leuk
Tavares et al., 1966	surg.	sect.	F	scan.	Deeley	int.	leuk (+ 10 %)
Valeri et al., 1967	biop.	sect.	F	plug	Lison	int.	ly
van Vloten et al., 1974	biop.	impr.	F	scan.	Zeiss	int.	norm. epidermis
Vokaer, 1951	currett.	sect.	F	plug	Lison	int.	?
Wagner and Richart, 1968	currett.	sect.	F	t.w.	Leitz	int.	ly
Wagner et al., 1968	currett.	sect.	F	plug	Leitz	int.	ly (+ 20 %)
Wagner et al., 1972	—	vag. sm.	F	flu.	Leitz	int.	norm. interm. cells
Wied et al., 1966	—	vag. sm.	F	scan.	Deeley	int.	ly
Wilbanks et al., 1967	biep.	sect.	F	t.w.	Leitz	int.	ly
Zank and Krug, 1970	aut.	susp. sm.	F	scan.	self constr.	int.	ly

Table 2. Total numbers of cases and of tissue specimen (in brackets) investigated from 10 different tumor categories (personal investigations)

	Number of cases	Number of tissue specimen investigated
1. Benign lesions	8	(8)
2. Bronchial carcinomas	17	(35)
3. Mammary carcinomas	14	(18)
4. Gastric carninomas	11	(16)
5. Carcinomas of the large intestine	12	(14)
6. Endometrial carcinomas	9	(14)
7. Hypernephroid renal carcinomas	6	(8)
8. Miscellaneous carcinomas	17	(31)
9. Mal. lesions of the hematopoetic syst.	4	(10)
10. Sarcomas	7	(11)
Total	105	(165)

Table 3. Histology, location and nuclear DNA content of benign tumor lesions as revealed from the literature. In Izuo's paper the cases marked with * did not develop into carcinomas, while the cases marked with † did develop into carcinomas during the follow up period

Histogram coding: The numbers in italics indicate the position of the main tumor cell population, while the normally printed digits mark secondary or minor peaks of the histogram. The dots roughly represent scattered measuring values and the numbers given in brackets indicate the highest DNA values obtained.

Histology and Location	Nuclear DNA (2 c-diploid)	Reference
Adenoma of the renal cortex	*2* 4	Leuchtenberger *et al.*, 1954
Polyps of the large intestine, 8 cases, metaphases only	*4* (8)	Stich *et al.*, 1960
Adenomatous polyp of the colon	*2*....4	Cole and McKalen, 1960
Adenomatous polyp of the colon	*2*	Cole and McKalen, 1960
Adenomatous polyp of the colon	*2*	Cole and McKalen, 1960
Adenomatous polyp of the colon	*2*	Cole and McKalen, 1960
Adenomatous polyp of the colon	*2* 4	Cole and McKalen, 1960
Cystic adenoma of the lungs	..*2*....(4)	Seidel and Sandritter, 1963
Cystic hyperplasia of the breast	.*2*...(4)	Emson and Kirk, 1966
Cystic hyperplasia of the breast	*2*–3	Emson and Kirk, 1966
Cystic hyperplasia of the breast	*2*...(4)	Emson and Kirk, 1966
Adamantinoma	.*2*.	Nitze, 1969
Adenofibroma of the breast	*2*....4..	Sachs, 1971
Cystic hyperplasia of the breast	*2*...	Sachs, 1971
Cystic hyperplasia of the breast	.*2*..	Sachs, 1971
Sclerosing adenosis	*2*...(4)	Sachs, 1971
Urinary bladder tumor, grade I	*2*...(4)	Lederer *et al.*, 1972
Benign phaeochromocytoma, 12 cases	..*2*...4..8..16	Lewis, 1971
*Mastopathia, blunt duct adenosis	*2*	Izuo *et al.*, 1971a
*Mastopathia, duct papillomatosis	*2*	Izuo *et al.*, 1971a
*Mastopathia, duct. papill., 3 diff. reg.	*2*	Izuo *et al.*, 1971a
*Mastopathia, duct papillomatosis (1)	*2*	Izuo *et al.*, 1971a
*Mastopathia, duct epithel. hyper- plasia (2)	*2* **4**	Izuo *et al.*, 1971a

Table 3 (continued)

Histology and Location	Nuclear DNA (2 c-diploid)	Reference
*Mastopathia, blunt duct adenosis (3)	*2 4*	Izuo et al., 1971a
*Mastopathia, duct epithel. hyper-plasia	*2*	Izuo et al., 1971a
*Mastopathia, blunt duct adenosis	*2*	Izuo et al., 1971a
*Mastopathia, duct papillomatosis	*2 4*	Izuo et al., 1971a
[†]Mastopathia, duct papillomatosis	*2*	Izuo et al., 1971a
[†]Mastopathia, blunt duct adenosis	*2 4*	Izuo et al., 1971a
[†]Mastopathia, duct papillomatosis (1)	*..3.....(10)*	Izuo et al., 1971a
[†]Mastopathia, duct papillomatosis (2)	*..3.........(16)*	Izuo et al., 1971a
[†]Mastopathia, duct papillomatosis (3)	*1,5....6*	Izuo et al., 1971a
[†]Mastopathia, duct papillomatosis (4)	*2 4*	Izuo et al., 1971a
[†]Mastopathia, blunt duct adenosis (5)	*2 4*	Izuo et al., 1971a
[†]Mastopathia, blunt duct adenosis	*2*	Izuo et al., 1971a
[†]Mastopathia, blunt duct adenosis	*2*	Izuo et al., 1971a
[†]Mastopathia, apocrine metaplasia	*..3....(6)*	Izuo et al., 1971a
[†]Mastopathia, duct papillomatosis	*2*	Izuo et al., 1971a
[†]Mastopathia, blunt duct adenosis	*2*	Izuo et al., 1971a
[†]Mastopathia, duct papillomatosis (1)	*1,5...4 (6)*	Izuo et al., 1971a
[†]Mastopathia, duct papillomatosis (2)	*..2,5...5 (6)*	Izuo et al., 1971a
[†]Mastopathia, sclerosing adenosis (3)	*2.. 4*	Izuo et al., 1971a
Mastopathia, apocrine metaplasia, 2 cases	*2*	Izuo et al., 1971b
Mastopathia, apocrine metaplasia, 6 cases	*2 4*	Izuo et al., 1971b
Mastopathia, apocrine metaplasia	*..3......(8)*	Izuo et al., 1971b
Hyperplasia of the prostate	*2*	Sprenger et al., 1974
Chordoma, physaliferous cells (1)	*2*	Mikuz and Mydla, 1974
Chordoma, starlike cells (2)	*2....4*	Mikuz and Mydla, 1974

Table 4. Histology and DNA content of human thyroid nodules. Slightly modified and translated from Haemmerli (1970) with kind permission of the author and the publishers

Histology	Number of cases	Relative DNA content			
		about 2c	about 2.5c	about 3c	about 3.5c and higher
Normal thyroid tissue	20	20	—	—	—
Fetal thyroid tissue	5	5	—	—	—
Normo-follicular nodules	70	70	—	—	—
Macro-follicular nodules	45	45	—	—	—
Normo-macrofollicular nodules	70	70	—	—	—
Micro-normofollicular nodules	53	33	12	5	3
Microfollicular nodules	65	16	24	17	8
Oncocytic nodules	26	5	8	8	5
Carcinomas	17	14	2	1	—
Total	371				

Table 5. Personal investigations of eight benign lesions
No. = Number of nuclei measured.

Num-bering	Age/Sex	Histology and Location	Ob-tained by	Nuclear DNA (2c = diploid)	No.
T 1	67 ♀	Leiomyoma of the uterus, prolif.	surg.	2 . . . . . . (4) . .	229
T 23	50 ♀	Leiomyoma of the uterus	surg.	2 (4)	73
T 14	70 ♂	Adenoma of the prostate	surg.	2	117
T 15	66 ♀	Mixed tumor of the parotid gland	surg.	2 (4)	152
T 17	55 ♀	Cystoma of the ovary	surg.	2	41
T 30	47 ♀	Cystic hyperplasia of the endometr.	surg.	2 (4)	120
T 46	60 ♀	Cystic hyperplasia of the breast	surg.	2	121
T 50	61 ♂	Papillary polyp of the rectum	surg.	2 . . . (4)	204

Table 6. Carcinomas of the large intestine. The histogram code of the nuclear DNA content is explained in the Legend of Table 3

Histology and Location	Nuclear DNA (2c = diploid)	Reference
Adenocarcinoma, coecum	2 . . . 4	Leuchtenberger et al., 1954
Well diff. adenocarcinoma, rectum	. . 4 . . . 8 .	Atkin, Richards, 1956
Carcinoma, telo- and metaphases only	2.5 6 (11)	Stich and Emson, 1959
Well diff. adenocarcinoma, metaphases	5 . .	Stich et al., 1960
Well diff. adenocarcinoma, metaphases	4–5 . . .	Stich et al., 1960
Poorly diff. adenocarcinoma, metaphases	5 . . . 7.5	Stich et al., 1960
Poorly diff. adeno-ca. metaphases	5 10	Stich et al., 1960
Poorly diff. adeno-ca. metaphases	5 10	Stich et al., 1960
Poorly diff. adeno-ca. metaphases	. . . 6–7 . . (8)	Stich et al., 1960
Poorly diff. adeno-ca. metaphases	. . . 7 . . . (13)	Stich et al., 1960
Poorly diff. adeno-ca. metaphases	. . . 7 . . . (13) (24)	Stich et al., 1960
Poorly diff. adeno-ca. metaphases	. . 7–8 . .	Stich et al., 1960
Poorly diff. adeno-ca. metaphases	. . 7–8 . .	Stich et al., 1960
Adenocarcinoma	2.5 8	Cole and McKalen, 1960
Adenocarcinoma	. . 3.5 . . . (17)	Cole and McKalen, 1960
Adenocarcinoma	. . 3.5 . . . (18)	Cole and McKalen, 1960
Adenocarcinoma	. . 2.5 . . . (4)	Cole and McKalen, 1960
Adenocarcinoma	. . 2.5 . . . (4)	Cole and McKalen, 1960
Adenocarcinoma	. . 2.5 . . . 7 . . . (12)	Cole and McKalen, 1960
Adenocarcinoma	. . 2.5 . . . (7)	Cole and McKalen, 1960
Adenocarcinoma, inter-, telo- and metaphases	3.5 . . . 7 . .	Stich and Steele, 1962
Adenocarcinoma, rectum	. . 2.5 . . . 5 . . .	Sandritter and Kleinhans, 1964
Adenocarcinoma, rectum	. . 2.5 . . . . (6)	Sandritter et al., 1966
Adenocarcinoma, rectum	3.5 . . . (8)	Sandritter et al., 1966
Adenocarcinoma, rectum	. 3 . (6)	Sandritter et al., 1966
Adenocarcinoma, rectum	. . 4.5 . . . . (10)	Sandritter et al., 1966
Adenocarcinoma, rectum	. . . 3.5 . . (6)	Sandritter et al., 1966
Adenocarcinoma, rectum	. . 3.5 . . . (8)	Sandritter et al., 1966
Adenocarcinoma, rectum	. . 3.5 . . 7 . .	Sandritter et al., 1966
Carcinoma, prim. les. (1)	. . 1.5 . . 3 .	Zank and Krug, 1970
Carcinoma, ly. met. (2)	3 . . 5 . . 9 . .	Zank and Krug, 1970
Carcinoma, rectum, prim. les. (1)	. . 5 . . . 9 .	Zank and Krug, 1970
Carcinoma, rectum, ly. met. (2)	3 . . 4 . . . 8	Zank and Krug, 1970

Table 7. Personal investigations of 12 carcinomas of the large intestine
    No. = Number of nuclei measured. The histogram code of the nuclear DNA content
is explained in the legend of Table 3.

Num-bering	Age/Sex	Histology	Obtained by	Nuclear DNA (2c = diploid)	No.
T 20	49 ♂	Adenocarcinoma, sigma, prim. les.	surg.	2.5...5	203
21		Adenocarcinoma, sigma, serosa met.	surg.	2.5...5	214
T 22	66 ♀	Adenocarcinoma, coecum, prim. les.	surg.	2.5...5	197
T 44	60 ♀	Adenocarcinoma, rectum, prim. les.	surg.	2.5...5...10...(13)	302
T 49	61 ♂	Adenocarcinoma, rectum, prim. les.	surg.	...2.5...(5)	383
T 51	? ♀	Adenocarcinoma, rectum, prim. les.	surg.	...4.5...9..	366
T 53	73 ♂	Adenocarcinoma, coecum, prim. les.	surg.	...3...7...	376
T 57	56 ♀	Adenocarcinoma, rectum, prim. les.	surg.	2.5...5...9	385
T 65	58 ♂	Adenocarcinoma, sigma, prim. les.	surg.	2.5...4...8...	422
T 64	63 ♀	Scirrhous adenocarcinoma, coecum, prim. lesion	surg.	....3...6...	356
T 54	75 ♀	Adenocarcinoma, transversum, prim. lesion	surg.	2.5..... (16)	295
T 59	65 ♀	Adenocarcinoma, sigma, prim. les. less differentiated, with giant cells	surg.	2.5...(6)	266
T 88	64 ♀	Adenocarcinoma, ascendens marg. region	surg.	2...3.5....(8)	406
89		Adenocarcinoma, ascendens centr. region	surg.	...3... (10)	315

Table 8. Histology and nuclear DNA content of endometrial carcinomas as revealed from
the literature. From 33 cases published by Atkin et al. (1959) "basic DNA values" are
reported only. Though the data were obtained cytophotometrically, no DNA histograms
are demonstrated. Therefore, no information is available about scatter or possible
bimodal DNA distribution of the individual tumors

Histology	Nuclear DNA (2c = diploid)	Reference
Diff. papillary adenoacanthoma	2.5 5	Atkin and Richards, 1956
Diff. adenocarcinoma	.4.5. ..9.. (12)	Atkin and Richards, 1956
Diff. papillary adenocarcinoma	..4.....(7)	Atkin and Richards, 1956
Well diff. adenocarcinoma (2 cases)	hypodiploid	Atkin et al., 1959
Well diff. adenocarcinoma (3 cases)	diploid	Atkin et al., 1959
Mod. diff. adenocarcinoma (10 cases)	diploid	Atkin et al., 1959
Poorly diff. adenocarcinoma (1 case)	diploid	Atkin et al., 1959
Well diff. adenoacanthoma (2 cases)	diploid	Atkin et al., 1959
Mod. diff. adenoacanthoma (3 cases)	diploid	Atkin et al., 1959
Mod. diff. adenocarcinoma (1 case)	hypotetraploid	Atkin et al., 1959
Mod. diff. adenocarcinoma (3 cases)	tetraploid	Atkin et al., 1959
Poorly diff. adenocarcinoma (2 cases)	tetraploid	Atkin et al., 1959
Poorly diff. adenoacanthoma, local recurr.	diploid	Atkin et al., 1959
Mod. diff. adenocarcinoma, local recurr.	tetraploid	Atkin et al., 1959
Poorly diff. adenocarcinoma, local recurr.	tetraploid	Atkin et al., 1959
Adenocarcinoma	.2....(4)	Ojima et al., 1960
Diff. adenocarcinoma	..2–2.5...5. (9)	Granberg et al., 1974
Diff. adenocarcinoma	(2).3..6...12.(18)	Granberg et al., 1974

Table 9. Personal investigations of 9 endometrial carcinomas. In some tumors measurements were derived from central and marginal regions of the tumor as well

No. = Number of nuclei measured. The histogram code of the nuclear DNA content is explained in the legend of Table 3.

Numbering	Age	Histology	Obtained by	Nuclear DNA-Content (2c = diploid)	No.
T 3	54	Well diff. adenocarcinoma, prim. les.	surg.	*2.5...5.*	240
T 56	60	Well diff. adenocarcinoma, prim. les.	surg.	*2.5...6.*	400
T 73	72	Well diff. adenocarcinoma, centr. reg.	surg.	*2.5...5*	190
74		Well diff. adenocarcinoma, marg. reg.	surg.	*2.5...5*	272
T 77	49	Well diff. adenocarcinoma, centr. reg.	surg.	*.3...6..*	342
78		Well diff. adenocarcinoma, marg. reg.	surg.	*2.5...4.5...*(7)	362
T 82	49	Well diff. adenocarcinoma, centr. reg.	surg.	*2.5...5...*(10)	328
81		Papillary adenocarcinoma, marg. reg.	surg.	*2.5...5...*(12)	381
T 94	66	Adenoacanthoma, centr. region	surg.	*2.5...4...7...*	478
95		Adenoacanthoma, marg. region	surg.	*2.5...5...*	213
T 125	60	Papillary adenocarcinoma, net. met.	autop.	*5...8...*(10)	491
126		Papillary adenocarcinoma, ly. met.	autop.	*5...8...*(10)	586
T 161	79	Undiff. adenocarcinoma, prim. les.	autop.	*...5...*(10)	597
T 41	?	Carcinosarcoma, prim. les.	surg.	*...4....* (13)	700

Table 10. Histology and nuclear DNA content of bronchial carcinomas. The histogram code of the nuclear DNA content is explained in the legend of Table 3

Histology	Nuclear DNA (2c = diploid)	Reference
Anaplastic carcinoma	*2.5* 5	LEUCHTENBERGER *et al.*, 1954
Poorly diff. adenocarcinoma	2 *4* 7	LEUCHTENBERGER *et al.*, 1954
Bronchogenic carcinoma, telo- and metaphases	*3* ...7..	STICH and EMSON, 1959
Bronchogenic carcinoma, telophases (1)	*1.5* 3 6 12	STICH and STEELE, 1962
Bronchogenic carcinoma, metaphases (2)	3 6 12 24	STICH AND STEELE, 1962
Bronchogenic carcinoma, prim. les. telo- and metaphases	6 ..12..	STICH and STEELE, 1962
Bronchogenic carcinoma, ly. met. telo- and metaphases	3.5 6.5	STICH and STEELE, 1962
Malignant adenomatosis, prim. lesion (1)	*..5–6...*(9)	SEIDEL and SANDRITTER, 1963
Malignant adenomatosis, lymphangiosis ca. (2)	*...6....*(10)	SEIDEL and SANDRITTER, 1963
Malignant adenomatosis, ly. met. (3)	3 *6–7...*(10)	SEIDEL and SANDRITTER, 1963
Squamous carcinoma	(2)*...4.5....*(10)	SANDRITTER and KLEINHANS, 1964
Squamous carcinoma, poorly diff.	*2....3.5...*	SANDRITTER and KLEINHANS, 1964
Squamous carcinoma, poorly diff.	*2.....*(6)	SANDRITTER and KLEINHANS, 1964

Table 10 (continued)

Histology	Nuclear DNA (2c = diploid)	Reference
Squamous carcinoma, poorly diff.	...3....(6)	Sandritter and Kleinhans, 1964
Small cell carcinoma	1.5.....(8)	Sandritter and Kleinhans, 1964
Squamous carcinoma	......4....(12)	Sandritter et al., 1965
Squamous carcinoma	4.....8....(12)	Sandritter et al., 1965
Squamous carcinoma	2–2.5...4...6...8	Sandritter et al., 1965
Epidermoid carcinoma	..4.5. (9)	Sandritter et al., 1966
Epidermoid carcinoma	..4.5..(10)	Sandritter et al., 1966
Epidermoid carcinoma	3..6.. (12)	Sandritter et al., 1966
Epidermoid carcinoma	3.5...5–7	Sandritter et al., 1966
Epidermoid carcinoma	2.5. 4.5..(9)	Sandritter et al., 1966
Oat cell carcinoma	..5...9.	Sandritter et al., 1966
Epidermoid carcinoma	2...4....(14)	Adams and Dahlgren, 1968
Epidermoid carcinoma	2...4....(14)	Adams and Dahlgren, 1968
Epidermoid carcinoma	2...4....(10)	Adams and Dahlgren, 1968
Epidermoid carcinoma	2....(12)	Adams and Dahlgren. 1968
Epidermoid carcinoma	2....7..	Adams and Dahlgren, 1968
Epidermoid carcinoma	.3 ..7..	Adams and Dahlgren, 1968
Epidermoid carcinoma	3 6	Adams and Dahlgren, 1968
Epidermoid carcinoma	2.5...(6)	Adams and Dahlgren, 1968
Epidermoid carcinoma	(2)...5...(10)	Adams and Dahlgren, 1968
Epidermoid carcinoma	2.5 ...8... (16)	Adams and Dahlgren, 1968
Epidermoid carcinoma	3.5 ....7.... ..(20)	Adams and Dahlgren, 1968
Epidermoid carcinoma	2...4.5....(12)	Adams and Dahlgren, 1968
Epidermoid carcinoma	3....(8)	Adams and Dahlgren, 1968
Adenocarcinoma	3...5...(10)	Adams and Dahlgren, 1968
Adenocarcinoma	3...(6)	Adams and Dahlgren, 1968
Adenocarcinoma	...5....(12)	Adams and Dahlgren, 1968
Adenocarcinoma	..5.. 10	Adams and Dahlgren, 1968
Adenocarcinoma	..5....(10)	Adams and Dahlgren, 1968
Adenocarcinoma	...5...(14)	Adams and Dahlgren, 1968
Adenocarcinoma	(2)...7......(18)	Adams and Dahlgren, 1968
Adenocarcinoma	10.....(21)	Adams and Dahlgren, 1968
Undiff. carcinoma	2...4.	Adams and Dahlgren, 1968
Undiff. carcinoma	3...(6)	Adams and Dahlgren, 1968
Undiff. carcinoma	3....(12)	Adams and Dahlgren, 1968
Undiff. carcinoma	..3..(6)	Adams and Dahlgren, 1968
Undiff. carcinoma	3....(12)	Adams and Dahlgren, 1968
Undiff. carcinoma	..3..(6)	Adams and Dahlgren, 1968
Undiff. carcinoma	2.5...(6)	Adams and Dahlgren, 1968
Undiff. carcinoma	3.5..(12)	Adams and Dahlgren, 1968
Undiff. carcinoma	3.5..6..(8)	Adams and Dahlgren, 1968
Undiff. carcinoma	4....(14)	Adams and Dahlgren, 1968
Undiff. carcinoma	..5...(9)	Adams and Dahlgren, 1968
Bronchial carcinoma, prim. les.	3 6	Zank and Krug, 1970
Bronchial carcinoma, metastasis	3 ...6	Zank and Krug, 1970
Bronchial carcinoma, prim. les.	2.5 ...5	Zank and Krug, 1970
Bronchial carcinoma, metastasis	2.5 ...(4)	Zank and Krug, 1970
Bronchial carcinoma, prim. les.	2 3.5...(9)	Zank and Krug, 1970
Bronchial carcinoma, metastasis	3.5...7	Zank and Krug, 1970
Giant cell carcinoma	2 3–4 6..8 (22)	Pfitzer, 1970

Table 10 (continued)

Histology	Nuclear DNA (2c = diploid)	Reference
Squamous carcinoma (6 cases)	diploid, near-diploid	GREISEN, 1971
Squamous carcinoma (7 cases)	triploid, near triploid	GREISEN, 1971
Adenocarcinoma (5 cases)	diploid, near-diploid	GREISEN, 1971
Adenocarcinoma (3 cases)	triploid, near-triploid	GREISEN, 1971
Small cell anaplastic carcinoma (5 cases)	diploid, near-diploid	GREISEN, 1971
Small cell anaplastic carcinoma (5 cases)	triploid, near-triploid	GREISEN, 1971
Bronchial carcinoid (6 cases)	*2.. ..(4)..*	GREISEN, 1971
Bronchial carcinoid (1 case)	*.3..*	GREISEN, 1971
Bronchial cylindroma (2 specimen) [a]	*2*	GREISEN, 1971
Bronchial cylindroma (2 specimen) [a]	*2.5*	GREISEN, 1971
Bronchial cylindroma (1 specimen) [a]	*2...4*	GREISEN, 1971

[a] All five specimens were obtained from the same patient, who developed multiple bronchial cylindromata, which all revealed a benign histological structure (bronchial adenomas).

Table 11. Personal investigations of 17 bronchial carcinomas and their metastases, predominantly obtained from autopsy cases

No. = Number of nuclei measured.

Numbering	Age/Sex	Histology and Location	Obtained by	Nuclear DNA (2c = diploid)	No.
T 28	56 ♀	Differentiated squamous carcinoma	surg.	*3.. .6. (12)*	257
T 72	51 ♂	Differentiated squamous carcinoma	surg.	*3... ..6....(12)*	357
T 106	59 ♂	Differentiated squamous carcinoma, prim. les.	autop.	*2.5...5...(6)*	377
107		Differentiated squamous carcinoma, liver met.	autop.	*2.5...(5)*	226
108		Differentiated squamous carcinoma, ly. met.	autop.	*.4....(8)*	336
109		Differentiated squamous carcinoma, pleura met.	autop.	*.4....(10)*	373
T 195	42 ♂	Undiff. and polymorphous squamous carcinoma	autop.	*...5–6....(12)*	706
T 140	64 ♂	Undifferentiated adenocarcinoma, kidney met.	autop.	*3.5..(6)*	266
T 149	66 ♂	Undifferentiated adenocarcinoma, liver met.	autop.	*3...4.5....(12)*	570
150		Undifferentiated adenocarcinoma, ly. met.	autop.	*3......(10)*	516

Table 11 (continued)

Num-bering	Age/Sex	Hystology and Location	Obtained by	Nuclear DNA (2c = diploid)	No.
T 167	62 ♂	Undifferentiated adenocarcinoma, prim. les.	autop.	..4.. (7)	496
169		Undifferentiated adenocarcinoma, pleura met.	autop.	..4.. (7)	421
T 174	73 ♀	Undifferentiated adenocarcinoma, prim. les.	autop.	...6....(12)	556
175		Undifferentiated adenocarcinoma, ly. met.	autop.	...6....(12)	449
176		Undifferentiated adenocarcinoma, ly. met.	autop.	...6....(12)	432
T 182	22 ♂	Undifferentiated adenocarcinoma, prim. les.	autop.	3.5 ...(6)	303
183		Undifferentiated adenocarcinoma, ly. met.	autop.	3.5...(7)	257
184		Undifferentiated adenocarcinoma, ly. met.	autop.	..5...(11)	367
185		Undifferentiated adenocarcinoma, kidney met.	autop.	..5...(11)	383
T 47	60 ♂	Small cell carcinoma	autop.	..5...10..	560
T 153	59 ♂	Small cell carcinoma, prim. les.	autop.	2.5..4...	363
156		Small cell carcinoma, ly. met.	autop.	3...4...	412
T 165	60 ♂	Small cell carcinoma, prim. les.	autop.	2...(4)	226
166		Small cell carcinoma, liver met.	autop.	2..3	196
T 170	56 ♂	Small cell carcinoma, liver met.	autop.	2.5..(4)	261
171		Small cell carcinoma, gallbladder met.	autop.	...3.5..(5)	296
T 178	59 ♀	Small cell carcinoma, pancreas met.	autop.	.....7.5..(10)	530
179		Small cell carcinoma, ly. met.	autop.	....7–9 (12)	713
T 189	61 ♂	Anaplastic carcinoma, prim. les.	autop.	.4....(10)	393
190		Anaplastic carcinoma, kidney met.	autop.	.4.....(10)	479
191		Anaplastic carcinoma, liver metastases	autop.	..6....(10)	499
T 197	68 ♀	Anaplastic carcinoma, prim. les.	autop.	(5)...9....(13)	717
199		Anaplastic carcinoma, liver met.	autop.	(6)...9....(13)	516
T 203	53 ♂	Anaplastic carcinoma, prim. les.	autop.	4...(8)	507
205		Anaplastic carcinoma, liver met.	autop.	4....(9)	333

Table 12. Histology and nuclear DNA content of carcinomas of the breast; data obtained from literature

Histology	Nuclear DNA (2c = diploid)	Reference
Adenocarcinoma	2.5	Leuchtenberger et al., 1954
Adenocarcinoma	2	Leuchtenberger et al., 1954
Adenocarcinoma	2	Leuchtenberger et al., 1954
Adenocarcinoma	2 4	Leuchtenberger et al., 1954

Table 12 (continued)

Histology	Nuclear DNA (2c = diploid)	References
Adenocarcinoma	2.5 4 6 9	Leuchtenberger et al., 1954
Adenocarcinoma	2.5 4 7	Leuchtenberger et al., 1954
Adenocarcinoma	3 6	Leuchtenberger et al., 1954
Adenocarcinoma	2 4 7	Leuchtenberger et al., 1954
Adenocarcinoma	2 4.5 8	Leuchtenberger et al., 1954
Adenocarcinoma	2 4	Leuchtenberger et al., 1954
Spheroidal cell carcinoma, skin met.	2.5 (4)	Atkin and Richards, 1956
Undiff. cell carcinoma, recurrence (1)	(2) 4.. .(8)	Atkin and Richards, 1956
Undiff. cell carcinoma, recurrence (2)	(2) 4...7...(12)	Atkin and Richards, 1956
? carcinoma, telo- and metaphases	5 ..10..	Stich and Emson, 1959
Adenocarcinoma	2......(8)	Rabotti, 1959
Adenocarcinoma, liver met.	...4..... (12)	Rabotti, 1959
Adenocarcinoma, bone met.	....6.....(10)	Rabotti, 1959
Anaplastic carcinoma, prim. les.	2.5 ......(6)	Meek, 1961
Anaplastic carcinoma, ly. met.	2.5.. 3–5 ..8...(16)	Meek, 1961
Breast-carcinoma, prim. les.	...4 (8)	Meek, 1961
Breast-carcinoma, ly. met.	(2) 4.. (9)	Meek, 1961
Diff. adenocarcinoma, prim. les.	2...4.5 .. 8 (10)	Meek, 1961
Diff. adenocarcinoma, ly. met.	2.5...4.5..(8)	Meek, 1961
? carcinoma, prim. les.	2.5–3..5.. (10)	Meek, 1961
? carcinoma, ly. met.	2.5 .5. (10)	Meek, 1961
? carcinoma, prim. les (4 cases)	2.5. 5	Meek, 1961
? carcinoma, ly. met. (4 cases)	2.5. 5	Meek, 1961
? carcinoma, prim. les.	3 6	Meek, 1961
? carcinoma, ly. met.	3 6	Meek, 1961
? carcinoma, prim. les.	4	Meek, 1961
? carcinoma, prim. les.	4	Meek, 1961
Adenocarcinoma, interphases	4 6 8....15....24	Stich and Steele, 1962
Adenocarcinoma, metaphases	8...11...16	Stich and Steele, 1962
Adenocarcinoma, telophases	6 (7)	Stich and Steele, 1962
Ductal carcinoma	4.5...(8)	Sandritter et al., 1966
Ductal carcinoma	..7.	Sandritter et al., 1966
Ductal carcinoma	..3.5...	Sandritter et al., 1966
Invasive adenocarcinoma	...5–6....(?)	Emson and Kirk, 1966
Invasive adenocarcinoma	2...4–6...(10)	Emson and Kirk, 1966
Invasive adenocarcinoma	3..5..	Emson and Kirk, 1966
Intraduct carcinoma	..3..	Emson and Kirk, 1966
Intraduct carcinoma	..3...(5)	Emson and Kirk, 1966
Intraduct carcinoma	..3...(6)	Emson and Kirk, 1966
Solid medullary carcinoma	(2)...4....(8)	Sachs, 1971
Ductal carcinoma	3... .....(10)	Sachs, 1971
Ductal carcinoma	2–4..... (8)	Sachs, 1971
Lobular carcinoma	2...3.5.	Sachs, 1971
Mucinous carcinoma	2 ...(4)	Sachs, 1971

Table 13. Personal investigations of 14 mammary carcinomas (and few metastases), predominantly obtained from surgical specimen
No. = Number of nuclei measured.

Numbering	Age/Sex	Histology	Obtained by	DNA-Content (2c = diploid)	No.
T 4	60 ♀	Scirrhous carcinoma, prim. les.	surg.	*3.5 ...7.. (10)*	272
5		Scirrhous carcinoma, ly. met.	surg.	*3.5 ...7.. (10)*	250
T 11	69 ♀	Medullary carcinoma, ly. met.	surg.	*2.5 ...5.. (10)*	260
T 32	41 ♀	Medullary carcinoma, prim. les.	surg.	*2.5 ...5.. (8)*	216
T 48	67 ♀	Scirrhous carcinoma, prim. les.	surg.	*2.5 ...5... (10)*	350
T 55	62 ♀	Scirrhous carcinoma, prim. les.	surg.	*4.5 ...(9)*	325
T 61	73 ♀	Scirrhous carcinoma, prim. les.	surg.	*...4.5... (12)*	431
T 68	82 ♀	Medullary carcinoma, prim. les.	surg.	*...4.5...9.. (17)*	434
T 114	78 ♀	Scirrhous carcinoma, ly. met.	autop.	*...5.. (9)*	482
115		Scirrhous carcinoma, bone met.	autop.	*...5. (10)*	494
T 158	66 ♀	Scirrhous carcinoma, prim. les.	autop.	*...4.. (8)*	465
159		Scirrhous carcinoma, pleura, met.	autop.	*3 ... (5)*	252
160		Scirrhous carcinoma, vertebra met.	autop.	*3...5.*	346
T 214	70 ♀	Medullary carcinoma, prim. les.	surg.	*4...6*	383
T 215	77 ♀	Anaplastic carcinoma, prim. les.	surg.	*...5.9.12...(15)*	403
T 232	35 ♀	Scirrhous carcinoma, prim. les.	surg.	*2–4......(12)*	568
T 234	48 ♀	Papillary adenocarcinoma, prim. les.	surg.	*3.5..6..(8)*	288
T 243	33 ♀	Scirrhous carcinoma, prim. les.	surg.	*..3–4...(9)*	416

Table 14. Histology and nuclear DNA content of *gastric carcinomas* as revealed from the literature

Histology	Nuclear DNA (2c = diploid)	Reference
Undiff. carcinoma	*...2...4*	Leuchtenberger *et al.*, 1954
Adenocarcinoma	*2...*	Leuchtenberger *et al.*, 1954
Adenocarcinoma, ly. met.	*...3...*	Leuchtenberger *et al.*, 1954
Adenocarcinoma	*(2)..4...(8)*	Atkin and Richards, 1956
Adenocarcinoma, interphases	*.. 4.5.....(24)*	Stich and Steele, 1962
Adenocarcinoma, telo- and metaphases	*4.5 9*	Stich and Steele, 1962
Adenocarcinoma acinosum (2 cases)	*2.5 ....(5)*	Inui and Oota, 1965
Adenocarcinoma gelatinonodulare (2 cases)	*..3....(5)*	Inui and Oota, 1965
Adenocarcinoma tubulare medullare (2 cases)	*...2.5....(6)*	Inui and Oota, 1965
Adenocarcinoma gelatinocellulare (2 cases)	*...3.5....(6)*	Inui and Oota, 1965
Adenocarcinoma papillotubulare (4 cases)	*...4.5.....(7)*	Inui and Oota, 1965
Adenocarcinoma scirrhosum (4 cases)	*...3–4....(7)*	Inui and Oota, 1965
Solid carcinoma	*3.5...7..(13)*	Sandritter *et al.*, 1966
? carcinoma	*(2) .4. ...8 (11)*	Zank and Krug, 1970
? carcinoma, ly. met.	*2 .4. (8)*	Zank and Krug, 1970
? carcinoma	*..3...(5)*	Zank and Krug, 1970
Adenocarcinoma	*2...4...8...(12)*	Sprenger *et al.*, 1974

Table 15. Personal investigations of 11 gastric carcinomas

Num- bering	Age/ Sex	Histology	Ob- tained by	Nuclear DNA-Content (2c = diploid)	No.
T 8	65 ♂	Diff. papillary adenocarcinoma, prim. les.	surg.	*4.5...9*	230
9		Diff. papillary adenocarcinoma, ly. met.	surg.	*4.5...9*	54
T 52	79 ♂	Diff. adenocarcinoma, prim. les.	surg.	*(2)...4...8.. 10*	410
T 62	74 ♀	Papillary adenocarcinoma, prim. les.	surg.	*...4.5.....(12)*	388
T 85	73 ♂	Differentiated adenocarcinoma, centr. reg.	surg.	*3..6...(12)*	365
86		Medullary adenocarcinoma, marginal, reg.	surg.	*5...(12)*	376
T 7	65 ♀	Undiff. adenocarcinoma, prim. les.	surg.	*.2...4.. (8)*	260
6		Undiff. adenocarcinoma, ly. met.	surg.	*.2...4.. (8)*	287
T 67	72 ♂	Scirrhous carcinoma, prim. les.	surg.	*3.5..5*	265
T 135	66 ♂	Undiff. adenocarcinoma, ly. met.	autop.	*...4...(7)*	401
T 206	58 ♀	Undiff. polymorph. ca., prim. les.	autop.	*3.5...6..9...(14)*	560
207		Undiff. polymorph. ca., ly. met.	autop.	*3.5...6..(9)*	413
T 162	80 ♂	Undiff. medullary carcinoma, prim. les.	autop.	*3.5...(9)*	367
T 120	67 ♂	Undiff. medullary carcinoma, ly. met.	autop.	*4...6...(9)*	432
T 213	59 ♂	Mucinous adenocarcinoma, prim. les.	autop.	*...4...7..(10)*	461
212		Undiff. polymorph. carcinoma, liver met.	autop.	*...7...(14)*	866

Table 16. Personal investigations of 6 hypernephroid carcinomas (renal tubule carcinomas).
All specimen were obtained from surgical material

No. = Number of nuclei measured.

Num- bering	Age/ Sex	Histology	Ob- tained by	Nuclear DNA (2c = diploid)	No.
T 12	59 ♂	Differentiated clear cell carcinoma, prim. les.	surg.	*..4...8...(15)*	200
T 96	56 ♂	Differentiated clear cell carcinoma, centr. reg.	surg.	*2...4*	115
97		Differentiated clear cell carcinoma, marg. reg.	surg.	*2... (4)*	113
T 75	65 ♂	Less diff. clear cell carcinoma, centr. reg.	surg.	*2.5...5...(7)*	315
76		Less diff. clear cell carcinoma, marg. reg.	surg.	*2.5...5...(8)*	345
T 63	71 ♂	Less diff. clear cell carcinoma, prim. les.	surg.	*...7... (16)*	299
T 34	56 ♀	Anaplastic carcinoma, prim. les.	surg.	*...5...(12)*	280
T 27	71 ♂	Anaplastic carcinoma, prim. les.	surg.	*...5...8...(16)*	285

Table 17. Histology and nuclear DNA content of carcinomas of the urinary bladder

Histology	Nuclear DNA (2c = diploid)	Reference
Transitional cell carcinoma	(2)..4–6 8–10 (12)	Leuchtenberger et al., 1954
Transitional cell carcinoma	..3...6... ...(14)	Leuchtenberger et al., 1954
Epidermoid carcinoma	2......(7)	Leuchtenberger et al., 1954
Anaplastic glandular carcinoma, prim. ?	2.5	Leuchtenberger et al., 1954
Well diff. pap. noninvasive	2.5 (5)	Levi et al., 1969
Well diff. pap. noninvasive (2 cases)	2	Levi et al., 1969
Well diff. pap. noninvasive	hypodiploid	Levi et al., 1969
Well diff. pap. invasion of fronds	..3....(6)	Levi et al., 1969
Mod. diff. noninvasive	4	Levi et al., 1969
Mod. diff. noninvasive	hyperdiploid	Levi et al., 1969
Mod. diff. pap. invasion of fronds	2	Levi et al., 1969
Mod. diff. invasive	hypotetraploid	Levi et al., 1969
Mod. diff. invasive of fronds	2	Levi et al., 1969
Well diff. pap. invasive	2.5 5	Levi et al., 1969
Well diff. pap. invasive (2 cases)	2	Levi et al., 1969
Well diff. pap. invasive (2 cases)	2 4	Levi et al., 1969
Mod. diff. pap. invasive	hyperdiploid	Levi et al., 1969
Mod. diff. pap. invasive (2 cases)	2	Levi et al., 1969
Poorly diff. pap. invasive	2 4	Levi et al., 1969
Poorly diff. pap. invasive	...3.5....(8)	Levi et al., 1969
Poorly diff. pap. invasive (2 cases)	..2....(5)	Levi et al., 1969
Poorly diff. pap. solid (2 cases)	aneuploid	Levi et al., 1969
Solid anaplastic	hypotetraploid	Levi et al., 1969
Solid anaplastic (2 cases)	....3.5	Levi et al., 1969
Solid anaplastic	..2..3...4....(9)	Levi et al., 1969
Solid anaplastic	2.5 ...6...(8)	Levi et al., 1969
Solid anaplastic	2	Levi et al., 1969
Solid undiff. invasive	2 4	Levi et al., 1969
Pap. and solid. invasive	2	Levi et al., 1969
Transitional cell tumor, grade I	2..	Lederer et al., 1972

Table 17 (continued)

Histology	Nuclear DNA (2c = diploid)	Reference
Transitional cell tumor, grade II	*2*... 4	LEDERER *et al.*, 1972
Transitional cell tumor, grade III	..*4*... ..*7*.. (10)	LEDERER *et al.*, 1972
Transitional cell tumor, grade IV	(2).. *4–5*....8....(12)	LEDERER *et al.*, 1972
Diff. transitional cell ca., WHO grade I (10 cases)	*2* ..*4*..	FOSSA, 1975
Diff. transitional cell ca., WHO grade I (1 case)	*4*	FOSSA, 1975
Mod. diff. transitional cell ca., WHO grade II (4 cases)	*2* ..*4*..	FOSSA, 1975
Mod. diff. transitional cell ca., WHO grade II (1 case)	*3* ..*6*..	FOSSA, 1975
Mod. diff. transitional cell ca., WHO grade II (2 cases)	..*4*......(10)	FOSSA, 1975
Mod. diff. transitional cell ca., WHO grade II (1 case)	..*6*.. ..(12)	FOSSA, 1975
Undiff. transitional cell ca., WHO grade III (4 cases)	*2* ..*4*..	FOSSA, 1975
Undiff. transitional cell ca., WHO grade III (1 case)	2 4 *6* ...12..(16)	FOSSA, 1975

Table 18. Personal investigations of 14 miscellaneous carcinomas

Numbering	Age/ Sex	Histology	Obtained by	Nuclear DNA-Content (2c = diploid)	No.
T 122	67 ♂	Anaplastic thyroid carcinoma, ly. supraclav.	autop.	*4.5*.. (7)	378
123		Anaplastic thyroid carcinoma, ly. paraaortal	autop.	..*4.5*. (8)	330
124		Anaplastic thyroid carcinoma, ly. inguinal	autop.	*4.5*...(9)	369
T 164	65 ♂	Undifferentiated thyroid carcinoma, prim. les.	autop.	...*3*...(7)	503
T 239	37 ♀	Anaplastic thyroid carcinoma, prim. les.	autop.	...*4*...*7*...(10)	459
241		Anaplastic thyroid carcinoma, kidney met.	autop.	..*4*....(8)	436
242		Anaplastic thyroid carcinoma, ly. met.	autop.	..*4.5*...(12)	604

Table 18 (continued)

Num-bering	Age/Sex	Histology	Ob-tained by	Nuclear DNA-Content (2c = diploid)	No.
T 101	68 ♂	Undiff. carcinoma of the urinary bladder	autop.	$..3.5....(8)$	415
T 26	58 ♀	Papillary adenocarcinoma of the ovary	surg.	$2.5...5...(16)$	371
T 244	53 ♀	Papillary adenocarcinoma of the ovary	surg.	$3...(6)$	311
T 157	54 ♂	Diff. adenocarcinoma of the prostate	autop.	$2.5...(5)$	268
T 117	66 ♂	Less diff. squamous Ca. of the esophagus, prim. les.	autop.	$3.5..4.5..(8)$	445
118		Less diff. squamous Ca. of the esophagus, lung. met.	autop.	$3.5..4.5...(10)$	517
119		Less diff. squamous Ca. of the esophagus, ly met.	autop.	$3.5.. 4.5...(8)$	442
T 200	60 ♀	Undiff. squamous Ca. of the esophagus, prim. les.	autop.	$. 4...(8)$	412
201		Undiff. squamous Ca. of the esophagus, ly. met.	autop.	$..4.5...9..(12)$	459
202		Undiff. squamous Ca. of the esophagus, liver met.	autop.	$4...9...(11)$	416
T 103	50 ♂	Diff. adenocarcinoma of the pancreas, prim. les.	autop.	$2.5...5..(8)$	397
104		Diff. adenocarcinoma of the pancreas, periton, met.	autop.	$2.5...5..(8)$	370
105		Diff. adenocarcinoma of the pancreas, liver met.	autop.	$..3...5...(8)$	293
T 192	73 ♂	Signet ring cell carcinoma of the pancreas, prim. les.	autop.	$...6–8...(13)$	785
193		Signet ring cell carcinoma of the pancreas, ly. met.	autop.	$...6–8...(13)$	765
194		Signet ring cell carcinoma of the pancreas, liver met.	autop.	$...6–8...(15)$	674
T 24	62 ♂	Diff. adenocarcinoma of the ileum	surg.	$2...4..(6)$	224
T 79	80 ♂	Epidermoid carcinoma of the lip, centr. area	surg.	$2.5...5..(8)$	199
80		Epidermoid carcinoma of the lip, marg. area	surg.	$2.5...$	248
T 40	79 ♀	Diff. adenocarcinoma of the gall bladder	surg.	$3.5...7..(10)$	372
T 223	61 ♀	Undiff. adenocarcinoma of the gall bladder, prim. les.	autop.	$..4...(9)$	497
224		Undiff. adenocarcinoma of the gall bladder, ly met.	autop.	$..4...(7)$	413
T 39	28 ♂	Seminoma	surg.	$2.5...5...(10)$	290
T 16	34 ♀	Trophoblastic carcinoma	surg.	$2.5....(16)$	210

Table 19. Histology and nuclear DNA-content of ovarian carcinomas, obtained from literature

Histology	Nuclear DNA (2c = diploid)	Reference
Papillary serous adenocarcinoma, interphase (1)	*2...4..* (8)	BADER, 1959
Papillary serous adenocarcinoma, metaphases (2)	(2)*..5....*(12)	BADER, 1959
Papillary serous adenocarcinoma, anaphases (3)	*2*	BADER, 1959
Papillary serous adenocarcinoma, interphases (1)	*2...4..* (13)	BADER, 1959
Papillary serous adenocarcinoma, metaphases (2)	*...4.* 8 (13)	BADER, 1959
Papillary serous adenocarcinoma, anaphases (3)	*2..*	BADER, 1959
Papillary serous adenocarcinoma, interphases (1)	*2...4...7...*(10)	BADER, 1959
Papillary serous adenocarcinoma, metaphases (2)	*...6....*(13)	BADER, 1959
Papillary serous adenocarcinoma, anaphases (3)	*2..*	BADER, 1959
Papillary serous adenocarcinoma, interphases (1)	*2...4* (6)	BADER, 1959
Papillary serous adenocarcinoma, metaphases (2)	*...4.. ..8*	BADER, 1959
Papillary serous adenocarcinoma, anaphases (3)	*2*	BADER, 1959
Papillary serous adenocarcinoma, interphases (1)	(2)*..4...*(8)	BADER, 1959
Papillary serous adenocarcinoma, metaphases (2)	*4...7....*(13)	BADER, 1959
Papillary serous adenocarcinoma, anaphases (3)	*1.5–3*	BADER, 1959
Papillary serous adenocarcinoma, grade I (4 cases)	*2...4*	BADER *et al.*, 1960
Papillary serous adenocarcinoma, grade II	*2...4..*	BADER *et al.*, 1960
Papillary serous adenocarcinoma, grade II	*..3..*(6)	BADER *et al.*, 1960
Papillary serous adenocarcinoma, grade II	*2..3...*(6)	BADER *et al.*, 1960
Papillary serous adenocarcinoma, grade II	*2...* (6)	BADER *et al.*, 1960
Papillary serous adenocarcinoma, grade II	*2....*(7)	BADER *et al.*, 1960
Papillary serous adenocarcinoma, grade II	*2....*(9)	BADER *et al.*, 1960
Papillary serous adenocarcinoma, grade II	*2.....*(10)	BADER *et al.*, 1960
Papillary serous adenocarcinoma, grade III	*2..3*	BADER *et al.*, 1960
Papillary serous adenocarcinoma, grade III	*..3...*(7)	BADER *et al.*, 1960
Papillary serous adenocarcinoma, grade III	*2....*(4) (7)	BADER *et al.*, 1960
Papillary serous adenocarcinoma, grade III	*2....* (8)	BADER *et al.*, 1960
Papillary serous adenocarcinoma, grade III	*....4.....* (8)	BADER *et al.*, 1960
Papillary serous adenocarcinoma, grade III	*2....* (10)	BADER *et al.*, 1960
Papillary serous adenocarcinoma, grade III	*2..3....6....*(10)	BADER *et al.*, 1960
Papillary serous adenocarcinoma, grade III	*2...4....*(10)	BADER *et al.*, 1960
Papillary serous adenocarcinoma, grade III	*..3.5....* (12)	BADER *et al.*, 1960
Papillary carcinoma	*..6...*(10)	SANDRITTER *et al.*, 1966
Papillary carcinoma	*4...8..*	SANDRITTER *et al.*, 1966

Table 20. *Histology (or cytology) and nuclear DNA content of preneoplastic and cancerous lesion of the cercix uteri*

Histology or Cytology	Nuclear DNA (2c = diploid)	Reference
Poorly diff. squamous cell carcinoma	*2..4..*	Atkin and Richards, 1956
Poorly diff. squamous cell carcinoma	*...4....8...(10)*	Atkin and Richards, 1956
Moderately diff. squamous cell carcinoma	*..4....8...(10)*	Atkin and Richards, 1956
"Metaplasia"	*2.. .4...8...(25)*	Reid and Singh, 1960
Invasive carcinoma	*3–6.....(20)*	Reid and Singh, 1960
Squamous cell carcinoma	*...2.5....(6)*	Ojima et al., 1960
Squamous cell carcinoma	*..2.5...(4)*	Ojima et al., 1960
Squamous cell carcinoma	*...3....(5)*	Ojima et al., 1960
Squamous cell carcinoma	*....4.5...(7)*	Ojima et al., 1960
Squamous cell carcinoma	*..3.5–4 .... (8)*	Ojima et al., 1960
Cervical adenocarcinoma	*...2...(4)*	Ojima et al., 1960
Basal cell carcinoma	*...2.5.. (4)*	Ojima et al., 1960
Mild dysplasia	*..2...(4)*	Grundmann et al., 1961
Moderate dysplasia	*..2...4...(8)*	Grundmann et al., 1961
Moderate dysplasia; basal cells only	*...2..*	Grundmann et al., 1961
Severe dysplasia	*...4...(8)*	Grundmann et al., 1961
Severe dysplasia; basal cells only	*..4..*	Grundmann et al., 1961
Carcinoma in situ	*..2..(4)*	Grundmann et al., 1961
Carcinoma in situ; basal cells only	*...2*	Grundmann et al., 1961
Invasive carcinoma	*...4...(8)*	Grundmann et al., 1961
Invasive carcinoma	*..2.5...(8)*	Grundmann et al., 1961
Dysplasia	*2....4..*	Sandritter and Fischer, 1962
Carcinoma in situ	*2.5....(5)*	Sandritter and Fischer, 1962
Carcinoma in situ	*..5–7...*	Sandritter and Fischer, 1962
Carcinoma in situ	*(2)....6....(12)*	Sandritter and Fischer, 1962
Carcinoma in situ, simple replacement (1)	*2.5...(5)*	Sandritter and Fischer, 1962
Carcinoma in situ, gland invasion (2)	*2.5....(5)*	Sandritter and Fischer, 1962
Carcinoma in situ, early stroma invasion (3)	*2.5...(6)*	Sandritter and Fischer, 1962
Carcinoma in situ, and microcarcinoma (4)	*2.5....(4)*	Sandritter and Fischer, 1962
Carcinoma in situ, simple replacement (1)	*..6...(8)*	Sandritter and Fischer, 1962
Carcinoma in situ, gland invasion (2)	*..5...(7)*	Sandritter and Fischer, 1962
Carcinoma in situ, early stroma invasion (3)	*..2.5..(4)*	Sandritter and Fischer, 1962
Carcinoma in situ, and microcarcinoma (4)	*..2.5...5*	Sandritter and Fischer, 1962
Carcinoma in situ	*3.5....7*	Kother and Sandritter 1964
Squamous carcinoma	*..2.5...(10)*	Sandritter and Kleinhans, 1964

Table 20 (continued)

Histology or Cytology	Nuclear DNA (2c = diploid)	Reference
Epidermoid carcinoma	2.5...5..	SANDRITTER and KLEINHANS, 1964
Carcinoma in situ, basal layer (1)	...3...(6)	SANDRITTER, 1963
Carcinoma in situ, intermediate layer (2)	..2.5....(6)	SANDRITTER, 1963
Carcinoma in situ, superficial layer (3)	...3....(6)	SANDRITTER, 1963
Carcinoma in situ	..1.5. 3...(5)	SANDRITTER, 1963
Well diff. squamous cell carcinoma, biopsy	..2...4	ATKIN, 1964
Well diff. squamous cell carcinoma, smear	..2 .4.	ATKIN, 1964
Mod. well diff. squamous cell carcinoma, biopsy	..2 ...4..	ATKIN, 1964
Mod. well diff. squamous cell carcinoma, smear	..2 ...4	ATKIN, 1964
Poorly diff. squamous cell carcinoma, biopsy	3.5 7	ATKIN, 1964
Poorly diff. squamous cell carcinoma, smear	3.5 7	ATKIN, 1964
Anaplastic cervical adenoacanthoma, biopsy	3	ATKIN, 1964
Anaplastic cervical adenoacanthoma, smear	3	ATKIN, 1964
Mod. well diff. squamous cell carcinoma, biopsy	..4. (8)	ATKIN, 1964
Mod. well diff. squamous cell carcinoma, smear	. 4.. (8)	ATKIN, 1964
Poorly diff. squamous cell carcinoma biopsy	..2...4..	ATKIN, 1964
Poorly diff. squamous cell carcinoma, biopsy 3.5 7 later	..2 ..4 (8)	ATKIN, 1964
Squamous carcinoma, cervical scrape after washing	..4.5..... (12)	CASPERSSON, 1964
Squamous carcinoma	..2–3 ....6....(10)	CASPERSSON, 1964
Squamous carcinoma	..3..(6)	CASPERSSON, 1964
Squamous carcinoma	..2..4	CASPERSSON, 1964
Squamous carcinoma	2...4....(8)	CASPERSSON, 1964
Dysplasia (pooled from 6 cases)	...5...	WIED et al., 1966
Carcinoma in situ (from 6 cases)	...7...(10)	WIED et al., 1966
Invasive squamous carcinoma (pooled from 6 cases)	....6...(10)	WIED et al., 1966
Epidermoid carcinoma	2.5 ...(5)	SANDRITTER et al., 1966
Epidermoid carcinoma	....(5)....(12)	SANDRITTER et al., 1966
Squamous cell carcinoma	...3.5...(9)	SANDRITTER et al., 1966
Squamous cell carcinoma	2.5...5..	SANDRITTER et al., 1966
Squamous cell carcinoma	2.5......(10)	SANDRITTER et al., 1966
Carcinoma in situ	.4...8.. (32)	VALERI et al., 1967
Invasive carcinoma	..4.5 ....9 (32)	VALERI et al., 1967
Mild dysplasia	..2.5...4...(6)	WILBANKS et al., 1967
Mild dysplasia	...3...6...(10)	WILBANKS et al., 1967
Mild dysplasia	....4–5..8.. ...(32)	WILBANKS et al., 1967

Table 20 (continued)

Histology or Cytology	Nuclear DNA (2c = diploid)	Reference
Moderate dysplasia	...6..8.. ...(32)	Wilbanks *et al.*, 1967
Moderate dysplasia	...4–6...8..(12)	Wilbanks *et al.*, 1967
Severe dysplasia	..2..4...(6)	Wilbanks *et al.*, 1967
Severe dysplasia	...3....(12)	Wilbanks *et al.*, 1967
Carcinoma in situ	...3–4....(12)	Wilbanks *et al.*, 1967
Carcinoma in situ	(2)..4 6....(32)	Wilbanks *et al.*, 1967
Poorly diff. squamous carcinoma, untreated (1)	2.5...5...(8)	Holzner and Golob, 1968
Poorly diff. squamous carcinoma, after radium irrad. (2)	2.5...5...8	Holzner and Golob, 1968
Poorly diff. squamous carcinoma, untreated (1)	2.5...(5)	Holzner and Golob, 1968
Poorly diff. squamous carcinoma, after 1.6 mg Trenimon (2)	2.5...(5)	Holzner and Golob, 1968
Poorly diff. squamous carcinoma, after radium irrad. (3)	2.5....(10)	Holzner and Golob, 1968
Mod. diff. squamous carcinoma, untreated (1)	2.5....5	Holzner and Golob, 1968
Mod. diff. squamous carcinoma, after 1.8 mg Trenimon (2)	2.5...(5)	Holzner and Golob, 1968
Mod. diff. squamous carcinoma, after telecobalt irrad. (3)	2.5 ..5 ....(8)	Holzner and Golob, 1968
Well diff. squamous carcinoma, untreated (1)	2.5...4.5 (6)	Holzner and Golob, 1968
Well diff. squamous carcinoma, after 1.4 mg Trenimon (2)	2.5...4.5 (6)	Holzner and Golob, 1968
Well diff. squamous carcinoma, after radium irrad. (3)	2.5...5...(8)	Holzner and Golob, 1968
Well diff. squamous carcinoma, untreated (1)	2.5...4.5..(6)	Holzner and Golob, 1968
Well diff. squamous carcinoma, after 1.6 mg Trenimon (2)	2.5...4.5..(10)	Holzner and Golob, 1968
Well diff. squamous carcinoma, after radium irrad. (3)	2.5...4.5–5.. 7(10)	Holzner and Golob, 1968
Dysplasia (3 cases)	..2.. ..4.. ..8	Brandao, 1969
Dysplasia (2 cases)	..2. 3.5.. (5)	Brandao, 1969
Dysplasia	...4...(7)	Brandao, 1969
Atypical cells, exfoliated (1)	..2.5....(8)	Hrushovetz, 1969
Atypical cells, exfoliated (2)	....3–3.5..(6)	Hrushovetz, 1969
Atypical cells, exfoliated	...2.5.... (10)	Hrushovetz, 1969
Atypical cells, exfoliated (1)	..1.5.... (10)	Hrushovetz, 1969
Atypical cells, exfoliated (2)	..2....(6)	Hrushovetz, 1969
Atypical cells, exfoliated	2..3–5......(8)	Hrushovetz, 1969
Atypical cells, exfoliated	.1.5–2 ....4...(7)	Hrushovetz, 1969
Atypical cells, exfoliated	..2.5...(5)	Hrushovetz, 1969
Atypical cells, exfoliated	..2..3.. (10)	Hrushovetz, 1969
Squamous carcinoma	2.5..	Zank and Krug, 1970
Squamous carcinoma, met.	2.5. 5	Zank and Krug, 1970
Mild dysplasia (4 cases)	2...4..(6)	Hrushovetz and Lauchlan, 1970
Mild dysplasia (2 cases)	2.5	Hrushovetz and Lauchlan, 1970

Table 20 (continued)

Histology or Cytology	Nuclear DNA (2c = diploid)	Reference
Mild dysplasia (2 cases)	.2.5...(4) (6)	HRUSHOVETZ and LAUCHLAN, 1970
Mild dysplasia	..3..	HRUSHOVETZ and LAUCHLAN, 1970
Severe dysplasia	2...4...(6)	HRUSHOVETZ and LAUCHLAN, 1970
Severe dysplasia	2.5...5	HRUSHOVETZ and LAUCHLAN, 1970
Carcinoma in situ	2...4...(6)	HRUSHOVETZ and LAUCHLAN, 1970
Carcinoma in situ (2 cases)	2...(5)	HRUSHOVETZ and LAUCHLAN, 1970
Carcinoma in situ	2.5..(6)	HRUSHOVEZT and LAUCHLAN, 1970
Carcinoma in situ	2.5....(11)	HRUSHOVETZ and LAUCHLAN, 1970
Microcarcinoma	2....(6)	HRUSHOVETZ and LAUCHLAN, 1970
Microcarcinoma	3....(6)	HRUSHOVETZ and LAUCHLAN, 1970
Mod. diff. carcinoma	3...(8)	NODSKOV-PEDERSEN, 1971
Mod. diff. carcinoma	..3.5..(18)	NODSKOV-PEDERSEN, 1971
Mod. diff. carcinoma	...3..(8)	NODSKOV-PEDERSEN, 1971
Mod. diff. carcinoma	..4.5...8..(11)	NODSKOV-PEDERSEN, 1971
Less. diff. carcinoma	(6)....12....(20)	NODSKOV-PEDERSEN, 1971
Dysplasia, Pap. IV	..4...8..	BÖHM et al., 1971
Dysplasia, Pap. IV	(4) 8...14 (16)	BÖHM et al., 1971
Carcinoma in situ, Pap. V	3. .6. (12)	BÖHM et al., 1971
Carcinoma in situ + dysplasia, Pap. V	..4..6.....(32)	BÖHM et al., 1971
Invasive carcinoma	3.5...7....(14)	BÖHM et al., 1971
Mild dysplasia	4...8...16...(30)	WAGNER et al., 1972
Moderate dysplasia	...4...8...(16)	WAGNER et al., 1972
Severe dysplasia	...4...8...(16)	WAGNER et al., 1972
Carcinoma in situ	...6...10...(18)	WAGNER et al., 1972
Dyscariotic cells, Pap. IVa (1)	2.. 4.5....(10)	SPRENGER et al., 1974b
Mild inflammation, Pap. II (2)	..2...(4)	SPRENGER et al., 1974b
Atypical cells, Pap. IVa (3)	..2...4...(8)	SPRENGER et al., 1974b
Dyscariotic cells, Pap. IVa (1)	2....(10)	SPRENGER et al., 1974b
Pseudodyscariotic cells, Pap. III (2)	..2....(12)	SPRENGER et al., 1974b
Pseudodyscariotic cells, Pap. III (3)	..2...4.	SPRENGER et al., 1974b
Mild inflamation, Pap. II (4)	2 (5)	SPRENGER et al., 1974b
Pseudodyscariotic and dyscariotic cells (Pap. III) (4 times)	2...4.5....(10)	SPRENGER et al., 1974b

Table 21. Histology and nuclear DNA content of precancerous lesions and malignant neoplasms of the skin

Histology	Nuclear DNA (2c = diploid)	Reference
Senile keratosis (2 cases)	..4...	Leuchtenberger et al., 1954
Senile keratosis	..4.5...	Leuchtenberger et al., 1954
Basal cell carcinoma	4.. .8.	Atkin and Richards, 1956
Epithelioma basocell. sol. med. (3 cases)	..2.5....(6)	Ehlers, 1968
Epithelioma basocell. sol. med. (2 cases)	.2.5....(8)	Ehlers, 1968
Epithelioma basocell. sol. med.	3...5..(8)	Ehlers, 1968
Epithelioma basocell. sol. med.	3...(5)	Ehlers, 1968
Epithelioma basocell cysticum	..4....(8)	Ehlers, 1968
Epithelioma basocell pigm.	..3.5...(5)	Ehlers, 1968
Epithelioma basocell pigm.	..3.5...(6)	Ehlers, 1968
Epithelioma basocell pigm.	...4–5..(6)	Ehlers, 1968
Epithelioma basocell. cyl.	..3.5...(6)	Ehlers, 1968
Epithelioma metatyp. interm. (2 cases)	..4...8	Ehlers, 1968
Basal cell carcinoma, metaphases (9 cases)	4..	Manocha, 1969
Basal cell carcinoma, anaphases	2	Manocha, 1969
Basal cell carcinoma, metaphases (2 cases)	4 ..8	Manocha, 1969
Basal cell carcinoma, metaphases (3 cases)	4....8...(10)	Manocha, 1969
Baso-squamous carcinoma, metaphases	2.. 3....8	Manocha, 1969
Senile keratosis (2 cases)	3.5 .....(8)	Manocha et al., 1969
Senile keratosis	2–4....(11)	Manocha et al., 1969
Senile keratosis	(2)...4 6 (8)	Manocha et al., 1969
Senile keratosis (2 cases)	2...5...(8)	Manocha et al., 1969
Senile keratosis, metaphases (2 cases)	4..	Manocha et al., 1969
Carcinoma in situ (metaphases)	(4)....5... ..(24)	Manocha et al., 1969
Carcinoma in situ (metaphases)	4...8.. ..18..	Manocha et al., 1969
Carcinoma in situ (metaphases)	4...8.. ..18..	Manocha et al., 1969
Carcinoma in situ (metaphases)	4 6...(20)	Manocha et al., 1969
Carcinoma in situ (metaphases)	5 8 (10)	Manocha et al., 1969
Carcinoma in situ (metaphases)	4....(8)	Manocha et al., 1969
Carcinoma in situ (metaphases)	4....8	Manocha et al., 1969
Carcinoma in situ (metaphases)	..5–6...(10) (16)	Manocha et al., 1969
Carcinoma in situ (metaphases)	..5.....(15)	Manocha et al., 1969
Carcinoma in situ (metaphases)	4.....(12)	Manocha et al., 1969
Carcinoma in situ (metaphases) (3 cases)	..4....(10)	Manocha et al., 1969
Squamous cell carcinoma (metaphases)	4...... (28)	Manocha et al., 1969
Squamous cell carcinoma (metaphases)	4...(10)	Manocha et al., 1969
Squamous cell carcinoma (metaphases)	4–6...(12)	Manocha et al., 1969
Squamous cell carcinoma (metaphases)	(4)....9.....(18)	Manocha et al., 1969
Squamous cell carcinoma (metaphases)	(5)....10....(16)	Manocha et al., 1969

Table 21 (continued)

Histology	Nuclear DNA (2c = diploid)	Reference
Squamous cell carcinoma (meta-phases)	6..5.....(14)	MANOCHA et al., 1969
Squamous cell carcinoma (2 cases) (metaphases)	(4)...7....(16)	MANOCHA et al., 1969
Squamous cell carcinoma (meta-phases)	(3)...5......(24)	MANOCHA et al., 1969
Squamous cell carcinoma (meta-phases)	4–6 ...(8)	MANOCHA et al., 1969
Squamous cell carcinoma (meta-phases) (1)	..4..	MANOCHA et al., 1969
Squamous cell carcinoma (meta-phases) (2)	3.5 5..7	MANOCHA et al., 1969
Squamous cell carcinoma (meta-phases) (3)	(4)..8...(12)	MANOCHA et al., 1969
Morbus Paget of the nipple	(2)..5...(10)	SACHS, 1970
Morbus Paget of the nipple	(2)..3...6...(12)	SACHS, 1970
Morbus Paget of the vulva	(4)..6–7...(15)	SACHS, 1970
Morbus Paget of the vulva	(2)...5..(10)	SACHS, 1970
Paget-carcinoma of the nipple	(4)...6–7...(14)	SACHS, 1970
Paget-carcinoma of the nipple	(3)...5..(7)	SACHS, 1970
Arsenical keratosis	...3...(6)	EHLERS and STEPHAN, 1972a
Senile keratosis	...3.5–4....(10)	EHLERS and STEPHAN, 1972a
Senile keratosis (2 cases)	...4...(6)	EHLERS and STEPHAN, 1972a
Senile keratosis	..2...5....(8)	EHLERS and STEPHAN, 1972a
Senile keratosis	3 ..6–7	EHLERS and STEPHAN, 1972a
Leukoplakia vegetans	...4....(8)	EHLERS and STEPHAN, 1972a
Leukoplakia vegetans	...5...(8)	EHLERS and STEPHAN, 1972a
Leukoplakia vegetans	...5...(7)	EHLERS and STEPHAN, 1972a
Leukoplakia vegetans	...4–5...(8)	EHLERS and STEPHAN, 1972a
Leukoplakia vegetans	..3...5...(8)	EHLERS and STEPHAN, 1972a
Cornu cutaneum	....4..(6)	EHLERS and STEPHAN, 1972b
Cornu cutaneum	....4..6..(8)	EHLERS and STEPHAN, 1972b
Cornu cutaneum	....4..6.. (18)	EHLERS and STEPHAN, 1972b
Cornu cutaneum	...5...(8)	EHLERS and STEPHAN, 1972b
Cornu cutaneum	(2)...6...(10)	EHLERS and STEPHAN, 1972b
M. Bowen	....4.....(12)	EHLERS and STEPHAN, 1972b
M. Bowen	...5... (10)	EHLERS and STEPHAN, 1972b
M. Bowen	....6....(10)	EHLERS and STEPHAN, 1972b
M. Bowen	....6.....(11)	EHLERS and STEPHAN, 1972b
M. Bowen	......7...(10)	EHLERS and STEPHAN, 1972b
Erythroplasia Queyrat	..2.5..5...8...(11)	EHLERS and STEPHAN, 1972b
Erythroplasia Queyrat	....4–7..	EHLERS and STEPHAN, 1972b
M. Paget	....4....(12)	EHLERS and STEPHAN, 1972b
M. Paget (2 cases)	....5....(10)	EHLERS and STEPHAN, 1972b
M. Paget	....5...(8)	EHLERS and STEPHAN, 1972b
Melanosis p.c. Dubreuilh	...4....(10)	EHLERS and STEPHAN, 1972b
Melanosis p.c. Dubreuilh (4 cases)	...5....(9)	EHLERS and STEPHAN, 1972b
Epidermoid carcinoma	..2...(4)	EHLERS and HERBSTREIT, 1973
Epidermoid carcinoma	..2.5...(6)	EHLERS and HERBSTREIT, 1973
Epidermoid carcinoma (2 cases)	..3...(6)	EHLERS and HERBSTREIT, 1973
Epidermoid carcinoma	..3....(8)	EHLERS and HERBSTREIT, 1973
Epidermoid carcinoma	..3...6...(9)	EHLERS and HERBSTREIT, 1973
Epidermoid carcinoma	..2.5...(5)	EHLERS and HERBSTREIT, 1973

Table 21 (continued)

Histology	Nuclear DNA (2c = diploid)	Reference
Epidermoid carcinoma	..2.5....(8)	Ehlers and Herbstreit, 1973
Epidermoid carcinoma (2 cases)	3...(6)	Ehlers and Herbstreit, 1973
Epidermoid carcinoma	..3.. 4 ...(7)	Ehlers and Herbstreit, 1973
Epidermoid carcinoma	...4.5....(20)	Ehlers and Herbstreit, 1973
Mycosis fungoides	2...4	van Vloten et al., 1974
Mycosis fungoides	2...(4)	van Vloten et al., 1974
Mycosis fungoides (2 cases)	2...4..(6)	van Vloten et al., 1974
Mycosis fungoides	2...4....(8)	van Vloten et al., 1974
Mycosis fungoides	2...4...(8)	van Vloten et al., 1974
Mycosis fungoides	2...4...(6)	van Vloten et al., 1974
Mycosis fungoides (2 cases)	2....(6)	van Vloten et al., 1974
Mycosis fungoides	(2) 3.5....(7)	van Vloten et al., 1974

Table 22. Nuclear DNA content of miscellaneous malignant neoplasmas of various origin

Histology and tumor location	Nuclear DNA (2c = diploid)	Reference
Adenocarcinoma of the pancreas	2...4	Leuchtenberger et al., 1954
Adenocarcinoma of the pancreas, liver met.	3...(10)	Leuchtenberger et al., 1954
Adenocarcinoma of the pancreas	1.5 ...4	Leuchtenberger et al., 1954
Seminoma	..3.. (7)	Leuchtenberger et al., 1954
Poorly diff. squamous cell ca. of the anus	2.5....5..	Atkin and Richards, 1956
Epidermoid carcinoma of the vagina	2.5...(5)	Atkin and Richards, 1956
Anapl. squamous cell carcinoma of the cheek	...4.....(8)	Atkin and Richards, 1956
Epidermoid carcinoma of the tongue	2...4....8	Atkin and Richards, 1956
Malignant melanoma of the vulva	2.5...5.	Atkin and Richards, 1956
Chorionepithelioma	(2)....4....(12)	Atkin and Richards, 1956
Adenocarcinoma of the pancreas	2.5....(5)	Sandritter et al., 1966
Seminoma	..4.5... (7)	Sandritter et al., 1966
Mucoepidermoid carcinoma of the palate	..3....(6)	Nitze, 1969
Epidermoid carcinoma of the larynx	..4.....(10)	Nitze, 1969
Epidermoid carcinoma of the tongue	..6....10. (18)	Nitze, 1969
Epidermoid carcinoma of the larynx before rad.	.2-3.. 4 ..	Nitze, 1969
Epidermoid carcinoma of the larynx after rad.	..3-5.....(20)	Nitze, 1969
Pseudoseminoma	..2.5....(5)	Ehlers and Soll, 1971
Polymorphous carcinoma of the palate	2..4...8....16....32..	Pfitzer and Pape, 1971
Malignant phaeochromocytoma (3 cases)	...3....(9)	Lewis, 1971

Table 23. Nuclear DNA content of various leukemias and myeloma

Hematologic or histologic diagnosis	Nuclear DNA (2c = diploid)	Reference
Chronic lymphocytic leukemia (6 cases)	2	PETRAKIS, 1953
Chronic lymphocytic leukemia (3 cases)	2.5...	PETRAKIS, 1953
Acute lymphocytic leukemia (5 cases)	...3...	PETRAKIS, 1953
Chronic myeloid leukemia	2. .4.	HALE and WILSON, 1959
Subacute myeloid leukemia	..2....4..	HALE and WILSON, 1959
Chronic lymphatic leukemia	2.. (4)	HALE and WILSON, 1959
Acute lymphatic leukemia	..2.....(4)	HALE and WILSON, 1959
Lymphosarcoma (leukemic)	2..	HALE and WILSON, 1959
Lymphosarcoma (leukemic)	2 (4)	HALE and WILSON, 1959
CML, primitive cells only	(2)....4... (6)	HALE and WILSON, 1959
Chronic myeloid leukemia (2 cases)	2.....4... (6)	HALE and WILSON, 1959
Acute myeloid leukemia (4 cases)	2.....(4–5)	HALE and WILSON, 1959
Chronic lymphatic leukemia	2	CHRISTOPHERSON et al., 1963
Chronic lymphatic leukemia	.2.5.	CHRISTOPHERSON et al., 1963
Chronic lymphatic leukemia	2..4. (6)	CHRISTOPHERSON et al., 1963
Acute lymphatic leukemia (2 cases)	2.....3.5	LAMPERT, 1967, 1968
Acute lymphatic leukemia (2 cases)	2.5.....(5)	LAMPERT, 1967, 1968
Acute lymphatic leukemia (3 cases)	3.....(6)	LAMPERT, 1967, 1968
Acute lymphatic leukemia (2 cases)	..3.5.....(8)	LAMPERT, 1967, 1968
Acute lymphatic leukemia	(2)....3.5....(6)	LAMPERT, 1967, 1968
Acute myeloid leukemia	2	MÜLLER, 1969
Acute myeloid leukemia	2..(3)	MÜLLER, 1969
Acute lymphoid leukemia	2 (3)	MÜLLER, 1969
Acute lymphoid leukemia	1.5	MÜLLER, 1969
Acute monocytoid leukemia	2.5	MÜLLER, 1969
Acute undiff. leukemia	2	MÜLLER, 1969
Acute undiff. leukemia	2....(4)	MÜLLER, 1969
Acute undiff. leukemia	1.5....(3)	MÜLLER, 1969
Acute myeloid leukemia peroxydase-type	2	OBRECHT et al., 1970
Acute myeloid leukemia peroxydase-type (3 cases)	2.5	OBRECHT et al., 1970
Acute myeloid leukemia peroxydase-type (3 cases)	2.5 ..5.	OBRECHT et al., 1970
Acute lymphoid leukemia, PAS-type	2	OBRECHT et al., 1970
Acute lymphoid leukemia, PAS-type	2...(4)	OBRECHT et al., 1970
Acute lymphoid leukemia, PAS-type	2–2.5...(4)	OBRECHT et al., 1970
Acute lymphoid leukemia, PAS-type (2 cases)	2.5....4	OBRECHT et al., 1970
Acute lymphoid leukemia, PAS-type	2.5..5 (10)	OBRECHT et al., 1970
Acute undiff. leukemia	4.5. (9)	OBRECHT et al., 1970
Myeloma (10 cases)	2	MUNDY, 1973
Myeloma (7 cases)	2.5	MUNDY, 1973
Myeloma (2 cases)	2.5.. .. (8)	MUNDY, 1973
Myeloma (3 cases)	(1) .2.	MUNDY, 1973
Myeloma	..2...4.. .8..	MUNDY, 1973

Table 24. Personal investigations of 4 malignant tumorous lesions of the hematopoetic system

Numbering	Age/ Sex	Histology	Obtained by	Nuclear DNA-content (2c = diploid)	No.
T 18	68 ♂	Hodgkin's disease, mixed type, cervically.	surg.	*3* 6 (12)	220
T 127	69 ♂	Chronic lymphadenosis, para-aortally.	autop.	*.3.* (6)	207
128		Chronic lymphadenosis, axillarly.	autop.	*2.5*	178
128		Chronic lymphadenosis, iliacally.	autop.	*2.5*	160
T 110	69 ♂	Plasmocytoma, lumbar vertebra	autop.	*3...6*	235
111		Plasmocytoma, thoracic vertebra	autop.	*3...6.*	386
112		Plasmocytoma, sternum	autop.	*3...6*	317
T 145	52 ♀	Plasmocytoma, extramedullary, rib serosa	autop.	*2.5...* (5)	283
146		Plasmocytoma, extramedullary, liver	autop.	*2.5...* (5)	271
147		Plasmocytoma, lumbar vertebra	autop.	*2–3...* (5)	387

Table 25. Nuclear DNA-content of sarcomas and malignant mixed tumor

Histology and Location	DNA-content (2c = diploid)	Reference
Leiomyosarcoma of the uterus	*2.5....* (7)	Atkin and Richards, 1956
Leiomyosarcoma of the colon (1)	*3.5.....* (16)	Stich and Steele, 1962
Leiomyosarcoma of the colon, metaphases (2)	7 12	Stich and Steele, 1962
Leiomyosarcoma of the colon, telophases (3)	3,5 6	Stich and Steele, 1962
Osteogenic sarcoma, telo- and metaphases (1)	*3* (5).....(21)	Stich and Steele, 1962
Osteogenic sarcoma, telo- and metaphases (2)	*3* ... *6*	Stich and Steele, 1962
Leiomyosarcoma of the uterus	(2) ....*4*.... (10)	Atkin, 1964
Angioblastic reticulosarcoma of the skin	....*5*.... (10)	Ehlers et al., 1971
Angioblastic reticulosarcoma of the skin	...*3*....6	Ehlers et al., 1971
Angioblastic reticulosarcoma of the skin	..*3*..*4*...7..(15)	Ehlers et al., 1971
Polymorphous osteogenic sarcoma	(2)....*5*....10.....(22)	Födisch et al., 1974
Polymorphous osteogenic sarcoma	(2) *5*...10.. (32)	Födisch et al., 1974
Osteoplastic osteosarcoma (1)	(2) ..*3.5*...7... (14)	Födisch et al., 1974
Osteoplastic osteosarcoma (2)	(2) ...*5*....10..(12)	Födisch et al., 1974
Chondrosarcoma (1)	*2*... (5)	Födisch et al., 1974
Chondrosarcoma (2)	*2*.... (8)	Födisch et al., 1974
Wilms tumor	*2.5*.... (5)	Sandritter et al., 1966

Table 26. Personal investigations of 6 malignant mesenchymal tumors (sarcomas) and one nephroblastoma

Num-bering	Age/ Sex	Histology	Ob-tained by	Nuclear DNA-content (2c = diploid)	No.
T 25	12 ♀	Desmoid of the thigh fascia	surg.	*2.5...5*	186
T 31	57 ♀	Diff. liposarcoma of the leg	surg.	*2.5 5*	196
T 33	37 ♀	Monomorphic spindlecell sarcoma of the thigh	surg.	*2.5 ..5.*	314
T 60	71 ♂	Rhabdomyosarcoma of the leg	surg.	*2.5...5...*(9)	335
T 172	31 ♀	Monomorphic leiomyosarcoma of the uterus	autop.	*..3..*	362
T 238	80 ♀	Undifferentiated endometrial sarcoma	surg.	*...4–6...* (10)	681
T 225	6 ♂	Nephroblastoma, predominantly sarcomatous (1)	autop.	*...4...*	449
226		Nephroblastoma, predominantly sarcomatous (2)	autop.	*...3...*	312
227		Nephroblastoma, predominantly sarcomatous (3)	autop.	*...4..*	375
228		Nephroblastoma, predominantly sarcomatous (4)	autop.	*...4..*	438
230		Nephroblastoma, predominantly sarcomatous (5)	autop.	*...4..*	357
231		Normal kidney parenchyma (6)	autop.	*2*	149

Table 27. Progression theory of cancer, demonstrated for example from consecutive lesions of the uterine cervix

Histogram	DNA ploidy	Histology of the cervical lesion
unimodal 2c ↓	euploid ↓	normal squamous epithelium ↓
unimodal, scattered values ↙ up to 4c	euploid, proliferating ↙	prolif. epithelium, inflammation ↙
bi- or trimodal doubling peaks up to 32c ↘	euploid-polyploid ↘	dysplasia ↘
unimodal, broad scatter (2–5c) no stemline ↓	aneuploid	carcinoma in situ
bimodal with stemline (2, 2.5, 3, 4.5c) ↓	aneuploid-polyploid	invasive carcinoma
unimodal broad scatter (3c) no stemline	aneuploid	late stage invasive carcinoma

References

Adams, L. R., Dahlgren, S. E.: Cytophotometric measurements of the DNA content of lung tumours. Acta path. microbiol. scand. **72**, 561–574 (1968).

Adler, C. P., Sandritter, W.: Polyploidisierung des Herzmuskels bei Herzhypertrophie. Verh. dtsch. Ges. inn. Med. **77**, 1252–1256 (1971).

Atkin, N. B.: The deoxyribonucleic acid content of malignant cells in cervical smears. Acta cytol. (Philad.) **8**, 68–72 (1964).

Atkin, N. B.: Modal DNA value and chromosome number in ovarian neoplasia. Cancer (Philad.) **27**, 1064–1073 (1971).

Atkin, N. B.: Modal deoxyribonucleic acid value and survival in carcinoma of the breast. Brit. med. J. **1972**, 271–272.

Atkin, N. B.: High chromosome numbers of seminomata and malignant teratomata of the testis: A review of data on 103 tumours. Brit. J. Cancer **28**, 275–279 (1973).

Atkin, N. B., Baker, M. C.: Chromosome abnormalities as primary events in human malignant disease: Evidence from marker chromosomes. J. nat. Cancer Inst. **36**, 539–551 (1966).

Atkin, N. B., Baker, M. C., Robinson, R., Gaze, S. E.: Chromosome studies on 14 near-diploid carcinomas of the ovary. Europ. J. Cancer **10**, 143–146 (1974).

Atkin, N. B., Mattinson, G., Baker, M. C.: A comparison of the DNA content and chromosome number of fifty human tumours. Brit. J. Cancer **20**, 84–101 (1966).

Atkin, N. B., Mattinson, G., Becak, W., Ohno, S.: The comparative DNA content of 19 species of placental mammals, reptiles and birds. Chromosoma (Berl.) **17**, 1–10 (1965).

Atkin, N. B., Richards, B. M.: Deoxyribonucleic acid in human tumours as measured by microspectrophotometry of Feulgen stain: A comparison of tumours arising at different sites. Brit. J. Cancer **10**, 769–786 (1956).

Atkin, N. B., Richards, B. M.: Clinical significance of ploidy in carcinoma of cervix: Its relation to prognosis. Brit. med. J. **1962**, 1445–1446.

Atkin, N. B., Richards, B. M., Ross, A.: The DNA content of carcinoma of the uterus. An assessment of its possible significance in relation to histopathology and clinical course based on data from 165 cases. Brit. J. Cancer **13**, 773–787 (1959).

Bader, S.: A cytochemical study of the stem cell concept in specimens of a human ovarian tumor. J. biophys. biochem. Cytol. **5**, 217–229 (1959).

Bader, S., Taylor, E., Engle, E.: Deoxyribonucleic acid (DNA) content of human ovarian tumors in relation to histological grading. Lab. Invest. **9**, 443–459 (1960).

Böhm, N.: Einfluß der Fixierung und der Säurekonzentration auf die Feulgen-Hydrolyse bei 28°C. Histochemie **14**, 201–211 (1968).

Böhm, N.: Fluorescence cytophotometric determination of DNA. In: Techniques of biochemical and biophysical morphology, vol. 1 (D. Glick, R. M. Rosenbaum, eds.), p. 89–141. New York: John Wiley and Sons 1972.

Böhm, N., Moser, B.: Reversible Hyperplasie und Hypertrophie der Mäuseleber unter funktioneller Belastung mit Phenobarbital. Verh. dtsch. Ges. Path. **59**, in preparation.

Böhm, N., Roka, S., Sprenger, E., Wagner, D.: Absorptions- und fluoreszenzzytophotometrische DNS-Bestimmungen an vaginalzytologischem Material. Acta histochem. (Jena), Suppl. X, 233–242 (1971a).

Böhm, N., Sprenger, E.: Fluorescence cytophotometry: A valuable method for the quantitative determination of nuclear Feulgen-DNA. Histochemie **16**, 100–118 (1968).

Böhm, N., Sprenger, E., Sandritter, W.: Die Feulgen-Reaktion mit Acriflavin-SO$_2$. Ein Vergleich zwischen Absorptions- und Fluoreszenz-Cytophotometrie anhand von Hydrolysekurven. Acta histochem. (Jena) **35**, 324–329 (1970).

Böhm, N., Sprenger, E., Sandritter, W.: Fluorescence cytophotometric Feulgen-DNA measurements of benign and malignant human tumors. Beitr. Path. **142**, 210–220 (1971b).

Böhm, N., Sprenger, E., Schlüter, G., Sandritter, W.: Proportionalitätsfehler bei der Feulgen-Hydrolyse. Histochemie **15**, 194–203 (1968).

Boivin, A., Vendreley, R., Vendreley, C.: L'acide désoxyribonucléique du noyau cellulaire, dépositaire des caractères héréditaires; arguments d'ordre analytique. C. R. Acad. Sci. (Paris) **226**, 1061–1063 (1948).

BRANDAO, H. J. S.: DNA content in epithelial cells of dysplasia of the uterine cervix, Histologic and microspectrophotometric observations. Acta cytol. (Philad.) 13, 232–237 (1969).

CASPERSSON, O.: Quantitative cytochemical studies on normal, malignant, premalignant and atypical cell populations from the human uterine cervix. Acta cytol. (Philad.) 8, 45–59 (1964).

CHRISTOPHERSON, W. M., BROCHAMER, W. L., SWARTZ, F. J.: Deoxyribonucleic acid and anhydrous nuclear mass values in leukemia and normal lymphocytes. Amer. J. Path. 42, 337–344 (1963).

COLE, J. W., MCKALEN, A.: Observations on the cytochemical composition of adenomas and carcinomas of the colon. Amer. J. Surg. 152, 615–620 (1960).

DEELY, E. M.: An integrating microdensitometer for biological cells. J. sci. Instrum. 32, 263–267 (1955).

EHLERS, G.: Vergleichende quantitativ-cytochemische Untersuchungen über den Desoxyribonucleinsäure- und Nucleohiston-Gehalt von Basalzellepitheliomen. Arch. klin. exp. Derm. 232, 102–118 (1968).

EHLERS, G.: Die Wirksamkeit von Bleomycin auf kutane Malignome. Dtsch. Ärztebl., Heft 4, 195–204 (1975).

EHLERS, G., HERBSTREIT, I.: Cytophotometrische Untersuchungen des Desoxyribonucleinsäure- und Nucleohiston-Gehaltes unterschiedlich differenzierter Plattenepithelcarcinome der Haut und der Übergangsschleimhaut. Arch. Derm. Forsch. 247, 125–144 (1973).

EHLERS, G., HERBSTREIT, A., KAMPFFMEIER, U.: Klinische, histologische und cytophotometrische Untersuchungen über primärcutane metastasierende angioblastische Reticulosarkome unter besonderer Berücksichtigung der Wirksamkeit von Cytostatica. Hautarzt 22, 245–252 (1971).

EHLERS, G., SOLL, C.: Bilaterale maligne Hodentumoren. Zugleich ein Beitrag über die DNS-Verteilung eines Pseudoseminoms. Hautarzt 22, 25–30 (1971).

EHLERS, G., STEPHAN, T.: Quantitativ-histochemische Untersuchungen über den DNS-Gehalt fakultativer und obligater Präkanzerosen der Haut. Zur DNS-Ausstattung sog. fakultativer Präkanzerosen. Arch. Derm. Forsch. 243, 114–132 (1972a).

EHLERS, G., STEPHAN, T.: Quantitativ-histochemische Untersuchungen über den DNS-Gehalt fakultativer und obligater Präkanzerosen der Haut. Zur DNS-Ausstattung sog. obligater Präkanzerosen. Arch. Derm. Forsch. 243, 133–152 (1972b).

EINARSON, L.: On the theory of gallocyaninchromalaun staining and its application for quantitative estimation of basophilia. A selective staining of exquisite progressivity. Acta path. microbiol. scand. 28, 82–102 (1951).

EMSON, H. E., KIRK, H. D.: Desoxyribonucleic-acid content of breast lesions. Lancet 1966I, 905–907.

FÖDISCH, H. J., MIKUZ, G., WALTER, D.: Cytophotometrische Untersuchungen an Knochengeschwülsten. Verh. dtsch. Ges. Path. 58, 425–429 (1974).

FOSSA, D.: Feulgen-DNA-values in transitional cell carcinoma of the human urinary bladder. Beitr. Path. 155, 44–55 (1975).

GARCIA, A. M.: Studies on DNA in leucocytes and related cells of mammals. III. The Feulgen-DNA content of human leucocytes. Acta histochem. (Jena) 17, 230–245 (1964).

GARCIA, A. M.: Cytophotometric studies on haploid and diploid cells with different degrees of chromatin coiling. Ann. N.Y. Acad. Sci. 157, 237–249 (1969).

GRANBERG, I., GUPTA, S., JOELSSON, I., SPRENGER, E.: Chromosome and nuclear DNA study of a uterine adenocarcinoma and its metastases. Acta path. microbiol. scand., Section A 82, 1–6 (1974).

GREISEN, O.: The bronchial epithelium. Nucleic acid content in morphologically normal, metaplastic and neoplastic bronchial mucosae. Acta oto-laryng., Suppl. 276, 1–110 (1971).

GRUNDMANN, E., HILLEMANNS, H. G., RHA, K.: Cytophotometrische Untersuchungen am menschlichen Portioepithel während der Krebsentwicklung. Z. Krebsforsch. 64, 390–402 (1961).

HÄHRER, H., KAFFENBERGER, H.: Vergleichende UV-photometrische Nukleinsäurebestimmungen an normalen und Tumorzellen des Menschen. Ann. Histochim., Suppl. 2, 19–24 (1962).

Haemmerli, G.: Zytophotometrische und zytogenetische Untersuchungen an knotigen Veränderungen der menschlichen Schilddrüse. Schweiz. med. Wschr. **100**, 633–641 (1970).

Hale, A. J.: The leucocyte as a possible exception to the theory of deoxyribonucleic acid constancy. J. Path. Bact. **85**, 311–326 (1963).

Hale, A. J., Wilson, S. J.: The deoxyribonucleic acid content of leucocytes in normal and in leukemic human blood. J. Path. Bact. **77**, 605–614 (1959).

Haour, P., Conti, C.: Advantages and disadvantages of the Feulgen reaction and histophotometric technique as applied to cervical smears. Acta cytol. (Philad.) **2**, 326–329 (1958).

Holzner, J. H., Golob, E.: Changes of the DNA content in cells from cervical cancer under cytostatic and radiation therapy. Acta cytol. (Philad.) **12**, 473–477 (1968).

Hrushovetz, S. B.: Two-wave length Feulgen cytophotometry of cells exfoliated from the uterine cervix. Acta cytol. (Philad.) **13**, 583–594 (1969).

Hrushovetz, S. B., Lauchlan, S. C.: Comparative DNA content of cells in the intermediate and parabasal layers of cervical intraepithelial neoplasia studied by two-wavelength cytophotometry. Acta cytol. (Philad.) **14**, 68–77 (1970).

Inui, N., Oota, K.: DNA content of human tumor cell nucleus: A study on gastric carcinoma with special reference to its histological features. GANN **56**, 567–574 (1965).

Izuo, M., Okagaki, T., Richart, R. M., Lattes, R.: Nuclear DNA content in hyperplastic lesions of cystic disease of the breast with special reference to malignant alteration. Cancer (Philad.) **28**, 620–627 (1971a).

Izuo, M., Okagaki, T., Richart, R. M., Lattes, R.: DNA content in "apocrine metaplasia" of fibrocystic disease of the breast. Cancer (Philad.) **27**, 643–650 (1971b).

Izuo, M., Okagaki, T., Richart, R. M., Lattes, R.: Nuclear DNA content of acinar cells of the human breast during lactation. Amer. J. clin. Path. **56**, 443–447 (1971c).

Jacobsen, A. E.: Prostataepithelkerners relative nucleinsyreinhold. København: Munksgaard 1968; p. 1–168, cited from O. Greisen, 1971.

James, J.: Extinction effects in Feulgen-DNA scanning photometry of human lymphocytes. Acta cytol. (Philad.) **17**, 15–18 (1973).

Kother, L., Sandritter, W.: DNA content of the carcinoma in situ. Gynaecologia (Basel) **157**, 9–19 (1964).

Lampert, F.: Kerntrockengewicht, DNS-Gehalt und Chromosomen bei akuten Leukämien im Kindesalter. Virchows Arch. Abt. B **1**, 31–48 (1968).

Lampert, F.: Chromosome alterations in human carcinogenesis. In: Advances in cell and molecular biology, vol. 1, p. 185–212. New York and London: Academic Press 1971.

Laumonier, R., Laquerrière, R., Nobecourt, J., Hemet, J.: L'histophotométrie de l'acide désoxyribonucléique (DNA) et le problème de l'épithélioma non invasif du col utérin. Ann. Anat. path. **8**, 275–291 (1963).

Lederer, B., Mikuz, G., Gütter, W., zur Nedden, G.: Zytophotometrische Untersuchungen von Tumoren des Übergangsepithels der Harnblase. Vergleich zytophotometrischer Untersuchungsergebnisse mit dem histologischen Grading. Beitr. Path. **147**, 379–389 (1972).

Leuchtenberger, C., Leuchtenberger, R., Davis, A.: A microspectrophotometric study of the desoxyribonucleic acid (DNA) content in cells of normal and malignant human tissues. Amer. J. Path. **30**, 65–85 (1954).

Levan, A., Hauschka, T. S.: Chromosome numbers of three mouse ascites tumors. Hereditas (Lund) **38**, 251–255 (1952).

Levi, P. E., Cooper, E. H., Anderson, C. K., Path, M. C., Williams, R. E.: Analyses of DNA content, nuclear size and cell proliferation of transitional cell carcinoma in man. Cancer (Philad.) **23**, 1074–1085 (1969).

Lewis, P.: A cytophotometric study of benign and malignant phaeochromocytomas. Virchows Arch. Abt. B **9**, 371–376 (1971).

Makino, S., Kano, K.: Cytological studies of tumors. IX. Characteristic chromosome individuality in tumor strain-cells in ascites tumor of rats. J. nat. Cancer Inst. **13**, 1213–1234 (1952).

Mandel, P., Métais, P., Cuny, S.: Les quantités d'acide désoxypentose-nucléique par leukocyte chez diverses espéces de mammifères. C. R. Acad. Sci. (Paris) **231**, 1172–1174 (1950).

MANOCHA, S. L.: The diploid deoxyribonucleic acid (DNA) content of basal cell carcinomas in man. Experientia (Basel) 25, 201–203 (1969).

MANOCHA, S. L., STEELE, H. D., STICH, H. F.: The mosaic composition of the DNA content of the epidermal carcinomas of man. Z. Krebsforsch. 72, 144–154 (1969).

MAYALL, B. H.: Variability in the stoichiometry of deoxyribonucleic acid stains. J. Histochem. Cytochem. 15, 762–763 (1967).

MAYALL, B. H.: Deoxyribonucleic acid cytophotometry of stained human leukocytes. J. Histochem. Cytochem. 17, 249–257 (1969).

MEEK, E. S.: The cellular distribution of deoxyribonucleic acid in primary and secondary growths of human breast cancer. J. Path. Bact. 82, 167–176 (1961).

MIKUZ, G., MYDLA, F.: Elektronenmikroskopische und zytophotometrische Untersuchungen des Chordoms. Verh. dtsch. Ges. Path. 58, 447–453 (1974).

MÜLLER, D.: Der DNS-Gehalt leukämischer Zellen und seine Beziehungen zur Zellmorphologie und zum Krankheitsverlauf. Acta histochem. (Jena), Suppl. IX, 201–206 (1971).

MUNDY, G. R.: DNA values in myeloma. Cancer (Philad.) 32, 61–68 (1973).

NG, A., ATKIN, B.: Histological cell type and DNA value in the prognosis of squamous cell cancer of uterine cervix. Brit. J. Cancer 28, 322–331 (1973).

NITZE, H. R.: Cytologische Untersuchungen an Tumoren mit unterschiedlichem klinischem Verhalten. Arch. klin. exp. Ohr.-, Nas.- u. Kehlk.-Heilk. 193, 112–120 (1969).

NØDSKOV-PEDERSEN, S.: Degree of malignancy of cancer involving the cervix uteri, judged on the basis of clinical stage, histology, size of nuclei and content of DNA. Acta path. microbiol. scand., Section A 79, 617–628 (1971).

OBRECHT, P., MERKER, H., HENNEKEUSER, H., MEURET, G., WESTERHAUSEN, M., SIMON, A.: Klinisch-pharmakologische, cytochemische und Feulgen-photometrische Untersuchungen bei unreifzelligen Erwachsenenleukosen unter kombinierter Chemotherapie mit Vincristin, Daunorubicin und Prednison. Klin. Wschr. 18, 1281–1291 (1970).

OJIMA, Y., INUI, N., MAKINO, S.: Cytochemical studies on tumor cells. V. Measurement of deoxyribonucleic acid (DNA) by Feulgen-microspectrophotometry in some human uterine tumors. GANN 51, 371–376 (1960).

ORNSTEIN, L.: The distributional error in microspectrophotometry. Lab. Invest. 1, 250–265 (1952).

PATAU, K.: Absorption microphotometry of irregular-shaped objects. Chromosoma (Berl.) 5, 341–362 (1952).

PETRAKIS, N. L.: Microspectrophotometric estimation of desoxyribonucleic acid (DNA) content of individual normal and leukemic human lymphocytes. Blood 8, 905–915 (1953).

PFITZER, P.: The DNA content of alveolar macrophages and so-called alveolar cell carcinoma. Acta cytol. (Philad.) 14, 479–485 (1970).

PFITZER, P.: Nuclear DNA content of human myocardial cells. Curr. Top. Path. 54, 125–168 (1971).

PFITZER, P., PAPE, D.: DNA values from cytology in a case of palatal carcinoma. Acta cytol. (Philad.) 15, 559–561 (1971).

POLLISTER, A. W.: Photomultiplier apparatus for microspectrophotometry of cells. Lab. Invest. 1, 106 (1951).

RABOTTI, G.: Ploidy of primary and metastatic human tumours. Nature (Lond.) 183, 1276–1277 (1959).

REID, B. L., SINGH, S.: Deoxyribonucleic acid values (Feulgen microspectrophotometry) in epithelium of human ectocervix, normal and cancerous. J. nat. Cancer Inst. 25, 1291–1299 (1960).

SACHS, H.: Cytophotometrische Messungen an Zellen des Morbus Paget der Mamille und der Vulva. Arch. Gynäk. 209, 256–261 (1970).

SACHS, H.: Zytophotometrische Untersuchungen bei Präkanzerosen der Mamma. Beitr. Path. 143, 360–377 (1971).

SACHS, H., STEGNER, H. E., BAHNSEN, J.: Cytophotometrische Untersuchungen an Epitheldysplasien des Collum uteri. Arch. Gynäk. 212, 97–129 (1972).

SANDBERG, A. A., SAKURAI, M.: Chromosomes in the causation and progression of cancer and leukemia. In: The molecular biology of cancer (H. BUSCH, ed.), p. 81–106. New York and London: Academic Press 1974.

Sandberg, A. A., Takagi, N., Sofuni, T., Crosswhite, L. H.: Chromosomes and causation of human cancer and leukemia. V. Karyotypic aspects of acute leukemia. Cancer (Philad.) 22, 1268–1282 (1968).

Sandritter, W.: Über den Nucleinsäurestoffwechsel in verschiedenen Tumoren. Frankfurt. Z. Path. 63, 423–446 (1952a).

Sandritter, W.: Über den Nucleinsäurestoffwechsel in Plattenepithel- und kleinzelligen Bronchialcarcinomen. Frankfurt. Z. Path. 63, 387–422 (1952b).

Sandritter, W.: Cytophotometrische Untersuchungen am Portiocarcinom und seinen Vorstufen. Verh. dtsch. Ges. Path. 48, 34–43 (1964).

Sandritter, W., Carl, M., Ritter, W.: Cytophotometric measurements of the DNA content of human malignant tumors by means of the Feulgen reaction. Acta cytol. (Philad.) 10, 26–30 (1966).

Sandritter, W., Cramer, H., Mondorf, W.: Zur Krebsdiagnostik an vaginalen Zellausstrichen mittels cytophotometrischer Messungen. Arch. Gynäk. 192, 293–303 (1960).

Sandritter, W., Fischer, R.: Der DNS-Gehalt des normalen Plattenepithels, des Carcinoma in situ und des invasiven Carcinoms der Portio. In: The Proceedings of the First International Congress of Exfoliative Cytology, p. 189–195. Philadelphia: Lippincott Co. 1962.

Sandritter, W., Kiefer, G., Rick, W.: Über die Stöchiometrie von Gallocyaninchromalaun mit Desoxyribonukleinsäure. Histochemie 3, 315–340 (1963).

Sandritter, W., Kleinhans, D.: Über das Trockengewicht, den DNS- und Histonproteingehalt von menschlichen Tumoren. Z. Krebsforsch. 66, 333–348 (1964).

Sandritter, W., Lobel, B. L., Kiefer, G.: Photometric cytodiagnosis of vaginal smears. J. nat. Cancer Inst. 32, 1221–1228 (1964).

Sandritter, W., Scomazzoni, G.: Deoxyribonucleic acid content (Feulgen photometry) and dry weight (interference microscopy) of normal and hypertrophic heart muscle fibres. Nature (Lond.) 202, 100–101 (1964).

Sandritter, W., Seidel, A., Kleinhans, D., Paddags, L., Dontenwill, W.: Cytophotometrische Messungen des DNS-Gehaltes an menschlichen und tierexperimentellen Bronchialepithelmetaplasien. Z. Krebsforsch. 67, 69–79 (1965).

Seidel, A., Sandritter, W.: Cytophotometrische Messungen des DNS-Gehaltes eines Lungenadenoms und einer malignen Lungenadenomatose. Z. Krebsforsch. 65, 555–559 (1963).

Sprenger, E., Böhm, N.: Eine Möglichkeit automatisierter Meßwerterfassung in der Fluoreszenzzytophotometrie. Acta histochem. (Jena), Suppl. X 243–246 (1971).

Sprenger, E., Böhm, N., Sandritter, W.: Durchflußfluoreszenzzytophotometrie für ultraschnelle DNS-Messungen an großen Zellpopulationen. Histochemie 26, 238–257 (1971a).

Sprenger, E., Hilgarth, M., Schaden, M.: Die Zellkern-DNS-Bestimmung bei Verlaufsbeobachtung unklarer zytologischer Befunde. Beitr. Path. 152, 58–65 (1974b).

Sprenger, E., Rossner, R., Otto, Ch., Schaden, M., Sandritter, W.: The mathematical evaluation of flow-through cytophotometric data in processing cervical cytology. Beitr. Path. 153, 289–296 (1974c).

Sprenger, E., Sandritter, W., Böhm, N., Schaden, M., Hilgarth, M., Wagner, D.: Durchflußfluoreszenzzytophotometrie: Ein Prescreening-Verfahren für die gynäkologische Zytodiagnostik. Beitr. Path. 143, 323–344 (1971b).

Sprenger, E., Sandritter, W., Böhm, N., Wagner, D., Hilgarth, M., Schaden, M.: Flow-through-cytophotometry—A step towards automated cytology? Acta cytol. (Philad.) 16, 297–303 (1972).

Sprenger, E., Schaden, M., Wagner, D., Hilgarth, M., Sandritter, W.: Durchflußfluoreszenzzytophotometrisches Prescreening in der Zervixzytologie — Ein Methodenvergleich. Beitr. Path. 151, 373–383 (1974a).

Sprenger, E., Volk, L., Michaelis, W. E.: The significance of nuclear DNA-measurements in the diagnosis of prostatic carcinoma. Beitr. Path. 153, 370–378 (1974d).

Sprenger, E., Witte, S., Schaden, M.: The differential diagnostic role of nuclear DNA contents in gastric cytology. In: Early gastric cancer (E. Grundmann, H. Grunze, S. Witte, eds.), p. 154–158. Berlin-Heidelberg-New York: Springer 1974e.

STANGEL, J. J., RICHART, R. M., TAKASHI, O., COTTRAL, G.: Nuclear DNA content of luteinized cells of the human ovary. Amer. J. Obstet. Gynec. **108**, 543–549 (1970).

STEELE, H. D., MANOCHA, S. L., STICH, H. F.: DNA content of epidermal in-situ carcinomas. Brit. med. J. **1969** II, 1314–1315.

STICH, H. F.: Mosaic composition of preneoplastic lesions and malignant neoplasms. Exp. Cell Res., Suppl 9, 277–285 (1963).

STICH, H. F., EMSON, H. E.: Aneuploid deoxyribonucleic acid content of human carcinomas. Nature (Lond.) **184**, 290–291 (1959).

STICH, H. F., FLORIAN, S. F., EMSON, H. E.: The DNA content of tumor cells. I. Polyps and adenocarcinomas of the large intestine of man. J. nat. Cancer Inst. **24**, 471–482 (1960).

STICH, H. F., STEELE, H. D.: DNA content of tumor cells. III. Mosaic composition of sarcomas and carcinomas in man. J. nat. Cancer Inst. **28**, 1207–1218 (1962).

STOWELL, E. R.: Nucleic acids in human tumors. Cancer Res. **6**, 426–435 (1946).

STOWELL, R. E., COOPER, Z. K.: The relative thymocucleic acid content of human normal epidermis, hyperplastic epidermis, and epidermoid carcinomas. Cancer Res. **5**, 295–301 (1945).

SUGIYAMA, T.: Specific vulnerability of the largest telocentric chromosome of rat bone marrow cells to 7.12 dimethylbenz (α) anthracene. J. nat. Cancer Inst. **47**, 1267–1275 (1971).

SULLIVAN, P., GARCIA, A. M.: Correlation between nuclear size and Feulgen-DNA value in lymphocytes. Acta cytol (Philad.) **14**, 104–110 (1970).

SWARTZ, F.: The development in the human liver of multiple desoxribose nucleic acid (DNA) classes and their relationship to the age of the individual. Chromosoma (Berl.) **8**, 53–72 (1956).

TAVARES, A. S., COSTA, J., CARVALHO, A. de, REIS, M.: Tumour ploidy and prognosis in carcinomas of the bladder and prostate. Brit. J. Cancer **20**, 438–441 (1966).

URASINSKI, I., HABICHT, W., GROSS, R.: Vergleichende Messungen der Nukleinsäuren an Paraleukoblasten vor und während zytostatischer Therapie. Acta histochem. (Jena), Suppl. IX, 207–210 (1971).

VALERI, V., CRUZ, A. R., BRANDAO, H. J. S., LISON, L.: Relationship between cell nuclear volume and deoxyribonucleic acid of cells of normal epithelium, of carcinoma in situ and of invasive carcinoma of the uterine cervix. Acta cytol. (Philad.) **11**, 488–496 (1967).

VENDRELEY, R., VENDRELEY, C.: La teneur du noyau cellulaire en acide désoxyribonucléique à travers les organes, les individus et les espèces animales. Experientia (Basel) **5**, 327–329 (1949).

VLOTEN, W. A. VAN, DUIJN, P. VAN, SCHABERG, A.: Cytodiagnostic use of Feulgen-DNA measurements in cell imprints from the skin of patients with mycosis fungoides. Brit. J. Derm. **91**, 365–371 (1974).

VOKAER, R.: Observations sur l'histologie, l'histométrie et l'histophotométrie de l'endométre humain. Gynéc. et Obstét. **50**, 373–385 (1951).

WAGNER, D., RICHART, R. M.: Polyploidy in the human endometrium with the Arias-Stella reaction. Arch. Path. **85**, 475–480 (1968).

WAGNER, D., RICHART, R. M., TERNER, J. Y.: DNA content of human endometrial gland cells during the menstrual cycle. Amer. J. Obstet. Gynec. **100**, 90–97 (1968).

WAGNER, D., SPRENGER, E., BLANK, M. H.: DNA-content of dysplastic cells of the uterine cervix. Acta cytol. (Philad.) **16**, 517–522 (1972).

WIED, G. L., MESSINA, A. M., ROSENTHAL, E.: Comparative quantitative DNA-measurements on Feulgen-stained cervical epithelial cells. Acta cytol. (Philad.) **10**, 31–37 (1966).

WILBANKS, G. D., RICHART, R. M., TERNER, J. Y.: DNA content of cervical intraepithelial neoplasia studied by two-wavelength Feulgen cytophotometry. Amer. J. Obstet. Gynec. **98**, 792–799 (1967).

ZANK, M., KRUG, H.: Zytophotometrische DNS-Bestimmungen an Primärtumoren und Metastasen. Arch. Geschwulstforsch. **36**, 343–359 (1970).

Index to Volumes 37—59

Ergebnisse der allgemeinen Pathologie und der pathologischen Anatomie

Current Topics in Pathology

GPSR Compliance
The European Union's (EU) General Product Safety Regulation (GPSR) is a set
of rules that requires consumer products to be safe and our obligations to
ensure this.

If you have any concerns about our products, you can contact us on

ProductSafety@springernature.com

In case Publisher is established outside the EU, the EU authorized
representative is:

Springer Nature Customer Service Center GmbH
Europaplatz 3
69115 Heidelberg, Germany